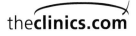
theclinics.com

SURGICAL CLINICS
OF NORTH AMERICA

Surgical Response to Disaster

GUEST EDITOR
LTC Robert M. Rush, Jr, MD

CONSULTING EDITOR
LTC Ronald F. Martin, MD

INVITED COMMENTARY
LTG Kevin C. Kiley, MD

June 2006 • Volume 86 • Number 3

SAUNDERS

An Imprint of Elsevier, Inc.
PHILADELPHIA   LONDON   TORONTO   MONTREAL   SYDNEY   TOKYO

W.B. SAUNDERS COMPANY
A Division of Elsevier Inc.

1600 John F. Kennedy Blvd., Suite 1800, Philadelphia, PA 19103-2899

http://www.theclinics.com

SURGICAL CLINICS OF NORTH AMERICA   Volume 86, Number 3
June 2006   ISSN 0039–6109
Editor: Catherine Bewick   ISBN 1-4160-3559-1

Reprints. For copies of 100 or more of articles in this publication, please contact the commercial Reprints Department Elsevier Inc., 360 Park Avenue South, New York, New York 10010-1710. Tel. (212) 633-3813, Fax: (212) 462-1935, email: reprints@elsevier.com

The ideas and opinions expressed in *The Surgical Clinics of North America* do not necessarily reflect those of the Publisher. The Publisher does not assume any responsibility for any injury and/or damage to persons or property arising out of or related to any use of the material contained in this periodical. The reader is advised to check the appropriate medical literature and the product information currently provided by the manufacturer of each drug to be administered to verify the dosage, the method and duration of administration, or contraindications. It is the responsibility of the treating physician or other health care professional, relying on independent experience and knowledge of the patient, to determine drug dosages and the best treatment for the patient. Mention of any product in this issue should not be construed as endorsement by the contributors, editors, or the Publisher of the product or manufacturers' claims.

Surgical Clinics of North America (ISSN 0039–6109) is published bimonthly by W.B. Saunders, 360 Park Avenue South, New York, NY 10010-1710. Months of publication are February, April, June, August, October, and December. Business and Editorial Offices: 1600 John F. Kennedy Blvd., Suite 1800, Philadelphia, PA 19103-2899. Accounting and Circulation Offices: 6277 Sea Harbor Drive, Orlando, FL 32887-4800. Periodicals postage paid at New York, NY and additional mailing offices. Subscription prices are $200.00 per year for US individuals, $315.00 per year for US institutions, $100.00 per year for US students and residents, $245.00 per year for Canadian individuals, $385.00 per year for Canadian institutions, $260.00 for international individuals, $385.00 for international institutions and $130.00 per year for Canadian and foreign students/residents. To receive student/resident rate, orders must be accompanied by name of affiliated institution, date of term, and the *signature* of program/residency coordinator on institution letterhead. Orders will be billed at individual rate until proof of status is received. Foreign air speed delivery is included in all *Clinics* subscription prices. All prices are subject to change without notice. POSTMASTER: Send address changes to *The Surgical Clinics of North America*, Elsevier Periodicals Customer Service, 6277 Sea Harbor Drive, Orlando, FL 32887-4800. **Customer Service: 1-800-654-2452 (US). From outside of the US, call 1-407-345-1000.**

The Surgical Clinics of North America is also published in Spanish by McGraw-Hill Interamericana Editores S.A., P.O. Box 5-237 06500 Mexico D.F. Mexico; and in Portuguese by Interlivros Edicoes Ltda., Rua Comandante Coelho 1085, CEP 21250, Rio de Janeiro, Brazil; and in Greek by Paschalidis Medical Publications, Athens Greece.

The Surgical Clinics of North America is covered in *Index Medicus, EMBASE/Excerpta Medica, Current Contents/Clinical Medicine, Current Contents/Life Sciences, Science Citation Index*, and *ISI/BIOMED*.

Printed in the United States of America.

CONSULTING EDITOR

LTC RONALD F. MARTIN, MD, Staff Surgeon, Department of Surgery, Marshfield Clinic, Marshfield, Wisconsin; Clinical Associate Professor of Surgery, University of Vermont, Burlington, Vermont; United States Army Reserves, Medical Corps

GUEST EDITOR

LTC ROBERT M. RUSH, JR, MD, Adjunct Assistant Professor of Surgery, Uniformed Services University of the Health Sciences, Bethesda, Maryland; Attending Surgeon, Department of Surgery, Madigan Army Medical Center, Tacoma, Washington; Clinical Instructor of Surgery, University of Washington School of Medicine, Seattle, Washington; Minimally Invasive Surgery Fellow, Mayo Medical School, Mayo Clinic, Scottsdale, Arizona

CONTRIBUTORS

MAJ ALEC C. BEEKLEY, MD, FACS, United States Army, Medical Corps; Trauma Medical Director, General Surgeon, Madigan Army Medical Center, Fort Lewis, Washington

SUSAN M. BRIGGS, MD, MPH, FACS, Associate Professor of Surgery, Harvard Medical School; Director, International Trauma and Disaster Institute, Massachusetts General Hospital, Boston, Massachusetts

JENNIFER BENCIE FAIRBURN, MD, MSA, Director, Emergency Medical Operations, Department of Health, Division of Emergency Medical Operations, Tallahassee, Florida

COL DANIEL F. FLYNN, MD, United States Army Reserves Medical Corps, Office of the Command Surgeon, Devens, Massachusetts; Visiting Faculty, Radiation Emergency Assistance Center and Training Site, Oak Ridge, Tennessee; New England Radiation Therapy Associates, Radiation Oncology Department, Holy Family Hospital, Methuen, Massachusetts

DONALD E. FRY, MD, Professor Emeritus, Department of Surgery, University of New Mexico, Albuquerque, New Mexico

RONALD E. GOANS, MD, PhD, Visiting Faculty, Radiation Emergency Assistance Center and Training Site, Oak Ridge Institute for Science and Education, Oak Ridge, Tennessee; MJW Corporation, University Park, Amherst, New York; Center for Applied Environmental Health, Tulane University School of Public Health and Tropical Medicine, New Orleans, Louisiana

COL STEPHEN P. HETZ, MD, FACS, Medical Corps, US Army (Retired), Department of Surgery, William Beaumont Army Medical Center, El Paso, Texas

LTC SETH IZENBERG, MD, United States Army Reserves, Medical Corps; Associate Director Trauma Services, Emanuel Hospital, Portland, Oregon

LTG KEVIN C. KILEY, MD, Surgeon General of the Army, United States Army

CAPT MARK LLEWELLYN, MD, MC USN, United States Navy, Medical Corps; Director for Medical Services, Naval Medical Center, San Diego, California; Commanding Officer, Medical Treatment Facility, USNS Mercy (T-AH 19)

COL EDWARD B. LUCCI, MD, FACEP, Chief, Emergency and Operational Medicine, Walter Reed Army Medical Center, Washington, DC; Adjunct Assistant Professor of Military and Emergency Medicine, Uniformed Services University of the Health Sciences, Bethesda, Maryland

Lt Col W. BRIAN PERRY, MD, United States Air Force, Medical Corps; Assistant Professor of Surgery, Uniformed Services University of the Health Sciences, Bethesda, Maryland; Assistant Professor of Surgery, University of Texas Health Science Center, San Antonio, Texas

COL RONALD J. PLACE, MD, United States Army, Medical Corps; Assistant Professor of Surgery, Uniformed Services University of Health Sciences; Deputy Commander (Outlying Clinics/Managed Care), Landstuhl Regional Medical Center, Landstuhl, Germany

LTC ROBERT M. RUSH, JR, MD, United States Army, Medical Corps; Adjunct Assistant Professor of Surgery, Uniformed Services University of the Health Sciences, Bethesda, Maryland; Attending Surgeon, Department of Surgery, Madigan Army Medical Center, Tacoma, Washington; Clinical Instructor of Surgery, University of Washington School of Medicine, Seattle, Washington; Minimally Invasive Surgery Fellow, Mayo Medical School, Mayo Clinic, Scottsdale, Arizona

MAJ JAMES SEBESTA, MD, United States Army, Medical Corps; Staff General Surgeon and Instructor, Department of Surgery, Madigan Army Medical Center, Tacoma, Washington

DAVID V. SHATZ, MD, FACS, Professor of Surgery, Division of Trauma, Burns, and Surgical Critical Care, Department of Surgery, University of Miami Miller School of Medicine, Miami; Medical Director, Federal Emergency Management Agency Urban Search and Rescue, Florida Task Force 1, Miami, Florida

LTC BENJAMIN W. STARNES, MD, United States Army, Medical Corps; Vascular and Endovascular Surgeon, Director of Endovascular Surgery, Madigan Army Medical Center, Tacoma, Washington; Assistant Professor of Surgery, Uniformed Services University of the Health Sciences, Bethesda, Maryland

KATHARINE WOLCOTT, MD, United States Army, Medical Corps; Resident, General Surgery, Department of Surgery, Madigan Army Medical Center, Tacoma, Washington

CONTENTS

Major earthquakes have the potential to be one of the most catastrophic natural disasters affecting mankind. Earthquakes of significant size threaten lives and damage property by setting off a chain
of events that disrupts all aspects of the environment and significantly impacts the public health and medical infrastructures of
the affected region. This article provides an overview of basic
earthquake facts and relief protocol for medical personnel.

Unlike most natural and man-made disasters, preparation and
planning for hurricanes is possible and effective. Medical needs
can be disparate, given the large geographic area involved and
the often-prolonged recovery phase. All aspects of medical
response, from first responders to hospitals, can directly and nega-
tively be affected by the storm. Planning and practice, however, can
drastically improve the outcome.

the ever-changing landscape of modern warfare and the devastating injuries produced. From the revamping of prehospital care to new applications of damage-control surgery, challenges have erupted, lessons have been learned, and lives are being saved.

Low-intensity conflicts and special operations present a wide range of injury scenarios for military and civilian surgeons alike. Harsh environments, difficult and high-risk missions, long lines of communication, and isolated locations are but some of the factors that create challenge in providing care for patients in this category. Often surgeons and other medical personnel are faced with many additional medical and nonmedical tasks outside their usual expertise because of the small number of support personnel and medical footprints brought forward in these missions.

Military surgeons serve a unique role in peacekeeping and stability operations and in response to natural disasters. Military medical units are the best medical resource to respond early in times of crisis but are often less equipped for prolonged missions and subsequent management of the chronic health care needs of the masses. Because endemic and host-nation diseases often add complexity to the management of these cases, military surgeons must perform operations outside the scope of their usual civilian practice. The primary medical mission is to treat the peacekeeping force, but the reality lies in eventually treating the refugees and victims of hostile conflict, including women, small children, and the elderly. This article explores the unique features of a surgeon's role in the support of these missions.

The recently reported abuses at Abu Ghraib prison have brought the issue of medical care for displaced persons (DPs) to greater prominence. Natural disasters in the United States (eg, Hurricane Katrina) and elsewhere also require significant medical resources in situations that lack basic infrastructure. Intimate knowledge of the basic tenets of international law is crucial to the care of DPs in any capacity. This article provides an introduction to the Geneva Conventions and the medical and administrative issues that form a framework on which to base DP care.

FORTHCOMING ISSUES

RECENT ISSUES

SURGICAL
CLINICS OF
NORTH AMERICA

ELSEVIER
SAUNDERS

Surg Clin N Am 86 (2006) xi–xv

Foreword

Surgical Response to Disaster

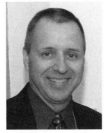

LTC Ronald F. Martin, MD
Consulting Editor

In times of crisis, surgeons are frequently called upon. And if you are a surgeon, that may mean you. Furthermore, the fact that surgeons are called upon is probably a good thing, because the very nature of the training of surgeons develops people who are generally more comfortable working in chaotic or highly fluid environments.

It used to be easier to imagine that the events that unfold in the world are distant and not that relevant to us individually. The people and places in the news were more of an intellectual concern or perhaps some strange theater— the original reality television, perhaps. It would be easier to believe that these events involve strangers but in fact, they involve you or your neighbor or your loved ones. These disastrous events, whether they are man-made or naturally occurring, involve very ordinary people just like us. And at times, these events might require that ordinary people be asked to do extraordinary things.

In recent years, the role of the military in response to war and disaster has been extremely visible. The active component of the military, the reserves, and the National Guard have been tasked with almost every mission imaginable. The medical components of all of these units have factored prominently into the missions. The nature of disaster response usually involves only a short time for preparation and a rapid execution of the mission with available assets. The mission of the reserves is to be prepared to stop what one is doing on a moment's notice and support the federal government in

The opinions stated in this foreword represent those of the author and do not necessarily reflect the views of the United States Army, the Department of Defense, or the United States Government.

achieving its objectives. Being a reservist can make personal planning challenging but there is, however, a tremendous advantage to being a reservist—one gets to *really* live in two parallel worlds, each with cultural strengths and weaknesses, physical and intellectual capacities, varying degrees of autonomy, and differing measures of success. Being able to function in both societies can offer tremendous advantages in times of change. I think it is fair to say that "the times, they are a changing."

The small details of what was done to and for whom in each of the many topics explored in this issue are not particularly germane to the discussion at hand. The small details will always change with circumstances. The broad concepts are important. Dr. Rob Rush has done our series and me a tremendous personal favor by Guest Editing this issue of the *Surgical Clinics of North America*. He has compiled in a concise and well-thought-out manner the breadth and depth of what the civilian, military, private, and public sectors have to offer when the nearly unimaginable happens. The original table of contents and topics for this issue were compiled long before Katrina was a name of national significance and even before most people could spell Banda Aceh. After the Indian Ocean tsunami struck, we agreed to rewrite the list of contributors. We have also upgraded the material since Hurricanes Katrina and Rita made landfall on the Gulf Coast and the occurrence of the Pakistani earthquake. We have taken every measure to enlist the help of the people who were and are closest to the actual events to add the dimension of personal understanding to theoretical framework.

The main theme of this issue is one of preparedness. In my opinion, it is imperative not to confuse preparedness with fear. It would be unreasonable to assert that we could truly prepare for every eventuality, or that even if we were able to do so, we could successfully implement the plans we had made. Unfortunately, bad things do occasionally happen to some of us, the root cause of which may be mal-intent or natural occurrence; that will never change. Our goals must therefore be to minimize risk while remaining mindful of the costs and limitations, both personal and financial, of such preparedness.

Redundancy probably offers the best, albeit expensive, mechanism of reduction of risk. Redundancy of personnel and supplies offers surge protection, but at the obvious cost of storing potentially non-utilizable products whose shelf lives expire, and of maintaining personnel who are sub-maximally employed. The military uses a concept of "force multipliers" that we in the civilian sector may be wise to adopt. There are many aspects of our day-to-day lives that could easily be changed to follow this concept. I shall expound a bit on these to avoid the risk of registering criticism without providing an alternative.

The first recommendation is to support a program or legislation that would consolidate the repository for documentation of health care workers. We have a National Credentials Verification Service, but its usage is not mandatory. Anyone who has applied for licensure in more than one state knows that the process of application is unnecessarily redundant—and expensive. The concept of "primary source verification" is valid, but not so the reinventing of wheels. For each of the health professions, there could be a mechanism for storage of information that will not change: proof of citizenship, place of birth, attendance and completion of schools, residencies and fellowships (when appropriate), prior issue of licenses, and so forth. National Practitioner Data Bank information and re-licensing data could be updated to this centralized data system on a periodic basis. This would eliminate the need for re-verification of the primary source data and would markedly streamline the process for varying states to issue new or temporary licenses under times of duress when a sudden influx of physicians or other health care workers are needed in a hurry. Establishing meaningful license reciprocity agreements between states would also be helpful. Personally, I would support the notion of creating only a Federal Medical Licensing Board, but I doubt that this idea would gain any traction, and it might incite a states' rights debate that would most likely be counterproductive.

Another aspect of redundancy refers to commercially acquired stocks and supplies. The individual stocking of supplies, particularly those with short expiration dates, is financially unsustainable for an individual private enterprise. Counties, states, regions, and the nation would be well served to work out a series of agreements and memoranda of understanding that would provide for a rational program for stockpiling critical items for an "all hazards" approach to disaster-related needs. This plan would require a mechanism for the appropriation of critically needed supplies, for the security to maintain their utility and to prevent theft or damage, and for emergent distribution, including plans for transportation and allocation. Agreements with commercial suppliers and vendors would be required to provide the availability of adequate supplies, with a reasonable shared risk between the suppliers and purchasers to avoid inequitable distribution of financial risk for excess non-reimbursed production or financial loss due to product non-usage for either side. Stock rotation policies and re-sale agreements must be considered carefully.

A review of the Emergency Medical Treatment and Active Labor Act rules must be considered and the conditions under which they may be altered taken into account. The mechanism for the transfer of patients from one facility to another may (and most likely will) be markedly altered by any calamity of significance. Again, cost sharing among and between facilities will need to be considered. Liability policies will also need to be examined in the setting of facilities and environments that are deemed to be overwhelmed. Specific language addressing the limits of liability (if any) during times of duly declared crisis should be incorporated into agreements or enacted into law to remove any potential barriers to appropriate quick reaction in times of need.

The citizenry, also known as our patients, colleagues, and families, will need to take part in this preparedness as well. An increased understanding of their personal responsibility in times of disaster is clearly required. It is said that charity begins at home—and probably so does preparedness. There will be financial burdens that the public will have to bear if the collective will is to increase our overall ability to respond to disaster. I have no intention of developing a line of thinking on tax policy in this foreword, so I shall leave this topic here. Patients may also need to accept a slightly reduced level of protection of personal information if strict adherence to Health Information Portability and Accountability Act policies were to significantly hamper a facility's ability to effectively respond to crisis. The reasons for reducing these protections and for limitations on these protections should be well considered along with their far-reaching implications in times when we are not actively engaged in a crisis.

Citizens and local governments also need to reassess our policies of the eco–human interface. Quite simply put, we cannot live just anywhere. The impact of building in and populating environmentally vulnerable areas has to be reckoned with. All the planning we can engage in will not make up for lack of prevention. Although being able to live on a muddy cliff with an ocean view may seem wonderful from an aesthetic point of view (don't worry—won't happen here in Wisconsin), it may not make sense from a public policy standpoint. Because disaster recovery is basically an insurance and re-insurance phenomenon, we cannot in good conscience expect the public to "re-insure" us if we make decidedly poor choices.

The implications of the Posse Comitatus Act and its subsequent provisions need to be deeply considered in regard to the ability of the United States Military to respond to crises on United States soil and the lawfulness of such responses. The law directs and limits the actions of the Army, Navy, and Marines and has come to include the Air Force. In brief, the Act prohibits the use of federal troops for law enforcement within the United States. There are exceptions for the maintenance of federal functions as defined by law, and there is no prohibition on logistical support. The Act does not regulate National Guard troops, who function under the command and authority of state governors. The current geopolitical commitments of the United States Armed Forces, the Federal Military Reserves, and the National Guard have all strained the ability of these forces to respond to domestic issues. It would appear that these commitments might persist for some time. Consideration of a nonmilitary "reserve force" to respond to domestic naturally occurring disasters may be advisable. Law enforcement personnel, health care workers, supply and logistics experts, utility workers, and construction experts (to name a few groups of people) might be more likely to be part of a "stand-by" force, ready to drop what they are doing in their own lives and suffer personal and financial hardship, including periodic training, if they were convinced that they were not going to be activated for war-related activities. In my opinion, volunteerism is alive and well in the United States, but the military is having difficulty with recruitment and retention. It is unreasonable to believe that the United States military is going to be the work force of last resort for any and every major catastrophe.

Each of you who read this issue should feel encouraged to consider how you can contribute to this need for preparedness. After all, the government is really an extension of the collective "us." Our ability to respond begins with each of us knowing what he or she can do to help if the unthinkable happens. At the bare minimum, we can educate ourselves as to the nature and science of the concerns that will become our responsibility in crisis. This issue of the *Surgical Clinics of North America* should help one to start with that. Organization, compromise, pro-active effort, and commitment will then need to follow. If the past few years are any predictor, there may be more hard times to come.

As was alluded to earlier, surgeons, collectively, tend to be well-suited by training to function in high-stress environments with rapidly changing and imperfect data. It is imperative that we personally engage in these planning efforts. The next major problem that occurs might result in a phone call to you.

I would like to beg your forgiveness for an indulgence as I close this foreword. There are a number of people that I should acknowledge in the development of this work. I would like to acknowledge and thank the following: the members of the 801st Combat Support Hospital, especially those who went forward, in particular our Commander, Colonel Craig Bugno, MD, USAR, who gave us his fullest support to care for those who needed us; the staff of Madigan Army Medical Center (many of whom have contributed directly to this issue), who are consummate professionals; the staff of the United States Embassy in Kuwait, who assisted us in innumerable ways and allowed us a broader vision into world events; the exceptional members of the United States Armed Forces everywhere, who do incredible things so that many of us can safely do ordinary things; the family members and loved ones, who do the really tough job of staying behind and maintaining our lives while some of us take off with little notice; and the colleagues who have absorbed the brunt of suddenly dropped workloads when we leave unexpectedly. Also, a very personal thanks to my "battle buddy," Colonel Patrick J. Sullivan, MD, USAR, whose support helped me preserve what occasionally passes for sanity during interesting times. Thanks as well to our publisher, Elsevier Science and, in particular, to Ms. Catherine Bewick, who have allowed us to broaden the scope of what we consider relevant to the general surgeon.

Most importantly, I would like us to remember all of those who have suffered or died as a result of these disasters or conflicts. It is in their memory that we try to learn what we can from the past to prevent its repetition in the future.

LTC Ronald F. Martin, MD
Department of Surgery
Marshfield Clinic
1000 North Oak Avenue
Marshfield, WI 54449, USA

E-mail address: martin.ronald@marshfieldclinic.org

Preface

Surgical Response to Disaster

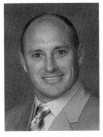

LTC Robert M. Rush, Jr., MD
Guest Editor

The past five years have witnessed extraordinary global eclipses in mass human suffering. Surely natural disasters, wars, and terrorist attacks have taken the lives of innumerable individuals throughout history, although the media projects catastrophes into an ever-increasing number of worldwide households of late, bringing these horrific events much-needed and deserved exposure. This issue of the *Surgical Clinics of North America* focuses on such events; disasters, whether man-made or acts of nature, the most cataclysmic events from tsunamis to war, are discussed with emphasis on educating the surgical community. The editors and authors have chosen a mechanistic/scenario-based focus to describe disaster and mass casualty management in this issue, along with special situations, such as the handling of displaced persons, the civilian application of military resources, and the framework of the military medical mass-casualty response. Many lessons learned are discussed by those with vast personal experience in their given topic. Although not all disaster scenarios are alike, an ever-adapting, systems-based approach (all-hazards approach) [1,2] to training and execution still holds true and is brought forth throughout.

In responding to any disaster, certain events must take place. Preparation must include attempts at nullifying the disaster's potential effects on human life and suffering, regardless of mechanism. This is a broad category that

0039-6109/06/$ - see front matter © 2006 Elsevier Inc. All rights reserved.
doi:10.1016/j.suc.2006.04.002

surgical.theclinics.com

includes pre-event evacuation (if we know it is coming), to building design, to hospital surge capacity plans to handle mass casualties. Disaster response also requires a paradigm shift, from taking care of the individual patient with every means necessary to doing the most good for the most people and looking at the situation as a whole, not just at each individual injured. Emergency personnel responding to the scene, city, or region in which the disaster has occurred must first set up incident/scene command and control, and reconnaissance, as well as scene safety measures to prevent rescuers and the uninjured from becoming casualties. Usually, scene command is a fire department and police department function in the United States. If there are many scenes to which to respond in a large disaster area, then there may be an incident commander, who can be a local official, a military unit commander, or the director of the Federal Emergency Management Agency, for large-scale disasters. Communication between the scenes of a disaster and the incident and hospital command systems is paramount. In all disaster responses, the lack of effective communication is a major problem area. Normal communication tools such as land lines and cell phones may be rendered ineffective, and the use of Web systems and satellite and long-range radio may be the only way to communicate effectively [1–4]. To tailor a response, information coming from the scene should include whether or not local capabilities for search and rescue, pre-hospital, and hospital care are adequate. This is an ongoing assessment, not a snapshot. Only when this information is known can external help be brought to the scene, area, or region affected. The military's system for battlefield mass casualty management is given in this issue as an example of this. Much can be learned from the interactions and cross-applications of military response to civilian response and vice versa.

A recent survey of members of the Eastern Association for the Surgery of Trauma found that only 33% of responding trauma surgeons felt prepared for mass casualties resulting from weapons of mass destruction and hazardous materials [5]. In this study, it was suggested that those surgeons with a military background were better prepared for disaster response and the handling of mass casualty incidents. Despite this, 93% of respondents were involved with external community response planning, showing that trauma surgeons are taking leading roles in disaster management and planning. Although trauma surgeons have an inherent interest in mass casualty management, all surgeons and physicians need to be included in the planning and education of disaster response. While disasters take most victims by surprise, so will they take by surprise those medical personnel cast into the fray simply by being in proximity. No longer can any surgeon or medical professional say, "That will not happen to me." Through the efforts of the American College of Surgeons, many groups, and many more individual efforts, tremendous strides have been made to improve overall disaster preparedness and the education and training of surgeons for such catastrophes in the United States [6]. There are many recent programs and short courses on disaster response that are provided at national medical conferences, in journals, on Web sites, and in hospitals and universities. The work presented herein simply represents an adjunct to this material and perhaps a different view, one based on specific mechanisms of disaster, injuries sustained, and preparedness needed.

In a recent address, Dr. Donald Trunkey pointed out the need for a pool of well-trained, experienced trauma/response teams that could be quickly mobilized in the event of war, terrorist attack, or natural disaster to respond to these events anywhere in the world [7]. This is certainly possible, and evident, inasmuch as many reserve medical/surgical units and personnel, mobilized from a variety of civilian practices, were or are actively participating in the Hurricane Katrina response and the wars in Iraq and Afghanistan. These reserve units are meshed into the complex and immense Department of Defense medical response framework. Civilian disaster response teams are also heavily engaged. The International Medical Surgical Response Team concept led by Dr. Briggs is an example. The concern that some reserve medical personnel may not be trained to the wartime status of their active-duty counterparts is slightly overstated. Many of the reserve surgeons have trauma and surgery experience that is sometimes greater than that of active-duty surgeons, especially at the beginning of wars, although active-duty surgeons may be more familiar with the military's deployment tactics and procedures. Either way, there is a learning curve all medical personnel must overcome in dealing with wartime and disaster casualties that can be shortened and straightened by pre-deployment courses and training currently mandated. The military and civilian trauma systems have certainly learned much from one another over the last century. The relationship between military and civilian physicians is continuing as, for example, military physicians develop protocols for blast injury that might apply to civilian terrorist events, and as civilian trauma database and collection systems are applied to the battlefield setting. Statewide trauma systems are ever-evolving entities that encompass more than just the inner-city level-one trauma centers, and are connecting state medical assets into a more coordinated response. There is more evidence building that national, state, and local assets should coordinate actions and communicate more thoroughly.

With this in mind, should national and military assets be available for local responses to disasters? For that matter, should local trauma assets, those with unimaginable experience in the care of the injured patient, from urban trauma centers be made available for international incidents such as war and disaster relief efforts inside and outside of our borders? As you read through the sections provided, you can form your own opinion as to the answers to these questions. Although I do not think that a complete "melding" of response assets is necessarily the answer to these questions, clearly, a coordinated response would benefit all. A response system that is rehearsed and involves, possibly, a tiered response, and one that has interchangeable parts is needed. After looking at action reviews of the response to hurricane

Katrina, those on the outside, as well as most of the victims, could not see an immediate, coordinated response. It cannot be assumed that level-one trauma centers will always be ready to take in casualties from local or distant disasters . There was no anticipation of the difficulty that might ensue if the level-one trauma centers in New Orleans were rendered near-ineffective in the aftermath of a major hurricane. A large systematic response does sometimes take days to coordinate, or worse chaos can ensue if everyone simply descends upon the disaster area with no overall scene command in place. Many individual teams just figured it out at first—as many Americans who have come before them have done when suddenly faced with a seemingly cataclysmic event. However, an emphasis on more preparation for such events is, without question, needed.

I am in awe of the authors here who have spent many hours researching and *living* the surgical response to disasters, those individuals who share these experiences with us not represented in this work, those guest editors coming before me who have contributed and constructed such intuitive and expert compilations of works of authors in past issues, and those who are both victims and care-givers placed in harm's way as a result of the catastrophes described herein. With continued exposure to disaster response and preparation provided in forums such as this, our understanding, experience, and heightened awareness of mass casualty management, no matter what the mechanism, will be seamless. I also would like to give many thanks to Dr. Martin, the consulting editor for SCNA, and to Catherine Bewick at Elsevier, our publisher, for their hard work and guidance through the editorial process.

LTC Robert M. Rush, Jr., MD, FACS
Uniformed Services University
Bethesda, MD, USA

Madigan Army Medical Center
Tacoma, WA 98431 USA

E-mail address: robert.rush@amedd.army.mil

References

[1] Briggs S. Editorial comments for Terrorism preparedness: Web-based resource management and the TOPOFF 3 exercise. J Trauma 2006;60:572.
[2] Frykberg ER. Editorial comments for Terrorism preparedness: Web-based resource management and the TOPOFF 3 exercise. J Trauma 2006;60:571–2.
[3] Jacobs LM, Burns KJ. Terrorism preparedness: Web-based resource management and the TOPOFF 3 exercise. J Trauma 2006;60:566–71.
[4] Hirshberg A, Frykberg ER. Surgeons and disasters: new challenges, new opportunities. Scand J Surg 2005;94:257–8.

[5] Ciraulo DL, Frykberg ER, Feliciano DV, et al. A survey assessment of the level of prepared-
    ness for domestic terrorism and mass casualty incidents among Eastern Association for the
    Surgery of Trauma members. J Trauma 2004;56:1033–9.
[6] Frykberg ER. Disaster and mass casualty management: a commentary on the American Col-
    lege of Surgeons position statement. J Am Coll Surg 2003;197:857–9.
[7] Dixon B. Registry boosts combat survival. Surgery News 2006;2(1):1–4.

**ELSEVIER
SAUNDERS**

SURGICAL
CLINICS OF
NORTH AMERICA

Surg Clin N Am 86 (2006) xxiii–xxiv

Invited Commentary

As our nation continues to defend democracy around the world and works with our allies to ensure the freedom of Iraqi and Afghan citizens, our military medical personnel at all levels are saving lives and restoring health. This issue of the *Surgical Clinics of North America* is an extremely important addition to the growing body of knowledge concerning military medical operations on the battlefield, the effect of weapons of mass destruction, and medical support for natural disasters. The authors are recognized experts in their fields and have hands-on experience in the topics they write about. I congratulate all of them on their efforts and encourage the readers of this issue of the *Clinics* to take the time to study and learn lessons hard-won on our battlefields and in recent disaster relief operations. There may be little or no time for study and preparation when the next event happens, and our medical community and its members are called upon to act and to lead.

On the battlefields of the Middle East, our fighting forces enjoy the highest survival rates in the history of combat. This brilliant record is a result of the combination of the exceptional clinical skills of our providers and the rapid fielding initiatives of equipment and pharmaceuticals. Combined with rapid turnaround of lessons learned, military medicine is making a big difference. No other nation in the world has the training, equipment, research, and capability of the medical systems of our US Armed Forces. EMT-B–trained combat medics are up front and trauma-trained surgical resuscitation teams are at our hospitals. Superb "CCAT" flying ICU teams composed of US Air Force doctors and nurses have brought back to the United States over 25,000 sick and injured soldiers, sailors, airmen, and marines. We have, in essence, brought the foxhole and the flight line back to our major military medical centers, including Walter Reed Army Medical Center and the National Naval Medical Center. Humanitarian medical relief operations have been equally magnificent, including support provided by the USNS Mercy and its staff of civilian and volunteer members after the 2004 tsunami and the emergency medical evacuation and clinical care provided at the Convention Center of New Orleans during relief operations for Hurricane Katrina.

Lessons learned in these efforts will improve our homeland defense and consequent management response. The threat of pandemic flu, the continued unrest around the world, or the arrival of this year's hurricane season may evoke the next great medical challenge. We have learned much about our

doi:10.1016/j.suc.2006.05.001

surgical.theclinics.com

medical capabilities and our shortfalls since the dawn of the twenty-first century. These lessons are both strategic, as in the nation's response to Hurricane Katrina, and tactical, as in the new aggressive use of tourniquets and factor VII on our nation's battlefronts. Trauma registries, coordinated community and federal consequence management tabletop exercises, and aggressive incorporation of the latest scientific and clinical knowledge into community and academic health care will improve our nation's medical readiness. I am very impressed with this issue of the *Surgical Clinics of North America* and encourage all to read it.

LTG Kevin C. Kiley, MD
United States Army
Lieutenant General
The Surgeon General

ELSEVIER
SAUNDERS

SURGICAL
CLINICS OF
NORTH AMERICA

Surg Clin N Am 86 (2006) 537–544

Earthquakes

Susan M. Briggs, MD, MPH

International Trauma and Disaster Institute, Massachusetts General Hospital,
8 Hawthorne Place, Suite 114, Boston, MA 02114, USA

Major earthquakes have the potential to be one of the most catastrophic natural disasters affecting mankind. Earthquakes of significant size threaten lives and damage property by setting off a chain of events that disrupts all aspects of the environment and significantly impacts the public health and medical infrastructures of the affected region. Accelerated urbanization in seismically active parts of the world dramatically increases the vulnerability of these regions to catastrophic numbers of earthquake-related injuries and fatalities (Fig. 1).

Earthquake zones

Worldwide, more than a million earthquakes occur each year, an average of two each minute [1–3]. The geographic and time distribution of earthquakes is referred to as seismicity. Some parts of the earth demonstrate greater seismicity than other areas. A large percentage of the world's earthquakes occur in one arching band, extending around the rim of the Pacific Ocean (Ring of Fire). Another distinct band of seismic activity extends through the Middle East and southern Europe [2]. Nine countries account for over 80% of earthquake fatalities (China, Japan, Pakistan, Chile, Russia, Turkey, Peru, Iran, and Italy) [1–5]. In the United States, there is an estimated 60% probability that an earthquake of Richter magnitude 7.5 or greater will occur on the San Andreas Fault in southern California, and a 40% to 63% probability of a Richter magnitude 6.0 earthquake occurring in the New Madrid seismic of the central US zone [1–3]. The state with the most earthquakes in the United States is Alaska [1–3].

Why earthquakes occur

The earth's surface is divided into about 15 tectonic or lithospheric plates that vary in size and move relative to one another over the earth's surface.

E-mail address: sbriggs@partners.org

surgical.theclinics.com

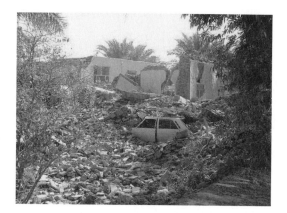

Fig. 1. Bam, Iran.

Tectonic plates move along at a slow, steady rate. Along their boundaries the plates do not slide smoothly. The fault(s) between the plates get stuck together or "locked" by friction. As a result, the surrounding crust bends or deforms. At some point, the strain becomes too great, friction is overcome, and the fault(s) literally snaps (elastic rebound). An earthquake occurs when the crust snaps, and the energy that has been built up and stored within is released as waves of vibration into the surrounding ground [1,2,4].

Earthquakes also can occur in association with active volcanoes. Earthquakes can immediately precede or accompany volcanic eruptions and may cause devastating mudslides. The eruption of Mount Pinatubo in the Philippine Islands in 1991 is an example of this phenomenon, triggering numerous small earthquakes for the next 2 to 3 months [1,2].

The most common causes of tsunamis (seismic sea waves) are submarine earthquakes. Tsunamis can travel thousands of miles at speeds up to 600 mph with little loss of energy and devastating results to low-lying regions. The Pacific coast of the United States is at greatest risk from tsunamis, resulting primarily from earthquakes in the Alaska/Aleutian Island region and South America. The 1964 Alaska earthquake generated tsunamis up to 20 feet in height along Washington, Oregon, and California and caused extensive damage in Alaska and Hawaii (Fig. 2) [1,2]. Human-generated factors or consequences of human activities are another cause of earthquakes (eg, underground explosion of nuclear devices or collapse of underground mine-workings).

Earthquake strength

Magnitude and intensity are two measures of the strength of an earthquake. The magnitude of an earthquake is a measure of the actual physical energy release at its source as estimated from instrumental observations. Magnitude refers to the force of the earthquake as a whole and does not vary from region to region. A number of magnitude scales are in usage,

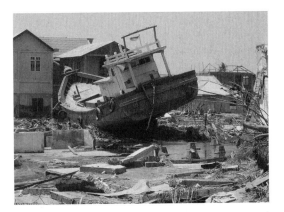

Fig. 2. Damage from tsunami.

but the most commonly used is the Richter magnitude scale, developed in 1936 by Charles Richter (scale 0–10). Two of the largest earthquakes occurring since the invention of the seismograph were a 9.5-magnitude quake in Chile (1960) and the Good Friday quake in Alaska (magnitude 9.2) in 1964. Earthquakes of a magnitude of 2.0 or less are weak and may not be noticed. Earthquakes above 7.0 are considered strong quakes, and quakes of 8.0 or more are known as severe quakes [1,2].

Intensity is a measure of the felt or perceived effects of a quake and is more relevant to the public health and medical consequences of the earthquake. Intensity refers to the effects of an earthquake at a particular site. The intensity is usually stronger close to the epicenter and weaker the farther a site is from the epicenter. The intensity of an earthquake at a particular site is on the basis of the visible consequences left by the earthquake and from individuals who experience the shaking. Many scales measuring intensity are in use, but the most common in the United States is the Modified Mercalli (MM) scale, a 12-point scale. The scale is meant to cover a range of observable impacts, from almost imperceptible shaking to catastrophic destruction. Low numbers are generally the effects of an earthquake felt by individuals, and high numbers characterize structural damage. The peak MM in the Northridge earthquake in California was X [2]. This type of earthquake often results in well-built wooden structures and most masonry and ordinary structures being destroyed; railroad tracks bent; landslides; and water spilling over banks of streams and lakes [1,2].

Factors influencing earthquake mortality and morbidity

Natural factors

Aftershocks

Earthquakes seldom occur alone. Most earthquakes are followed by numerous aftershocks, and some are preceded by foreshocks. Aftershocks are a continuation of the process known as "elastic rebound" and may be as strong as the main shock. Thirty-six percent of aftershocks occur in the first month. Aftershocks usually have an orderly and steady rate of decay, which means that they become less frequent with time. During the Northridge, California, earthquake in 1994, the main shock had a magnitude of 6.7. There were no foreshocks, but immediately after the main shock, and for the next 5 years, more than 14,000 aftershocks occurred in the region [2].

Landslides

Earthquake-triggered landslides and mudflows account for significant number of fatalities and injuries. Landslides were a significant feature in earthquakes that killed 100,000 in China in 1920 and in Peru in 1970 (66,000 fatalities) [1,6].

Hazardous materials

Industrial complexes contain chemical, biological, and radioactive products that may explode or leak during an earthquake, leading to widespread contamination. Pipelines carrying water, sewage, and natural gas may be seriously damaged during an earthquake [7]. Toxic materials were responsible for about 20% of the after-earthquake injuries following the Loma Prieta earthquake in northern California in 1989 [8,9].

Fires

Fires are a significant cause of mortality and morbidity following earthquakes. Data from Japan has shown that earthquakes in Japan that trigger urban fires cause 10 times the number of fatalities as those earthquakes not associated with fires [10]. The tremendous fire that occurred after the 1906 San Francisco earthquake contributed to much of the death toll. During the 1994 Northridge earthquake in southern California, the vibrations caused significant damage to underground fuel lines and gas connection points with spill of toxic materials and resultant fires. During the 1989 Loma Prieta earthquake in northern California, San Francisco had 27 structural fires and more than 500 reports of incidents of fire in 12 hours. The city's water supply was severely damaged, limiting the ability to fight these fires [11].

Dams

Flooding from dams with structural damage from earthquakes is common. Rapid reduction of water pressures and visual inspection of dams is now standard procedure after earthquakes.

Structural factors

Trauma caused by partial or complete collapse of masonry buildings is overwhelmingly the most common cause of injury and death in most earthquakes. It is estimated that 75% of earthquake fatalities are caused by the collapse of buildings that were not earthquake resistant, were built with in-adequate materials, or were poorly constructed [12,13]. The earthquake in Armenia in 1988 was a classic example of substandard construction leading to significant fatalities, many of which were children in schools [12,14,15]. Crush injuries and crush syndrome are common entities encountered by disaster medical responders.

Individual risk factors

Demographic characteristics associated with increased risk for death and injury are individuals over 60 years of age, children between 5 and 9 years of age, and chronically ill individuals [16]. Lack of mobility, exacerbation of underlying diseases, and inability to withstand major traumatic injury con-tribute to the increased vulnerability of these groups. Entrapment, the occu-pant's location within a building, the occupant's behavior during the earthquake, and time until rescue are factors impacting mortality and mor-bidity. Entrapment appears to be the most significant prognostic factor. Death rates for entrapped victims were 67 times higher than nonentrapped victims in the Armenia earthquake (1988) [14,17,18]. Injury rates were 11 times higher for entrapped victims. Time of rescue is important, not only for rescue teams but also for victim survival. Review of major earthquakes throughout the world has shown that the success of extricating survivors drops dramatically 24 hours after the quake [19].

Medical response to earthquakes

Similar to the ABCs of trauma care, disaster medical response includes basic elements that are similar in all disasters. The difference is the degree to which these responses are used in a specific disaster and the degree to which outside assistance is needed to perform the ABCs of disaster care. The mass casualty response to earthquakes includes the four essential ele-ments of disaster medical response: (1) search and rescue; (2) triage and initial stabilization; (3) definitive medical care; and (4) evacuation [20].

The requirements for search and rescue and definitive care are signifi-cantly increased in earthquake disasters as opposed to other natural disas-ters because of the severity of damage and complexity of injuries.

Search and rescue

The local population near any disaster site is the immediate search-and-rescue resource. In disasters involving large numbers of victims trapped in collapsed structures, the local response may be unsophisticated and haphaz-ard, lacking the technical equipment and expertise to facilitate extraction. Many countries have developed specialized search-and-rescue teams as an integral part of their national plans. Members of these teams receive special-ized training in "confined space environments," a common situation in earthquake disasters (Fig. 3) [17,20–22]. Search-and-rescue teams generally include a cadre of medical specialists, generally surgical specialties and emergency medicine physicians; technical specialists knowledgeable in hazardous material, structural engineering, heavy equipment operation, and technical search and rescue methodology (sensitive listening equipment, remote cameras); and trained canines and their handlers.

Triage and initial stabilization

When the scope of an earthquake disaster is large either in geographic scale or in number of injuries, the objective of triage is to do the greatest good for the greatest number of individuals (field medical triage). Triage many occur at three levels and is a dynamic process [20].

On-Site triage (level 1)

This is the rapid categorization of victims with potentially severe injuries "where they are lying" or at a triage site.

Medical triage (level 2)

Medical triage involves the rapid categorization of victims at a casualty site by the most experienced medical personnel available to identify the level of medical care. Knowledge of earthquake injury patterns (eg, crush and burns) is critical.

Evacuation triage (level 3)

Level 3 triage assigns priority to disaster victims for transfer to medical facilities.

Definitive care

Crush injury and crush syndrome are common earthquake injury patterns. Crush injury is defined as compression of extremities and body parts that

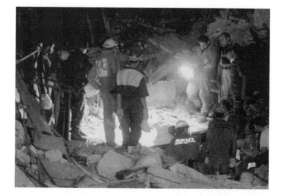

Fig. 3. Search and rescue efforts, Turkish earthquake, 1999.

causes muscle swelling or neurologic disturbances in the affected parts of the body. Typically affected body parts include lower extremities (74%), upper extremities (10%), and trunk (9%). Crush syndrome is localized crush injury with systemic manifestations. These systemic effects are caused by a traumatic rhabdomyolysis (muscle breakdown) and release of potentially toxic muscle cell components and electrolytes into the circulation. Crush syndrome can cause local tissue injury, organ dysfunction, and metabolic abnormalities, such as acidosis, hyperkalemia, and hypocalcemia. Much has been learned regarding the prehospital and hospital management of crush syndrome from experience with earthquake victims [20,21]. Previous experience with earthquakes that caused major structural damage demonstrated [20–23]:

- The incidence of crush syndrome was 2% to 15%.
- Approximately half of those with crush syndrome developed acute renal failure.
- Approximately half of those with acute renal failure needed dialysis.
- A significant number of patients (greater than 50%) with crush syndrome needed fasciotomy. Sudden release of a crushed extremity may result in acute hypovolemia and metabolic abnormalities (reperfusion syndrome). This may cause lethal cardiac arrhythmias and sudden death. Further, the sudden release of toxins from necrotic muscle into the circulation leads to myoglobinuria with subsequent renal failure if untreated. Thus, the key principles of management are the following:
  1. Pretreat casualties with prolonged crush (greater than 4 hours) as well as those who demonstrate abnormal neurologic or vascular exams with 1 to 2 liters of normal saline before releasing crush object whenever possible.
  2. If pretreatment with intravenous fluids is not possible before releasing the crushing object, apply a tourniquet the crushed limb until hydration can be initiated. Field amputation is an operation that can be life-saving, especially with entrapped earthquake victims, victims with severely crushed or mangled extremities, and in the case of prolonged limb ischemia following entrapment [20,24,25].

Summary

Earthquakes continue to be a major cause of traumatic disaster injuries. In addition to the full spectrum of traumatic injuries, hypothermia, secondary wound infections, gangrene requiring amputation, adult respiratory distress syndrome, multiple organ failure, and crush syndrome have been identified as major medical complications in past earthquakes. Early recognition of crush syndrome and associated injuries is important in reducing mortality and morbidity.

Further efforts in earthquake disaster mitigation are needed, as ultimately this will be the most significant factor in decreasing death and disability from earthquake disasters.

References

[1] Noji EK, editor. The public health consequences of disasters. New York: Oxford University Press; 1997.

[2] Prager EJ. Furious earth, the science and nature of earthquakes, volcanoes, and tsunamis. New York: McGraw-Hill; 1999.

[3] Hays WW. Perspectives on the international decade for natural reduction. Earthquake Spectra 1990;6:125–43.

[4] Perez E, Thompson P. Natural hazards: causes and effects. Lesson 2—earthquakes. Prehospital Disaster Med 1994;9:260–71.

[5] US Geological Survey. Scenarios of possible earthquakes affecting major California population centers, with estimates of intensity and ground shaking. Open-file report 81–115. Menlo Park (CA): USGS; 1981.

[6] Blake P. Peru earthquake, May 31, 1970. Report of the CDC epidemiologic team. Atlanta (GA): Center for Disease Control; 1970.

[7] Showalter PS, Myers MF. Natural disasters in the United States as release agents of oil, chemicals, or radiological materials between 1980–1989: analysis and recommendations. Risk Anal 1994;14:169–82.

[8] Durkin ME, Thiel CC, Schneider JE, et al. Injuries and emergency medical response in the Loma Prieta earthquake. Bull Seismological Society of America 1991;81:2143–66.

[9] Haynes BE, Freeman C, Rubin JL, et al. Medical response to catastrophic events: California's planning and the Loma Prieta earthquake. Ann Emerg Med 1992;21:368–474.

[10] Coburn AW, Murakami HO, Ohta Y. Factors affecting fatalities and injury in earthquakes. Internal Report. Engineering Seismology and Earthquake Disaster Prevention Planning. Hokkaido, Japan: Hokkaido University; 1987.

[11] EQE Engineering. The October 17, 1989 Loma Prieta earthquake: a quick look report. San Francisco: EQE Engineering; 1989.

[12] Coburn A, Spence R. Earthquake protection. New York: John Wiley & Sons; 1992. p. 2–12, 74–80, 277–84.

[13] Coburn AW, Spence RJS, Pomonis A. Factors determining human casualty levels in earthquakes: mortality prediction in building collapse. Reston (VA): US Geological Survey 1992.

[14] Aznaurian AV, Haroutunian GM, Atabekian AL, et al. Medical aspects of the consequences of earthquake in Armenia. Yerevan (Armenia): Armenian Ministry of Health; 1990. p. 9–10.

[15] Frechets CN. Rescuing earthquake victims in Armenia. Plast Reconstr Surg 1989;84:838–40.

[16] Class RI, Urrutia JJ, Sibony S, et al. Earthquake injuries related to housing in a Guatemalan village. Science 1977;197:638–43.

[17] Noji EK, Kelen GD, Armenian HK, et al. The 1988 earthquake in Soviet Armenia: a case study. Ann Emerg Med 1990;19:891–7.

[18] Durkin ME, Murakamia HO. Casualties, survival and entrapment in heavily damaged buildings. Tokyo: Japan Association for Earthquake Disaster Prevention; 1988. p. 977–82.

[19] Noji EK. Medical consequences of earthquakes: coordinating medical and rescue response. Disaster Management 1991;4:32–40.

[20] Briggs SM, editor. Advanced disaster medical response manual for providers. Boston: Harvard Medical International; 2003.

[21] Sheng ZY. Medical support in the Tangshan earthquake: a review of the management of mass casualties and certain major injuries. J Trauma 1987;27:1130–5.

[22] Noji EK, Armenian HK, Oganessian A. Issues of rescue and medical care following the 1988 Armenian earthquake. Int J Epidemiol 1993;22:1070–6.

[23] Noji ER. Acute renal failure in natural disasters. Ren Fail 1992;14:245–9.

[24] Eknoyan G. Acute renal failure in the Armenian earthquake. Kidney Int 1993;44:241–4.

[25] Pretto EA, Angus DC, Abrams JI, et al. An analysis of prehospital mortality in an earthquake. Prehospital Disaster Med 1994;9:107–24.

SURGICAL
CLINICS OF
NORTH AMERICA

Surg Clin N Am 86 (2006) 545–555

Response to Hurricane Disasters

David V. Shatz, MD[a,b,*], Katharine Wolcott, MD[c],
Jennifer Bencie Fairburn, MD, MSA[d]

[a]Division of Trauma, Burns, and Surgical Critical Care, Department of Surgery,
University of Miami Miller School of Medicine, PO Box 016960 (D-40),
Miami, FL 33101, USA
[b]Federal Emergency Management Agency Urban Search and Rescue,
Florida Task Force 1, 9300 NW 41 Street, Miami, FL 33178, USA
[c]Department of Surgery, Madigan Army Medical Center, Building 9040,
Fitzsimmons Drive, Tacoma, WA 98431-1100, USA
[d]Emergency Medical Operations, Department of Health,
Division of Emergency Medical Operations, 4052 Bald Cypress Way,
Bin C-18, Tallahassee, FL 32399-1739, USA

Hurricane season is the time of year when the tropical ocean waters warm and the atmospheric winds moisten. It is during this period that the eastern seaboard and gulf coast communities of the United States hope for a quiet season while governmental agencies prepare for the worst. Unlike natural disasters such as earthquakes and wildfires, the destructive paths of hurricanes can be predicted to some degree. Preparedness and adherence to recommended evacuation orders can and do save lives. Like other disasters, however, nature is an unpredictable force that can result in significant destruction, injury, and loss of life [1]. Systems at multiple levels, not the least of which is medical, may be stressed and must execute well-designed and practiced plans to function optimally. Plans are built on experience and on what to expect. For medical systems, these plans include the prehospital emergency medical systems, hospitals, and individual physicians. Although medical needs can vary as much as the strength of the storm, similarities exist across all windstorms. Knowledge of and preparation for these needs are what build effective plans.

* Corresponding author. Division of Trauma, Burns, and Surgical Critical Care, Department of Surgery, University of Miami Miller School of Medicine, PO Box 016960 (D-40), Miami, FL 33101.

  E-mail address: dshatz@miami.edu (D.V. Shatz).

0039-6109/06/$ - see front matter © 2006 Elsevier Inc. All rights reserved.
doi:10.1016/j.suc.2006.02.010

surgical.theclinics.com

What is a hurricane?

A hurricane is a tropical storm with winds that have reached a sustained speed of 74 miles per hour (mph) or more. Hurricane winds blow in a large spiral around a relatively calm center known as the "eye." The eye is generally 20 to 30 miles wide, and the storm may extend outward 400 miles. As a hurricane nears land, it can bring torrential rains, high winds, and storm surges. A single hurricane can last for more than 2 weeks over open waters and can run a path across the entire length of the eastern seaboard. August and September are peak months during the hurricane season, which lasts from June 1 through November 30.

Windstorms are classified by category based on the speed of the sustained winds (Saffir-Simpson Hurricane Scale). Tropical depressions are organized systems of clouds and thunderstorms with a defined circulation and maximum sustained winds of 38 mph or less. A tropical storm is an organized system of strong thunderstorms with a defined circulation and maximum sustained winds of 39 to 73 mph. Intense tropical weather systems with a well-defined circulation and maximum sustained winds of 74 mph or higher become hurricanes. Hurricanes are called typhoons in the western Pacific, whereas similar storms in the Indian Ocean are called cyclones.

Although the most destructive hurricanes affecting the United States form in the Atlantic Ocean, hurricanes can also form in the Gulf of Mexico, the Indian Ocean, the Caribbean Sea, and the Pacific Ocean. Hurricane winds in the Northern Hemisphere circulate in a counterclockwise motion around the hurricane's eye, whereas hurricane winds in the Southern Hemisphere circulate clockwise. Natural phenomena that affect a storm include temperature of the water, the Gulf Stream, and steering wind currents. Powered by heat from the sea, storms are steered by the easterly trade wind, the temperate westerlies, and by their own ferocious energy. Around their core, winds grow with great velocity, generating violent seas. Moving ashore, they sweep the ocean inward while spawning tornadoes and producing torrential rains and floods. In addition to the violent winds, the storm surge, which generates subsequent flooding, is the major source of destruction on land.

Although the damage inflicted by a hurricane differs with the terrain it encounters, the structural integrity of the buildings hit, the population density, the tide levels at the time of landfall, and the potential property damage and flooding expected along the coast can be estimated. Category 1 storms, with winds of 74 to 95 mph, produce no real damage to building structures; damage is limited primarily to unanchored mobile homes, shrubbery, and trees. Some coastal road flooding and minor pier damage may occur. Category 2 storms (winds 96–110 mph) result in some roofing material, door, and window damage. Considerable devastation to vegetation, mobile homes, and piers can be expected. Coastal and low-lying escape routes flood 2 to 4 hours before the arrival of the center of the storm, and small craft in unprotected anchorages break their moorings. Category 3 hurricanes (winds

111–130 mph) cause some structural damage to small residences and utility buildings, with a minor amount of curtainwall (non–weight-bearing panels suspended on the exterior of multistory structures between supporting columns) failures. Mobile homes are destroyed. Flooding near the coast destroys smaller structures, with larger structures damaged by floating debris. Terrain lower than 5 feet above sea level may be flooded 8 miles or more inland. As the winds increase to 131 to 155 mph (category 4), more extensive curtainwall failures occur, with some complete roof structure failure on small residences. Major erosion of the beach and major damage to lower floors of structures near the shore can be expected. Terrain lower than 10 feet above sea level may be flooded, requiring massive evacuation of residential areas as far as 6 miles inland. Top-level hurricanes (category 5: sustained winds >155 mph) produce complete roof failure on many residences and industrial buildings. Some complete building failures, with small utility buildings blown over or away, can be seen. Major damage occurs to lower floors of all structures located less than 15 feet above sea level and within 500 yards of the shoreline, which may require massive evacuation of residential areas on low ground within 5 to 10 miles of the shoreline.

Prestorm medical issues

With current-day communications, an approaching storm should be a surprise to no one. The National Hurricane Center, located in Miami, Florida, tracks storms from their inception, and has performed well in predicting the power and anticipated landfall location of most recent storms. With these predictions comes the ability to prepare, which for most involves the accumulation of supplies (water, food, flashlights, batteries), the securing of property (debris removal and placement of hurricane shutters), and evacuation. An adequate supply of prescription medications and supplies (syringes for diabetics, dressings for those who have recent wounds) must be anticipated and obtained. For those planning to weather the storm at home, placing these supplies in a safe room (away from windows and outside doors) should be done. Adequate supplies of fuel for personal vehicles and generators (in the event of power loss) need to be obtained before the storm arrives. These activities, representing only a partial list of the immediate preparation required, produce a very stressful environment.

As anxiety levels mount, errors occur that can lead to medical emergencies. Hurricane shutters can cause serious injury. These shutters are made of aluminum with very sharp edges and, in bulk, can be very heavy. Falling shutters have resulted in extensive lacerations and even death from head injuries. As people rush to accomplish their goals, motor vehicle accidents are also a concern.

As the storm approaches, emergency medical support disappears. Helicopters are typically grounded when wind speeds approach 45 mph. Operation of high-profile ground ambulances becomes risky at wind speeds of

45 mph, and dispatch of fire suppression units may terminate at wind speeds of 55 mph. Persons who have serious illness and injuries at this point become nontransportable.

Weathering the storm

The excitement of increasing winds and rain can be quickly replaced by substantial concern when that rain becomes torrential and the winds rattle structures. Fear that those structures may fail begins to mount. As power lines are downed, communication with relatives and news agencies is lost, and protective structures are left in darkness. Structures built to hurricane standards often do well; however, for structures not typically in hurricane-prone areas and those not built to the stringent standards of hurricane building codes, structure failure can occur. Total roof failure exposes those inside to flying debris. Many have been injured or killed when falling trees struck and collapsed houses. Reports of people wishing to go outside to experience the storm and being struck by flying debris (often with fatal results) are frequent.

Poststorm problems

As the storm passes, a sense of relief is quickly followed by one of awe or one of despair at first sight of the resulting damage. Here is where the real medical problems begin.

Power outages may be limited to neighborhoods or entire counties, lasting hours to months. With the lack of power comes the loss of refrigeration of food and medications, air conditioners, and lights. Those fortunate enough to have generators (17.5% in Florida following hurricanes Charley, Frances, Ivan, and Jeanne) [1] can spare some of these inconveniences, but generators are a risk unto themselves. Standard generators run on gasoline. Spilling gasoline onto a hot engine while attempting to refill the tank can lead to a burned victim. Despite the seemingly appropriate placement of generators away from living quarters, carbon monoxide is still a cause of fatal and nonfatal poisonings after hurricanes. One hundred sixty-seven such poisonings (including six fatalities) were treated in Florida in the aftermath of the four hurricanes of the summer of 2004 [2]. Although common knowledge might predict otherwise, 5% of those using generators placed them indoors [2]. Fifty-one cases of carbon monoxide poisoning were reported following Hurricane Katrina in 2005 in the states of Louisiana, Mississippi, and Alabama. Burns resulting from alternate sources of heat for cooking, such as barbeques and butane/propane stoves, are also frequent.

Downed power lines are also a source of injury. Contact with any structures charged by these lines leads to electrocution injury. In areas flooded by the storm, those entering the water to work or play are subject to lethal electrocution if that water is energized by a downed power line.

Clearing and repairing the damage to one's property can be arduous work. As noted, hurricanes occur during the summer months when the heat and humidity are at their highest. Many people are not accustomed to heavy workloads in these environments and, as a result, suffer heat disorders. Cardiac events also increase in frequency. Roof and tree damage leads to people climbing to heights not frequented by most. Falls from roofs and ladders are commonly seen in the aftermath of a storm. For some, only a home remedy is required, but for others, the injury is a significant laceration, fracture, or worse, brain injury or other form of life-threatening internal injury.

The debris after a hurricane is frequently in the form of shrubbery and fallen trees. Clearing these often requires knives, handsaws, machetes, and chain saws. Many people rent chain saws but have little or no experience using them. As one might imagine, a spectrum of lacerations, some quite severe, results from the use of these tools.

Preparation is key

Preparation is the key to minimizing injury and death from the destructive forces of a hurricane; however, as witnessed in the days surrounding the approach of Hurricanes Katrina and Rita toward the cities within Louisiana and Texas, and Hurricane Wilma in Florida during the summer of 2005, preparation can be formidable on a public health level. Evacuation plans must include those unable to evacuate themselves, including the healthy who do not have personal transportation and the residents and patients of nursing homes, group homes, hospices, and hospitals. Despite mandatory evacuation orders by local officials to those in predicted high-risk areas, a significant percentage of these residents do not heed these orders. As a result, call volumes for prehospital providers increase markedly. Although some patients acquire only minor injuries, many suffer chronic problems and have nowhere to go. The elderly are deposited in hospital emergency departments by family members, expecting a safe refuge—all this at a time when the hospitals themselves may be trying to evacuate. As seen during the hurricanes of 2005, many nursing homes had evacuation plans that included agreements with transportation companies, but because those companies had contracted with several nursing homes simultaneously, they did not have the capability of evacuating all of the patients in time.

Hospital disaster plans usually include a plan to discharge or transfer less acute patients to nonaffected facilities. Critical patients, however, are frequently not able to be transferred due to their acuity, and are rightfully left in place. Hurricanes can bring storm surges, heavy rains, and flooding, and hospitals with ground-based helipads are unable to evacuate patients by air if those helipads are under water. Most hospitals have ground-level or basement emergency generators that can similarly flood and become nonoperational. Although the Joint Commission for the Accreditation of Health

Care Organizations requires that hospitals have fuel for those generators, no minimum amount is specified. The American Institute of Architects guidelines state that hospitals should have a minimal storage capacity to permit continuous operation for at least 24 hours [3] in accordance with National Fire Protection Association (NFPA) 99, NFPA 101, and NFPA 110. Florida Building Code specifies a requirement for a fuel supply stored on-site to fuel generators for 100% load for 72 hours of actual demand load for all patient areas (Florida Building Code Section 419.4.2.9.2) for nursing homes (Florida Building Code Section 420.3.25) and hospitals (Florida Building Code Section 419.3.18). (NFPA 110 Section 2-2.3 requires a Class 48 generator, defined as having a fuel tank size of 48 hours, with an additional 33% over the 48 hours required as per Section 3-4.2.3. This requirement equates to 64 hours of fuel, but for simplicity, 72 hours is the standard). What if evacuation resources are not available until after that fuel is exhausted? Some health care facilities in New Orleans following Hurricane Katrina had accumulated a supply of food and water but had stored them in basement facilities, only to have them destroyed by floodwaters [4]. Even generator power can fail, leaving ventilators that lack backup batteries without a power source and, therefore, nonoperational. The usual 1:2 ICU nurse-to-patient ratio suddenly becomes unmanageable when ventilated patients require human-assisted ventilation with bag-valve-masks.

Special needs, hospice, nursing home, and hospitalized patients should probably be evacuated in larger storms, but many older adults requiring no special needs choose to remain in the area. During and after the storm, however, barriers to medical care for pre-existing needs can prove fatal [5]. Food, water, and medications can be destroyed in the storm, and isolation because of flooding or area destruction can prevent access to medical care. Because hurricanes tend to be summertime events, excessive heat can prove to be fatal in those who have frail health. As seen in Hurricane Katrina, even those in a normal state of health can succumb to the high temperatures produced in attics during attempts to escape rising floodwaters.

Although hospitals are on the high-priority list for restoration of support, lower-profile hospices, assisted living facilities, and skilled nursing facilities are often delayed in regaining necessary power and supplies. Outpatient dialysis centers are another significant area of need. Most hospitals are not equipped to handle a large number of chronic dialysis patients if the outpatient centers should become nonfunctional. For this reason, if advance warning is available, these patients should be dialyzed at their respective centers before the event occurs and be prepared to not be dialyzed for up to 3 days after; adherence to a proper emergency renal diet is necessary [6]. All Medicare-certified outpatient dialysis centers are required to have at least one backup facility [7], and this information must be passed on to the patients. Similar arrangements need to made for chemotherapy patients and other chronic needs patients. Oxygen supplies for health care facilities and those on home oxygen must also be kept current.

Coordination of the poststorm medical needs response should occur through the local and state Emergency Operations Centers. Emergency Support Function (ESF) 8 is the designated group within the disaster response organization responsible for this coordination and should be updated regularly with the functional status of all health care facilities within the affected areas. These facilities include all emergency medical services ground and air systems, bed surge capacities of hospitals, burn beds, acute care beds, skilled nursing and assisted living facilities, and a listing of all blood centers, dialysis centers, and outpatient chemotherapy and radiation centers.

Anticipation of blood needs is yet another task for hospitals. One of the many challenges facing resumption of clinical surgical services is blood product availability. All community-wide blood drives are usually suspended, which means that all blood products need to be delivered from remote locations. This delay in delivery is especially problematic for platelets, which have a shelf life of only 5 days.

Local and state disaster response

As outlined previously, hurricanes may pass into the history books as nothing more than a stressful threat or as the most devastating natural disaster in United States history. The degree of poststorm response is dictated by the degree of destruction.

Area hospital emergency rooms can quickly become busy. In the early hours and days after the storm, many of the visits are for injuries. In the authors' experience, these patients can be taken to areas of the hospital other than the emergency room (for instance, the recovery room if elective surgical cases are suspended) in an effort to offload the increasing surge on the emergency department. Because hospital registration is often the bottleneck to rapid care, wounds can be triaged and addressed first by surgeons brought in specifically for this reason, patients can be given a supply of antibiotics, and registration can be handled as the patients exit the area. In any large-scale disaster, medical care must be streamlined and sometimes inventive.

Medical licenses are issued by the state, which should allow personnel to practice anywhere within that state. The limitations to outside physician and nursing assistance, therefore, are at the individual hospital level. Emergency suspension of the requirement of hospital privileges allows personnel from unaffected areas to fill positions in the hospital temporarily vacated by medical personnel whose own lives have been disrupted by the storm. This waiver allows for the reopening of hospitals and much needed medical care in the immediate vicinity of the affected area.

Knowledge of the operational status of near and distant area facilities allows for expedited transfer or transport of patients to functional medical care facilities. Figs. 1 and 2 from the Department of Health and Human

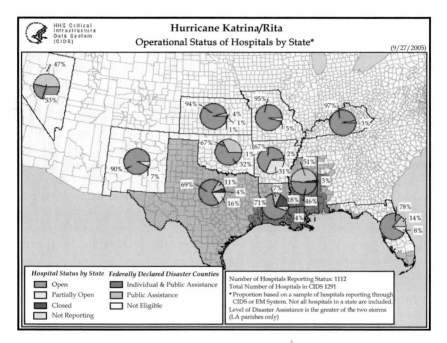

Fig. 1. Operational status of hospitals by state following Hurricane Katrina/Rita. (*From* US Department of Health and Human Services, Washington, DC.)

Services Critical Infrastructure Data System demonstrate the local, state, and national availability of medical care for hurricane victims following Hurricane Rita in 2005. A means of rapidly assessing the needs of the affected area also allows proper resource deployment and use [8].

Federal disaster assistance

In December 2004, the National Response Plan (NRP) [9] became operational, with a 4-month phase-in period, after which the previous Federal Response Plan, the US Government Domestic Terrorism Concept of Operations Plan, and the Federal Radiological Emergency Response Plan became obsolete. This document, based on the National Incident Management System, provides a framework within which disaster response can operate at all levels (local, state, tribal, federal, private sector, and nongovernmental organizations) and is designed to function in an all-hazards environment. With this plan comes definitions of roles and responsibilities of key authorities.

Although hurricanes allow for more planning and preparation than other natural disasters, much of the initial poststorm response lies in the hands of local authorities who are usually first on scene. This response includes an initial damage assessment, the subsequent restoration of power outages,

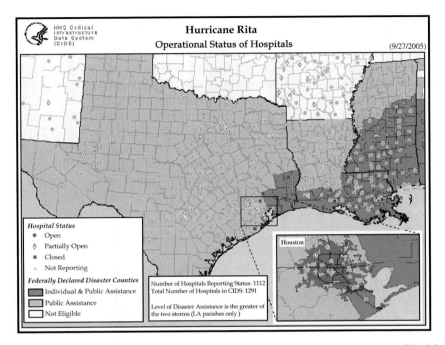

Fig. 2. Operational status of hospitals during Hurricane Rita. (*From* US Department of Health and Human Services, Washington, DC.)

the clearing of roads to allow the safe movement of traffic and rescue personnel, and the establishment of a law enforcement presence to prevent unlawful acts. In the event that local resources are overwhelmed, state assistance is requested. As outlined in the NRP, the governor, as the state's chief executive officer, is responsible for coordinating the state's resources "to address the full spectrum of actions to prevent, prepare for, respond to, and recover from incidents in an all-hazards context" [9]. If and when it becomes clear that state assets have been exceeded or exhausted, federal assistance can be requested by the governor. The process for this request and assistance is outlined in the Robert T. Stafford Disaster Relief and Assistance Act [10]. This federal assistance can be extensive and can include medical care.

Within the NRP are 15 ESFs. These ESFs, in their partial or full activation, provide a coordinated assistance mechanism for local, state, and tribal governments for recovery from any and all disasters. Two of these 15 ESFs provide medical assistance. Activation of ESF 9 (Urban Search and Rescue) mobilizes elite teams trained in the specialized area of heavy structure collapse. These teams provide primarily search and rescue capabilities but include a component of medical personnel for the treatment of rescued victims; however, their supplies and capabilities are limited. Within ESF 8 (Public Health and Medical Services) is the National Disaster Medical

System and the network of Disaster Medical Assistance Teams (DMATs). These DMATs consist of medical personnel from all areas of emergency medical care, including physicians, nurses, radiology and respiratory therapy technicians, and laboratory personnel. These teams deploy with their personnel and equipment and are capable of independent function as a field hospital in a parking lot or in filling personnel positions in existing hospitals. These teams were used extensively in the hurricanes of 2004 and especially in those of 2005. Over 64,000 patients were treated by the deployed DMAT teams in the 6 weeks following the landfall of Hurricanes Katrina and Rita in 2005 [11]. Military assets have also been successfully deployed following major storms [12] and can provide supplies, air support, manpower, and law enforcement resources.

The future

Every disaster carries with it new challenges that have never been seen or perhaps never been considered. As such, every disaster provides a teaching environment from which we can and should learn. Hurricane Katrina provided a significant classroom from which we can change future policy.

Few disasters in the United States have brought the infrastructure of an entire city to its knees as occurred in New Orleans in the summer of 2005. Few have produced the numbers of victims of that storm. A considerable amount of time and brainpower has been devoted over the years to preparing for disasters, but more postincident planning should be stressed. Although communication has long been a recognized problem in the postdisaster setting, transportation becomes a formidable issue in a large-scale disaster that affects thousands and eliminates the basic support structures. Before and after a storm, huge numbers of people must be evacuated by public and private transportation. Even those who heed evacuation demands find themselves caught in interminable traffic jams. Effective plans that allow for proper evacuation must be developed, and adequate numbers of vehicles used for postevent evacuation must be rapidly mobilized.

After victims are removed from immediate danger, they are frequently deposited in areas while awaiting definitive evacuation. Mass care of these potential thousands must be prepared for. Casualty collection points must be identified before the event and must be staffed and equipped properly with basic-needs medical care. These collection points can range in function from treatment areas to morgues. Mass casualty triage must be used effectively. Although most physicians are accustomed to treating the most severely sick and injured first, it is difficult for this practice to happen in these settings. Those in need of advanced medical care may fall into triage categories in which care will not be rendered, and physicians must be trained to deal with this scenario. Shelters should be identified for prestorm evacuees and the potential hundreds or thousands displaced from their homes after the storm.

Summary

The preparation and rebuilding in the wake of a devastating hurricane can be a challenge at all levels. The summer of 2004 proved how frequently these preparations might need to happen, and the hurricanes of 2005 demonstrated how extensive these preparations should be and the cost of inadequate preparation. Medical care is a very large component of the disaster plan for hurricanes and must include not only supplies but also personnel. Personal and professional limitations can impede the response of valuable personnel to distant sites, but one must remember that the local response falls in the hands of those first on site (ie, those who reside in the area). Proper planning and effective drills can mitigate the extent of damage to structures and human life, and when deemed necessary, effective evacuation of at-risk areas is crucial. In the end, nature is much too powerful a force for us to fight—we can only be prepared to respond to and bend with the potentially devastating forces directed our way.

References

[1] Epidemiologic assessment of the impact of four hurricanes—Florida, 2004. MMWR Morb Mortal Wkly Rep 2005;54(28):693–7.

[2] Carbon monoxide poisoning from hurricane-associated use of portable generators—Florida, 2004. MMWR Morb Mortal Wkly Rep 2005;54(28):697–700.

[3] Guidelines for design and construction of hospital and health care facilities. Washington, DC: American Institute of Architects; 2001. Chapter 7.

[4] Rohde D, McNeil DG, Abelson R, et al. Storm and crisis. The victims: vulnerable, and doomed in the storm. New York Times. Section A, page 1, column 1. September 19, 2005.

[5] Rapid assessment of the needs and health status of older adults after Hurricane Charley—Charlotte, DeSoto, and Hardee Counties, Florida, August 27–31, 2004. MMWR Morb Mortal Wkly Rep 2004;53(36):837–40.

[6] Preparing for emergencies: a guide for people on dialysis: Department of Health and Human Services, Center for Medicare and Medicated Services; 2002. Publication #CMS 10150. Available at: http://new.cms.hhs.gov/MLNProducts/downloads/10150.pdf or http://medicare.gov/Publications/Pubs/pdf/10150.pdf. Accessed March 29, 2006.

[7] Code of Federal Regulations, Title 42, Volume 2, Section 405.2160, Conditions for Coverage of Suppliers of End-Stage Renal Disease (ESRD) Services–Affiliation agreement or arrangement. Revised October 1, 2003. U.S. Government Printing Office. Washington DC.

[8] Waring S, Zakos-Feliberti A, Wood R, et al. The utility of geographic information systems (GIS) in rapid epidemiological assessments following weather-related disasters: methodological issues based on the Tropical Storm Allison experience. Int J Hyg Environ Health 2005;208(1–2):109–16.

[9] National Response Plan. Available at: http://www.dhs.gov/interweb/assetlibrary/NRP_FullText.pdf. Accessed March 29, 2006.

[10] Robert T. Stafford Disaster Relief and Assistance Act. Pub L No. 93-288, 88 Stat 143 (1974) (codified as amended at 42 USC §5121-5206, and scattered sections of 12 USC, 16 USC, 20 USC, 26 USC, 38 USC [2002]).

[11] National Disaster Medical System Resource Status Report, October 15, 2005.

[12] D'Amore AR, Hardin CK. Air Force expeditionary medical support unit at the Houston floods: use of a military model in civilian disaster response. Mil Med 2005;170(2):103–8.

SURGICAL CLINICS OF NORTH AMERICA

Surg Clin N Am 86 (2006) 557–578

Floods and Tsunamis

CAPT Mark Llewellyn, MD

Clinical Investigation Department (KCA), Naval Medical Center San Diego,
34800 Bob Wilson Drive, Suite 5, San Diego, CA 92134-1005

Floods and tsunamis cause few severe injuries, but those injuries can overwhelm local areas, depending on the magnitude of the disaster. Most injuries are extremity fractures, lacerations, and sprains. Because of the mechanism of soft tissue and bone injuries, infection is a significant risk. Aspiration pneumonias are also associated with tsunamis. Appropriate precautionary interventions prevent communicable disease outbreaks. Psychosocial health issues must be considered.

The events of the past year and a half have rewritten the history of destructive natural disasters. On December 26, 2004, a massive earthquake and subsequent tsunami in the Indian Ocean killed more than 200,000 people; on August 29, 2005, the most destructive hurricane in United States history devastated New Orleans and the Gulf Coast; and on October 8, 2005, a large earthquake in the Kashmir area of Pakistan killed more than 50,000 people. Disaster and disaster preparedness are on everyone's mind and television. Several publications, written before these recent events (including the destructive hurricanes that punished Florida in 2004), provide excellent reviews of disaster preparedness and management [1–4]. A more recent review provides an historical summary of disaster preparedness, describing the National Disaster Medical System (NDMS) and President Carter's creation of the Federal Emergency Management Agency (FEMA) in 1979 [5].

History, Epidemiology, and Basic Science

Floods are the most common natural disasters that affect developed and developing countries [6]. Mortality statistics are usually readily available, as

---

The views expressed in this article are those of the author and do not reflect the official policy or position of the Department of the Navy, Department of Defense, or the United States Government.

E-mail address: dmllewellyn@nmcsd.med.navy.mil

opposed to more specific information on injuries and illnesses that is essential for clinicians to optimally prepare for these events [6]. Mortality alone is not a sensitive indicator of health risk [7]. This article reviews the available data and extrapolates from recent experiences.

According to the OFDA/CRED International Disaster Database [8], the tsunami of December 26 was undoubtedly the most lethal natural disaster that occurred in 2004 (Table 1). Among the top disasters of 2004, determined by the number of resulting deaths, floods were the most common, and as shown in Box 1, occurred most frequently.

Clearly, people living in developing countries are more vulnerable to floods, and flood size and populations at risk are variable. What is being seen today seems to be what Dr. Noji [9] predicted 10 years ago: "The future seems to be even more frightening. Increasing population density in flood plains, along vulnerable coastal areas, and near dangerous faults... point to the probability of catastrophic natural disasters."

According to the National Oceanographic and Atmospheric Administration (NOAA), "In most years, flooding causes more deaths and damage than any other hydro- meteorological phenomena. In many years it is common for three-quarters of all federally declared disaster declarations to be due, at least in part, to flooding" [10]. Table 2 shows the United States fatalities from floods in recent years.

In 2004, deaths were reported from flash, river, and urban/small-stream floods. The 0- to 9- and 20- to 29-year-old age groups had the most deaths at 14 each, of which 62% were men. In recent years, 50% or more of all flood-related deaths have occurred in automobiles.

Approximately 8000 people died in 1900 when a large hurricane hit Galveston, Tex. In 1928, 1836 people died from another hurricane around Lake Okeechobee in Florida. Most of these deaths were believed to be caused by the large storm surge associated with powerful hurricanes. Deaths from

Table 1
Top disasters by deaths in 2004

Rank	Disaster	Month	Country	Number of deaths
1	December 26 Tsunami	December	12 countries	226,408
2	Hurricane Jeanne	September	Haiti	2,754
3	Flood	May/June	Haiti	2,665
4	Typhoon Winnie	November	Phillipines	1,619
5	Flood	June/August	India	900
6	Flood	June/August	Bangladesh	730
7	Flood	May/June	Dominican Republic	688
8	Dengue epidemic	January/April	Indonesia	658
9	Earthquake	February	Morocco	628
10	Meningitis epidemic	January/March	Burkina Faso	527
11	Cyclone Galifo	March	Madagascar	363

Data from EM-DAT: THE OFDA/CRED International Disaster Database. Available at: www.em-dat.net. Université Catholique de Louvain; Brussels, Belgium.

> **Box 1. Most frequent natural disasters of 2004**
>
> 1. Floods: 128 occurrences
> 2. Wind storms: 121 occurrences
> 3. Epidemic: 35 occurrences
> 4. Earthquake: 30 occurrences
>
> ---
>
> *Data from* EM-DAT: The OFDA/CRED International Disaster Database. Available at: www.em-dat.net. Université Catholique de Louvain; Brussels, Belgium.

Hurricane Katrina are estimated to be more than 1300, making 2005 the third deadliest year in United States history for flood deaths, and by far the worst in recent years. The storm surge, produced by the high winds and vacuum effect of low-pressure systems, can produce dramatically high seas. These large storm surges that are so destructive and fatal are believed to account for an estimated 90% of deaths before a warning and evacuation system is implemented [11]. According to NOAA, the storm surge "is unquestionably the most dangerous part of a hurricane," acting "like a giant bulldozer sweeping everything in its path" [10]. The slope of the continental shelf can influence the effects of the storm surge's coastal inundation, and a normal high tide can add to the raised water level. The storm surge of category 5 Hurricane Camille that pounded the Gulf Coast in 1969 measured 25 feet.

In the United States, as much as 90% of the damage from natural disasters (excluding droughts) is caused by floods, costing $3.7 billion annually between 1988 and 1997. Between 1940 and 1999 an average of 110 deaths per year occurred in the United States, mostly from flash floods. A flash flood is defined as flooding that occurs within 6 hours of the inciting event, such as a heavy rainfall or a levee or dam failure. Flooding occurs in known floodplains. "Conversion of land from fields and woodlands to roads and parking lots" has resulted in "loss of ability to absorb water and has increased run off" leading to increased flood risk in some areas [12].

Table 2
United States fatalities from floods in recent years

Year	Flooding deaths	Flood deaths in automobiles
2004	82	45
2003	99	47
2002	50	31
2001	66	31
2000	41	20
1999	77	40
1998	136	86

Data from NOAA, National Weather Service Available at: http://www.nws.noaa.gov.

The power of water, especially moving water, is astounding. For example, "Two feet of water will carry away most automobiles...The lateral force of a foot of water moving at 10 mph is about 500 pounds on the average car. And every foot of water displaces about 1,500 pounds of car weight. So two feet at 10 mph will float virtually every car" [12].

In recent years, Continental Europe has experienced increased flooding. The 2002 flooding was caused by record rainfall combined with record warm months resulting in glacier melting. Dams could not withstand the surges of water pressure. According to the World Health Organization (WHO), flooding is the most common natural disaster in Europe [13]. "The number of deaths associated with flooding is closely related to the life-threatening characteristics of the flood (rapidly rising water, deep flood waters, objects carried by the rapidly flowing water) and by the behavior of the victims" [13], such as being in automobiles. Injuries are likely to occur during the aftermath or cleanup stage, particularly sprains and strains, lacerations, and contusions. As in the United States, vulnerable groups include the elderly, the very young, and individuals who have disabilities. Unfortunately, a "comprehensive surveillance of morbidity following floods is limited" [14].

Injuries and illnesses related to floods

What morbidity information exists? In 1992, Alson and colleagues [15] reported on the experience of an NDMS Special Operations Response Team after Hurricane Andrew. The team, consisting of one surgeon, three emergency department physicians, one physician assistant, four registered nurses, one psychologist, one pharmacist, 19 emergency medicine technicians/paramedics, six support personnel, and one public health preventive medicine specialist, saw 1203 adult and 336 pediatric patients. Only five injuries were directly caused by the hurricane; 285 injuries were sustained during the cleanup. Most of the care was routine and provided to those whose source of care was destroyed or not accessible. Supplies of tetanus antitoxin, antibiotics, and insulin were depleted in 24 hours. Many visits were to obtain prescription refills. Of the patients seen, 54 were pregnant, 13 were in active labor, and 10 had obstetric complications, such as suspected ectopic pregnancy or placenta previa. Twenty cases of simple corneal abrasions or corneal foreign bodies were seen, with one penetrating globe injury. In descending order, the most common procedures were: cardiac monitoring, intravenous therapy, laceration repair, abscess drainage, extremity splinting, abrasion debridement, and foreign body removal. Major lessons learned were that the unit must be self-sustaining for 72 hours, and communications, supplies, and record keeping are vital functions.

D'Amore and Harin [16] reported their experiences with an Air Force Expeditionary Medical Support Unit (EMEDS) that deployed to Houston,

Tex, in 2001 when Tropical Storm Allison deposited 40 inches of rain on the city between June 6th and 10th. "The city's medical infrastructure bore the brunt of the storm's damage". Nine of the city's hospitals were closed or severely limited in services. The EMEDS +25 deployed from Wilford Hall with an 87-person staff. It had 10 ED beds, 2 OR tables, 3 ICU beds, 14 in-patient beds; and digital radiology, dental, and laboratory capabilities. It worked in coordination with a FEMA-operated Disaster Medical Assis-tance Team (DMAT). The DMAT performed most of the primary and re-ferral care, while the EMEDS functioned as the hospital. One thousand thirty-six cases were seen over 11 days. Five hundred seven were "general medicine" and 232 were "trauma." There were 16 operation room cases: 4 I/Ds, 3 ORIFs, 2 closed fracture reductions, 2 laceration repairs, 2 hernias, 1 DPL/ex-lap for multiple trauma with mesenteric tear, 1 peri-rectal abscess I/D, and one exploration for foreign body.

Numerous Centers for Disease Control and Prevention (CDC) Morbidity and Mortality Weekly Reports (MMWRs) have provided data on flood and hurricane/flood injuries. In 1999, flooding from Hurricane Floyd's 20 inches of rain resulted in 52 deaths, with drowning in cars the leading cause; 10% of deaths were rescue workers. Four conditions accounted for 63% of emer-gency department visits: orthopedic and soft tissue injuries (28%), respira-tory illnesses (15%), gastrointestinal illnesses (11%), and cardiovascular diseases (9%). Other conditions included 10 cases of carbon monoxide poi-soning, and hypothermia. Increases in suicide attempts, dog bites, febrile ill-nesses, basic medical needs, and dermatitis occurred in the first week after the floods, whereas increases in arthropod bites, diarrhea, violence, and asthma were seen 1 month later [17].

Other CDC MMWRs provide essentially the same information on in-juries in or around the home in the aftermath of these events. Most injuries are mild, predominantly consisting of cuts, lacerations, puncture wounds, and strains/sprains to extremities. Winds from Hurricane Charley in 2004 caused blunt trauma that resulted in more deaths than did drowning. Preex-isting conditions such as cardiovascular diseases and diabetes were exacer-bated [18–23].

Carbon monoxide poisonings are caused by placing generators indoors, in garages, or outdoors but near windows. After the 2004 hurricanes in Flor-ida, 157 persons were treated from 51 exposure incidents, with six reported deaths [23]. Carbon monoxide poisonings were recently associated with Hurricane Katrina. Of the 167 cases, 48.5% were treated and released with-out undergoing hyperbaric oxygen therapy (HBOT), 43.7% were released after undergoing HBOT, and 7.8% were hospitalized (most for just 1 day). Among the patients, 80% complained of headache, 51.5% nausea, 51% dizziness, 31.5% vomiting, and 16.4% dyspnea, and 14.5% experi-enced loss of consciousness. The mean carboxyhemoglobin level was 19.8%, with a range of 0.2% to 45.1%. Practitioners must be aware of this risk and how to prevent, recognize, and treat it.

The CDC Katrina updates provide excellent summaries and recommendations for prevention, recognition, and treatment of conditions associated with hurricanes, floods, and disasters. These can be found at www.cdc.gov/od/katrina.

The clinician must consider a wide spectrum of illnesses in the aftermath of a disaster; common illnesses are still most common among the conditions seen (Table 3).

Infectious diseases associated with flooding

When the incidence of an infectious disease increases after a natural disaster, usually that agent was present in the environment before the disaster. Therefore, because the victims may be "exposed to potentially contaminated flood waters and crowded living conditions, and have had many opportunities for traumatic injury," a broad differential diagnosis must be formed. Diseases associated with contaminated water include leptospirosis and *Vibrio vulnificus*. Leptospirosis is a zoonosis that has many wild and domestic animal reservoirs, including rats. Humans become infected after contact with contaminated water, whereby the organism enters skin abrasions or the conjunctiva. *V vulnificus* is a halophilic gram-negative bacterium found in salt water. Eighteen wound-associated cases of *V vulnificus* were reported after Hurricane Katrina. Workers with exposure to brackish waters should take precautions. Patients who have immunosuppression or chronic liver diseases are at increased risk. The wound infection begins with increased redness and local swelling and rapidly progresses, with characteristic findings such as vesicles and hemorrhagic bullae. Late-stage infections may result in gangrene, necrotizing fasciitis, systemic illness, and, potentially, sepsis. Treatment is with antibiotics (doxycycline and a third-generation

Table 3
Top 10 conditions: from limited needs assessments among persons staying in evacuation centers between September 10 and 12, 2005

Condition	Incidence per 1000 residents
Hypertension/cardiovascular	108.2
Diabetes	65.3
New psychiatric condition	59.0
Preexisting psychiatric condition	50.0
Rash	27.6
Asthma/Chronic obstructive pulmonary disease	27.5
Flu-like illness of pneumonia	26.3
Toxic Exposure	16.0
Other infections[a]	15.6
Diarrhea	12.8

Data from Centers for Disease Control and Prevention. Available at: www.cdc.gov/od/katrina/09-19-05.htm.

[a] Pertussis, varicella, rubella hepatitis, tuberculosis, and other communicable illness of outbreak concern.

cephalosporin) or fluoroquinolone [24]. Aggressive wound-site therapy may be needed. The CDC provides further recommendations for managing *V vulnificus* infection at www.bt.cdc.gov/disasters/hurricanes/katrina/vibrio-faq.asp, information on wound injury and emergency management of wounds at www.bt.cdc.gov/disasters/emergwoundhcp.asp, and recommendations for prevention and treatment of immersion foot at www.bt.cdc.gov/diasaters/trenchfoot.asp. Additional diagnoses to consider are provided at www.bt.cdc.gov/disasters/hurricanes/katrina/medcare.asp. Table 4 summarizes the direct and indirect effects of floods on human health.

Heating, ventilation, and air-conditioning (HVAC) systems may be submerged after floods and become health hazards from microorganism contamination. Either replacement or proper cleaning and disinfection are required to prevent respiratory allergic manifestations. The CDC provides recommendations for proper cleaning at www.cdc.gov/niosh/topics/flood/cleaning-flood-HVAC.html. *Legionella pneumophila* may occur in HVAC systems and lead to Legionellosis, either a severe form with pneumonia, or a milder form (Pontiac Fever).

Finally, molds present a significant hazard in houses after floodwater exposures. Fungal infections are possible in individuals who are immune suppressed. Allergic manifestations such as cough, hay fever, rash, or asthma exacerbation are most likely. Molds can produce toxins that are hazardous if eaten or taken internally.

The number of deaths that resulted from the tsunami of December 26, 2004, will never be certain because the exact number of people who were in many areas is unknown; Fig. 1 provides an estimated summary. In the World Disaster Report of 2005, the International Federation of the Red Cross and Red Crescent Societies (IFRC) reported 164,000 dead or missing and more than 400,000 homeless In Aceh, Indonesia alone [25].

Regardless of the numbers, this tsunami is of unprecedented enormity (Tables 5, 6a, and 6b). "It rapidly became the most reported and well-funded disaster in history. Over 200 humanitarian organizations—plus 3,000 military troops from a dozen countries—arrived to offer aid" [25]. By one to two orders of magnitude, this tsunami caused more deaths than any other in the past 100 years (Fig. 2).

History

The mythical Atlantis may have been a real site destroyed by a tsunami, perhaps one produced when Santorini exploded. Other famous tsunamis include the one produced by the explosive destruction of Krakatoa in 1883, which Killed 36,000 persons. The 1700 Cascadia Earthquake in Vancouver, Canada, caused the subsequent distant tsunami in Japan and a local tsunami that was recorded in Native American oral tradition. In 1755, approximately 100,000 people died in Lisbon, Portugal, from earthquake, tsunami,

Table 4
Effects of floods on human health

Direct effects

Causes	Health implications
Stream flow velocity; topographical features; absence of Warning; rapid speed of flood onset; deep flood waters; Landslides; risky behaviour; fast-flowing waters carrying boulders and fallen trees	Drowning; injuries
Contact with water	Respiratory diseases; shock; hypothermia; cardiac arrest
Contact with polluted water	Wound infections; dermatitis; conjunctivitis; gastrointestinal illnesses; ear, nose and throat infections; possible serious waterborne diseases
Increase in physical and emotional stress	Increased susceptibility to psychosocial disturbances and cardiovascular incidents

Indirect effects

Causes	Health implications
Damage to water supply systems; damage to sewerage and disposal systems; insufficient supply of drinking-water; insufficient supply of water for washing	Possible waterborne infections sewage (enteropathogenic *E. coli, Shigella,* hepatitis A, leptospirosis, giardiasis, Campylobacteriosis); dermatitis; conjunctivitis
Disruption of transport systems	Food shortages; disruption of emergency response
Disruption of underground piping; dislodgment of storage Tanks; overflow of toxic waste sites; release of chemicals; Disruption of petrol storage tanks, possibly leading to fire	Potential acute or chronic effects of chemical pollution
Standing water; heavy rainfall; expanded range of vector Habitats	Vectorborne diseases
Rodent migration	Possible rodent-borne diseases
Disruption of social networks; loss of property, jobs and family members and friends	Possible psychosocial disturbances
Clean-up activities following flooding	Electrocution; injuries; lacerations; puncture wounds
Destruction of primary food products	Food shortages
Damage to health services; disruption of "normal" health Services activities	Decrease in "normal" health care services; insufficient access to medical care

Data from Menne B, Pond K, Noji EK, et al. Floods and public health consequences, prevention and control measures. UNECE/MP.WAT/SEM.2/1999/22, discussion paper presented at the United Nations Economic Commission for Europe (UNCE) seminar on flood prevention, Berlin, 7–8 October, 1999. WHO European Centre for Environment and Health, Rome, Italy.

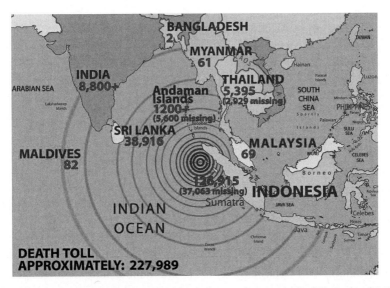

Fig. 1. Map showing death toll resulting from the massive tsunami of December 26, 2004. *From* the Pacific Disaster Management Information Network. Indian Ocean Earthquake and Tsunami Emergency Update, December 29, 2005. The Center of Excellence in Disaster Management and Humanitarian Assistance, Honolulu HI; with permission.

and fire. Tsunamis caused 40,000 deaths in the South China Sea in 1782, and 27,000 deaths in Japan in 1826. And in 1868, 25,000 deaths in Chile were tsunami-related. Two Hilo Hawaii tsunamis have occurred, one in 1960 that killed 61 people, caused by the largest earthquake (magnitude 9.5)

Table 5
The United States Agency for International Development data

Region	Individuals Dead/Missing	Individuals Displace/Affected
Indonesia (12/26/04 tsunami)	128,645 dead, 37,063 missing	532,898 displaced
Indonesia (3/28 earthquake)	39–626 dead	34,000 displaced
Sri Lanka	31,147 dead, 4,115 missing	519,063 displaced
India	10,749 dead, 5,640 missing	647,599 displaced
Maldives	82 dead, 26 missing	21,663 displaced
Thailand	5,395 dead, 2,845 missing	N/A
Malaysia	68 dead, ±6 missing	±8,000 displaced
Somalia	±150 dead	±5,000 displaced, 54,000 affected
Seychelles	±3 dead	40 households displaced

Data from the US Agency for International Development; Bureau for Democracy, Conflict and Humanitarian Assistance; Office of U/S Foreign Disaster Assistance; Bureau for Asia and the Near East; Government of Indonesia, 04/28/05; Government of Indonesia, 3/31/05; U.N. Office of the Humanitarian Coordinator for Indonesia; Government of Sri Lanka, 04/28/05; Government of India, 04/28/05; Maldives National Disaster Management Center, 04/28/05; U.N. Office for the Coordination of Humanitarian Affairs (OCHA), 1/18/05; Government of Thailand, 04/19/05; U.N. Consolidated Appeal, 1/06/05; U.N./Seychelles and USAID, 1/12/05.

Table 6a
Top 10 countries affected by wave/surge sorted by number of people killed

Country	Date	Killed
Indonesia	26 Dec 2004	165,708
Sri Lanka	26 Dec 2004	35,399
India	26 Dec 2004	16,389
Thailand	26 Dec 2004	8345
Japan	3 mar 1933	3000
Soviet Union	4 Nov 1952	2300
Papua New Guinea	17 Jul 1998	2182
Japan	1 sep 1923	2144
Japan	7 mar 1927	1100
Indonesia	18 Jul 1979	539

Data from EM-DAT: The OFDA/CRED International Disaster Database. Available at: www.em-dat.net. Universtié Catholique de Louvain; Brussels, Belgium.

ever recorded, and one in 1946 that killed 159 people [25a]. More recently, a 1998 tsunami in Papua, New Guinea, killed more than 2000 people. Since 1850, more than 420,000 deaths have been caused by tsunamis [25b]. "Most of these casualties were caused by local tsunamis that occur about once per year somewhere in the world" [26].

Basic science

The word *tsunami* is Japanese and means "harbor wave." The word may have been created when fishermen did not notice the open-ocean tsunami waves while in their boats and only realized the destructive power when they returned to port.

Tsunamis are generated when a massive amount of water is displaced, usually by an underwater earthquake. Volcanic eruptions or large

Table 6b
Top 10 countries affected by wave/surge sorted by number of people affected

Country	Date	Affected
Sri Lanka	26 Dec 2004	1,019,306
India	26 Dec 2004	654,512
Indonesia	26 Dec 2004	532,898
Somalia	26 Dec 2004	105,083
Thailand	26 Dec 2004	67,007
Korea Dem P Rep	21 Aug 1997	29,000
Maldives	26 Dec 2004	27,214
Myanmar	26 Dec 2004	12,500
Bangladesh	30 Aug 2000	12,010
Papua New Guinea	17 Jul 1998	9867

Data from EM-DAT: The OFDA/CRED International Disaster Database. Available at: www.em-dat.net. Universtié Catholique de Louvain; Brussels, Belgium.

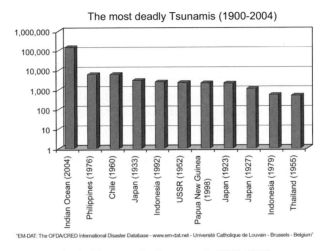

The most deadly Tsunamis (1900-2004)

"EM-DAT: The OFDA/CRED International Disaster Database - www.em-dat.net - Université Catholique de Louvain - Brussels - Belgium"

Fig. 2. The most deadly tsunamis (1900–2004).

underwater landslides can also produce tsunamis. The tsunami of December 26, 2004, was caused by an earthquake occurring 255 km SSE of Banda Aceh, Indonesia. Events leading up to that earthquake began "about 50 million years ago when the Indian Subcontinent collided with Asia raising the Himalayas." Parts of China and Southeast Asia are still being forced eastward. A plate boundary exists along the west coast of Sumatra where the heavier Indian plate is subducting beneath a lighter continental plate, the "Burma plate, which is a microplate between the Indian Plate and the Sunda Plate that contains much of Southeast Asia...Strain builds up and eventually the accumulated strain exceeds the frictional strength of the fault, and it slips in a great earthquake. The overriding plate that is dragged down rebounds and displaces a great volume of water" [27]. The magnitude 9.0 to 9.3 earthquake occurred along a 1200-km rupture on the ocean floor, causing the 2004 tsunami. "The fault slide was up to as much as 15 meters near Banda Aceh...The earthquake lasted at least 10 minutes—longer than any earthquake ever recorded" [28]. Along the entire 1200-km fault, the average vertical movement of the ocean floor was 4 meters. Lay and colleagues [28] warn that "there will be more earthquakes of this type, and with more humans exposed to the hazard there will be more devastating losses of life."

Once the entire water column is displaced, the initial tsunami splits into a "distant tsunami" that travels into open ocean and a "local tsunami" that moves toward the shore. The distant tsunami travels faster, because the speed of a tsunami is proportional to the square root of the water depth. Wave heights in deep water can only be tens of centimeters high, but move very quickly, up to 800 km per hour. However, the energy in the wave essentially goes to the bottom of the ocean and very little energy is lost as it moves large distances. The tsunami waves typically come in trains of 3 to 10 waves, separated by minutes. As the waves move closer to shore, they slow down to about 30 to 40 kilometers per hour, compress, and build in height. Finally the waves run ashore like a very strong and fast-moving tide, traveling much further inland than a normal wave [28a]. Tsunami waves do not look like a curling surfer's dream wave, but rather like a wall of water or "bore." Eyewitnesses often describe the tsunami as being black (Fig. 3). The waves can scour away the shoreline and anything in its path. Large objects, such as large boats, can be carried a few kilometers inland, as was seen in Banda Aceh. A negative wave may reach shore first, as it did on Sumatra, causing the waterline to recede and coax some people to venture out to retrieve stranded fish, only to be followed by a devastating incoming tsunami wave of ferocious strength (9–15 m high in Banda Aceh).

Tsunamis are most common in the Pacific basin and usually require an earthquake with a magnitude of at least 7.0 for generation. The U.S. Geological Survey's earthquake magnitude policy is to use the term *magnitude* alone. *Moment magnitude* is currently the preferred method of recording earthquakes, but information can be confusing to non–earth scientists. The famous logarithmic Richter scale was devised by Charles Richter of Cal Tech in 1935 to measure local Southern California earthquakes of moderate size (3 to 7 on the Richter scale) using a seismograph to measure movement [29]. (A 3 on the Richter scale is the smallest that can be felt by humans.) The Richter scale is usually used by the lay media, "But Richter's original method is no longer used because it doesn't give reliable results for larger earthquakes and for those far away [29]." Newer methods, designed to be consistent with Richter's logarithmic scale, measure movement from zero on a seismograph. The energy of an earthquake is proportional to the square root of the cube of the amplitude, or approximately 31.6 times more energy for each step of the Richter scale. The newer moment magnitude scale, devised in 1979, was "designed to be consistent with Richter's

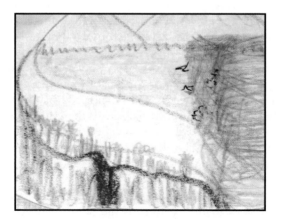

Fig. 3. Tsunami waves pictured by young witness.

logarithmic scale [29]" and is related to the dimensions of the earthquake and the energy released. Intensity scales are also used in some parts of the world to describe earthquake effects in the local area; however, the term *magnitude* avoids confusion [29].

Illnesses and injuries related to tsunamis

On July 17, 1998, a tsunami caused by a magnitude 7.0 earthquake that generated an underwater landslide devastated the north coast of Papua, New Guinea. Waves of 7 to 15 meters hit the coast within 10 minutes of the earthquake. Three coastal villages were swept away completely, 16 villages were destroyed, and 2200 people died [30].

The Australian Defense Force (ADF) responded to this disaster and reported their experiences [31,32]. Over 10 days, 251 patients were treated and 209 surgical procedures were performed. Only two deaths occurred, both related to aspiration pneumonitis and near-drowning. The Australian unit had two operating tables (with a third for minor wound debridement) and 20 beds. The ADF arrived 52 hours after the tsunami and reported that they "treated no patients with intracranial, intrathoracic, abdominal or spinal injuries as these patients had already succumbed before our deployment. Furthermore, few infants and elderly people had survived [31]." Every patient the ADF treated on the first day had some aspiration pneumonitis from near-drowning. Injuries consisted of lacerations, including numerous large-flap scalp lacerations, and open and closed fractures and dislocations.

"All wounds were grossly septic and contaminated with foreign material...Many victims had been impaled upon the mangroves [32]." The ADF performed many wound debridements and 14 amputations. They saw "patients with every imaginable limb injury [33]." Necrotizing fasciitis was common. "All surgical wounds were left open, using ample absorbent gauze dressings." Delayed primary closure of wounds occurred approximately 5 days later. As expected, many patients had underlying respiratory diseases and anemia secondary to malaria or intestinal parasites, which were prevalent. Dehydration compounded blood loss; blood transfusions were available but limited. Patients who had long bone fractures were transported unsplinted to the ADF because the medical capabilities in the villages had been destroyed.

In many ways the experiences after the December 26 tsunami were similar, but on a much larger scale. Tragically, a huge number of people washed out to sea and drowned. Some were likely killed or injured by the large earthquake that hit Sumatra before the tsunami, and many were killed by blunt or penetrating trauma from objects in the fast-moving water. Notwithstanding lessons from the past, the number of serious injuries was much lower than many emergency medical teams expected. Many of the injured suffered extremity trauma.

Maegele and colleagues [33] reported on 17 tourists who were severely injured in this tsunami and were returned to Germany. Of the 17 patients, 15 had large soft tissue injuries of the leg or hip; 7 had thoracic trauma with rib fractures, 3 with hemopneumothoraces; 6 had closed fractures; 5 had large soft tissues injuries of the arm; 4 had open fractures; and 3 had head lacerations. All patients had clinical and radiologic evidence of pneumonitis. The wounds were grossly contaminated and cultures grew bacteria common to the marine environment. Wound infection with sewage contamination was suspected. Also, wounds grew highly resistant organisms that are uncommon to an aquatic environment, such as *Acinetobacter*, beta-lactamase producing *Escherichia coli*, methicillin-resistant *Staphylococcus aureus* (MRSA), and *Candida*.

In an accompanying editorial, Masur and Murray [34] comment on and provide additional information about infectious organisms associated with the tsunami. Seawater may contain *Vibrio* spp, *Aeromonas*, and *Mycobacterium marinum*. Sewage contamination would add enteric organisms. Furthermore, other organisms, including *Pseudomonas* spp, *Aeromonas*, *Legionella*, *Burkholderia*, *Chromobacterium*, and *Leptospira*, present risks for those patients who were swept inland and landed in freshwater. (In Banda Aceh, the Aceh River flows right through the middle of the city and empties into the sea where the tsunami hit the city.) Traditional nosocomial pathogens could be contracted, such as MRSA and *Enterococcus*, especially in overwhelmed and damaged hospitals. *Acinetobacter*, with multiple drug resistances, was reported in 20% of the patients. Respiratory and contact isolation were recommended until infectious agents could be identified.

The infectious disease specialists on the USNS Mercy in Banda Aceh observed drug resistance to be "remarkably prevalent," including an extremely high incidence of MRSA and multiply-resistant gram-negative pathogens and a very high rate of fluoroquinolone resistance. The specialists found it "surprisingly hard to distinguish between nosocomially acquired multiply resistant organisms and true community-acquired resistance" (Ed Ryan, MD, and Mark Pasternack, MD, unpublished material). Antibiotics are much more casually prescribed in some parts of the world, which may have contributed to this effect.

Tsunami-related aspiration pneumonia was not uncommon in individuals who were exposed to the deluge. Allworth [35] reported a case of "tsunami lung." He reported on the Australian experience, with 1 specific case and 10 similar cases [36] presenting with cavitary, necrotizing pneumonia approximately 1 month after immersion. Some patients developed empyemas and pneumothoraces. These patients did not experience response to many broad-spectrum antibiotics, but did experience response to carbapenems, and therefore carbapenems became first-line or early second-line treatment for immersion-related respiratory infections. Allworth reports that *B pseudomallei* were cultured from pleural fluid in four patients, and because many patients described a "black wave," muddy water aspiration was suspected, making *B pseudomallei* a likely causal agent of the infections. However, polymicrobial infections or other agents could have caused the pneumonias. Chierakul and colleagues [37] described their experience in Thailand, reporting on six cases of melioidosis in tsunami survivors. All six cases had aspirated tsunami water, and four also had significant lacerations. One patient had major anterior and posterior tibial artery damage, severe bleeding, and extensive wound contamination, eventually necessitating a below-the-knee amputation. Three of the six patients had diabetes mellitus. One patient died. All presented with signs and symptoms of pneumonia 3 to 38 days after the tsunami. *B pseudomallei*, which is a gram-negative bacillus found in the soil and water of endemic areas, was cultured from three blood samples and four respiratory secretions. These patients were treated with ceftazidime or a carbapenem for 2 weeks, followed by oral trimethoprim-sulfamethoxazole plus doxycycline to complete a 20-week treatment course.

Kao and colleagues [38] reported on one experience of the USNS Mercy involving an aspiration pneumonia. This patient also developed a brain abscess with a dense hemiparesis that responded to aggressive antibiotic therapy, which favorably reviews the pulmonary, neurologic, and infectious disease possibilities. One of Mercy's first patients was a 12-year-old boy with aspiration pneumonia. He spent 1 week in the intensive care unit, followed by 1 week in one of Mercy's wards. His story was typical of many: he was washed out to sea by the tsunami and survived by holding onto floating debris. His immediate family had all been killed. After he was rescued at sea, an uncle eventually found him.

Andersen and colleagues [39] reported on a case of mucormycosis in an Australian survivor of the tsunami who had been pushed a kilometer from his beach hut through debris. He had a large deep soft tissue injury on his thigh and hip, and many other smaller lacerations and abrasions. After he was evacuated to Sydney, he was treated with meropenem, ciprofloxacin, and doxycycline, and tetanus immunoglobulin. He developed widespread necrotizing fasciitis on his chest and arm and was treated with debridement, amphotericin B (lipid formulation), and hyperbaric oxygen. His wounds were suspected to have become contaminated when his injuries occurred or during his early resuscitative care.

An increase in tetanus occurred in Aceh, with 106 cases and 20 deaths reported [40]. Before the tsunami, Aceh had approximately 30 cases of tetanus per year. Most of the new cases developed between January 9 and January 17, 2005 [41]. The Injury Control Research Center hospital saw 15 cases, mostly men; more than required ICU care, with 100% survival [41].

Vaccination coverage for Aceh was lower than for the rest of Indonesia, with approximately 60% for children and 20% to 30% for adults. The toxin tetanospasmin is produced when the vegetative form of *Clostridium tetani* germinates in wounds contaminated with soil, dirt from the street, or feces.

The toxin is then taken up by the nerve terminals and transported intra-axonally to the spinal neurons. It then causes a presynaptic inhibition of an inhibitory transmitter, glycine. This loss of inhibition causes rigidity, accounting for the classic trismus (lockjaw), and other symptoms such as opisthotonos from back-muscle rigidity. The autonomic nervous system can also be affected, leading to conditions such as severe dysrhythmias, hyperthermia, blood pressure fluctuations, and urinary retention.

Treatment involves respiratory support; benzodiazepines or vecuronium for spasms, if necessary; passive immunization with human tetanus immunoglobulin; active immunization with tetanus toxoid at a site separate from the immunoglobulin site; antibiotic therapy with penicillin G; treatment of autonomic dysfunction; and surgical debridement of wounds [42].

No cases of cholera were confirmed in the 4 months after the tsunami [41]. This pathogen does not survive well in saltwater, and proactive preventive measures were enacted by the international medical teams to further mitigate the risk factors associated with potable water shortage, crowding, and lack of sanitation. Also, no increases occurred in the incidence of malaria or dengue fever, which are both mosquito-borne illnesses. Although endemic, the baseline rates of these illnesses are not as high in Aceh as they are in other Indonesian provinces. However, tuberculosis was extremely widespread and prevalent. Intestinal parasites were also common and patients often passed *Ascaris* worms, particularly when under anesthesia.

Lim and colleagues [43] reported on the observations of two Korean medical relief teams working in Sri Lanka, noting that adequate potable water significantly mitigated transmission of diarrheal illnesses. Respiratory diseases and chronic conditions were prevalent in the displaced persons camps. Skin infections and minor skin trauma were particularly common.

International collaboration, communication, cooperation

The USNS Mercy arrived more than a month after the disaster struck. The WHO, the IFRC, non–governmental organizations (NGOs), and foreign militaries working with the host nations had already collaborated to help those in need. Mercy came with a floating tertiary capability that did not exist anywhere near Banda Aceh. It had a CT scanner, angiography, an extensive pharmacy, a full laboratory and blood bank, fully equipped ICU beds, and four staffed operating rooms. The treatment team consisted of volunteer nurses and doctors from the NGO Project HOPE, commissioned officers from the United States Public Health Service (particularly strong in valuable mental health resources), and Medical staff from the US Navy. Some patients had injuries (mostly orthopedic or maxillofacial) directly related to the tsunami that only the Mercy had resources to evaluate and treat. Aspiration pneumonia cases were also treated, as were some trauma cases that occurred in the damaged city. However, most patients were seen by Mercy staff because they had lost everything and had limited access to medical care.

The local hospital in Banda Aceh, Zainoel Abidin Hospital, lost more than 50% of its staff; it had just received a CT scanner a few months before being destroyed by the tsunami. Routine illnesses became urgent. The Mercy's first patient was a boy who had appendicitis and was brought in by his father; his mother and other siblings were dead or missing and presumed dead. Mercy's experience was unique in that it had more than enough work for its surgeons because it had the complete infrastructure to support almost any surgery needed. Mercy performed 285 operations in Banda Aceh, mostly onboard. The most procedures performed onshore were cataract surgeries. Surgeries performed were predominantly orthopedic; oromaxillofacial/ear, nose, and throat (OMFS/ENT); and general surgery cases: 40 patients underwent 65 orthopedic procedures, including 25 incision and drainage; 14 intramedullary nail; and 9 open reduction internal fixation. General surgery cases, including pediatric and plastics, ranged from thoracotomy to wound drainage. Fractures and a wide range of head and neck masses dominated the OMFS/ENT workload.

Although Mercy arrived more than 5 weeks after the event, the crew still saw disaster-related injuries. However, disaster-related injuries had mostly diminished by the fourth week [41], testifying to the success of the combined efforts of the civilian and military health care providers. However, getting the right resources to the right people at the right time did not always occur. A huge gift of goodwill was bestowed by the world community, which "reflects the universality of the humanitarian impulse" [44]. However, matching the assistance with the needs was not easy. Some assistance was considered inappropriate and "the overabundance of helpers added to the problems of coordination [44]." For example, some children were given up to four measles vaccinations. The IFRC reported that one United Nations witness in Meulaboh (south of Banda Aceh on the devastated west coast of Sumatra) saw "20 surgeons competing for a single patient...Yet midwives and nurses were in short supply. Women had to give birth without medical assistance" [25]. And, alas, we are reminded that we neglect "the forgotten emergencies" – the millions, mostly children, who die each year from malnutrition and preventable diseases.

People who witnessed the December 26 tsunami and became friends with those who suffered have difficulty not getting emotional when reflecting on the disaster. The magnitude, or denominator, of the devastation is difficult to fathom; physicians and surgeons are more inclined to look at the numerator, reflected by the individual sitting on the examination table or under the drape on the operation table. A disaster by definition overwhelms the resources, and therefore the denominator must be considered so that more individual patients can be helped. For tsunamis and floods, although the deaths may be many and the destruction widespread, the number of injuries requiring sophisticated care is relatively few. Adequate water, sanitation, clothing, nutrition, and shelter are early priorities [45].

Summary

The CDC provides the following review and summary of the health effects of tsunamis [46]:

Immediate health concerns

- After the rescue of survivors, the primary public health concerns are clean drinking water, food, shelter, and medical care for injuries.
- Flood waters can pose health risks such as contaminated water and food supplies.
- Loss of shelter leaves people vulnerable to insect exposure, heat, and other environmental hazards.
- Most deaths associated with tsunamis are related to drownings, but traumatic injuries are also a primary concern. Injuries such as broken limbs and head injuries are caused by the physical impact of people being washed into debris, such as houses, trees, and other stationary items. As the water recedes, the strong suction of debris being pulled into large populated areas can further cause injuries and undermine buildings and services.
- Medical care is critical in areas where little medical care exists.

Secondary effects

- Natural disasters do not necessarily cause an increase in infectious disease outbreaks. However, contaminated water and food supplies and the lack of shelter and medical care may have a secondary effect of worsening illnesses that already exist in the affected region.
- Decaying bodies create very little risk for major disease outbreaks.
- The people most at risk are those who handle the bodies or prepare them for burial.

Long-lasting effects

The effects of a disaster are long-lasting. In the months after a disaster, a greater need exists for financial and material assistance, including

- Surveying and monitoring for infectious and water- or insect-transmitted diseases
- Diverting medical supplies from nonaffected areas to meet the needs of the affected regions
- Restoring normal primary health services, water systems, housing, and employment

- Helping the community recover mentally and socially after the crisis has subsided

One sad and unusual statistic from the Indian Ocean tsunami disaster is that many more women than men were killed. Another sad fact is that the number of children killed was disproportionately high.

The mental health needs of the victims must be addressed. Addressing these psychologic needs, De Jong and colleagues [47] wrote: "In Banda Aceh we found that most people have a strong desire to move forward and to rebuild their lives." The crew on the Mercy observed great resiliency and strength in the Acehnese people. Although most people exposed to a disaster do well and only have transient symptoms, some individuals develop psychiatric illnesses [48]. Post-traumatic stress disorder clearly increases in the disaster-affected areas.

Table 7 provides a comparison of the consequences of various disasters, including floods and tsunamis. Earthquakes cause many injuries. The working rule of thumb is to calculate three injuries for every death. Floods and tsunamis, on the other hand, do not typically cause a large number of injuries compared with deaths. This observation of 25 years ago is still valid today.

For the United States to have been part of the international humanitarian response to the 2004 tsunami disasters was an honor and a privilege. The cooperation and coordination that occurred, though it may not have been perfect, gives reason to be optimistic about the future, for the world is truly a much smaller place than it used to be and the future depends on communication and mutual respect.

Table 7
Comparison of disaster consequences

Likely effects	Complex emergencies[a]	Earthquakes	High winds without flooding	Hurricanes, floods	Flash floods, tsunamis
Deaths	Many	Varies	Few	Few	Many
Severe injuries	Varies	Many	Moderate	Few	Few
Risk of communicable disease outbreaks[b]	High	Small	Small	Varies	Varies[c]
Food scarcity	Common	Rare	Rare	Varies	Varies
Population displacements	Common	Rare[d]	Rare	Common	Varies

Adapted from Pan American Health Organization, Emergency Health Managements After Natural Disaster. Washington (DC): Office of Emergency Preparedness and Disaster Relief Occordination; 1981. Scientific Publication No. 47.

[a] Complex emergencies not in original table published in 1981. Complex emergency = human disaster situation that can follow war or civil strife.

[b] "Risk of communicable diseases is potential after all major disasters. Probability rises with overcrowding and deteriorating sanitation".

[c] Epidemics are not inevitable after every disaster.

[d] Population displacements may occur in heavily damaged urban areas.

Acknowledgments

I wish to thank and acknowledge my shipmates: civilian volunteers from Project HOPE, Officers from the USPHS, Civilian Mariners from the Military Sealift Command, and sailors from the US Navy. And special thanks to Ms. Susana Hazelden for her administrative assistance with this manuscript.

Further reading

Winchester S. Krakatoa: the day the world exploded: August 27, 1883. New York: Harper Collins; 2003.

References

[1] Schult C, Koenig K, Noji E. Disaster preparedness. In: Marx JA, Hockberger RS, Walls RM, editors. Rosen's emergency medicine: concepts and clinical practice. 5th edition. St. Louis (MO): Mosby, Inc.; 2002. p. 2631–40.
[2] Noji E. Natural disaster management. In: Auerbach PS, editor. Wilderness medicine. 4th edition. St. Louis (MO): Mosby, Inc.; 2001. p. 1603–21.
[3] Reed S. Natural and human-made hazards: mitigation and management issues. In: Auerbach PS, editor. Wilderness medicine. 4th edition. St. Louis (MO): Mosby, Inc.; 2001. p. 1622–61.
[4] Noji E. Disasters: introduction and state of the art. Epidemiol Rev 2005;27:3–8.
[5] Dara SI, Ashton RW, Farmer JC, et al. Worldwide disaster medical response: an historical perspective. Crit Care Med 2005;33(1 suppl):S2–6.
[6] Ahern M, Kovats RS, Wilkinson P, et al. Global health impacts of floods: epidemiologic evidence. Epidemiol Rev 2005;27:36–46.
[7] One world, one response–needed, but not yet forthcoming. Lancet 2005;365:95–6.
[8] OFDA/CRED international disaster database from 1900 to present. Emergency events database (EM-DAT). Available at: www.em-dat.net. Accessed October 2, 2005.
[9] Noji E. Progress in disaster management [commentary]. Lancet 1994;343:1239–40.
[10] NOAA's national weather service. Natural hazard statistics. Available at: http://www.nws.noaa.gov/om/hazstats.shtml. Accessed October 2, 2005.
[11] Shultz J. Epidemiology of tropical cyclones: The dynamic of disaster, disease, and development. Epidemiol Rev 2005;27:21–35.
[12] The American National Redcross. Flood and flash flood. Available at: http://www.redcross.org/services/disaster/keepsafe/flood.html. Accessed October 7, 2005.
[13] WHO Europe fact sheet 05/02. Flooding: health effects and preventive measures. Available at: www.euro.who.int. Accessed October, 2005.
[14] Hajat S, Ebi KL, Kovats S, et al. The human health consequences of flooding in Europe and the implications for public health: a review of the evidence. Applied Environmental Science and Public Health 2003;1(1):13–21.
[15] Alson R, Alexander D, Leonard RB, et al. Analysis of medical treatment at a field hospital following Hurricane Andrew, 1992. Ann Emerg Med 1993;22:1721–8.
[16] D'Amore AR, Harin CK. Air Force Expeditionary Medical Support Unit at the Houston flood: use of a military model in civilian disaster response. Mil Med 2005;170:103–8.
[17] Bramon S, Boone C, Bowman S, et al. Morbidity and mortality associated with Hurricane Floyd–North Carolina, September–October 1999. MMWR Morb Mortal Wkly Rep 2000;49(17):369–72.

[18] Centers for Disease Control and Prevention. Preliminary medical examiner reports of mortality associated with Hurricane Charley—Florida, 2004. MMWR Morb Mortal Wkly Rep 2004;53(36):835–7.

[19] Kelso K, Wilson S, McFarland L. Injuries and illnesses related to Hurricane Andrew–Louisiana, 1992. MMWR Morb Mortal Wkly Rep 1993;42(13):242–3, 250–1.

[20] George-McDowell N, Hendry AB, Sewerbridges-Wilkins LB, et al. Surveillance for injuries and illnesses and rapid health-needs assessment following Hurricanes Marilyn and Opal, September–October 1995. MMWR Morb Mortal Wkly Rep 1996;45(4):81–5.

[21] Little B, Gill J, Schulte J, et al. Rapid assessment of the needs and health status of older adults after Hurricane Charley–Charlotte, Desoto, and Handee Counties, Florida August 27–31, 2004. MMWR Morb Mortal Wkly Rep 2004;53(36):837–40.

[22] Schmidt W, Skala M, Donelson I, Donnell HD. Morbidity surveillance following the Midwest flood–Missouri, 1993. MMWR Morb Mortal Wkly Rep 1993;42(41):797–8.

[23] Bailey MA, Glover R, Huang Y. Epidemiologic assessment of the impact of four hurricanes–Florida, 2004. MMWR Morb Mortal Wkly Rep 2005;54(28):693–7.

[24] Engelthelar D, Lewis K, Anderson S, et al. Vibrio illness after Hurricane Katrina–Multiple states, August–September 2005. MMWR Morb Mortal Wkly Rep 2005;54(37):928–31.

[25] World Disasters Report 2005—Chapter 4. Available at: www.ifrc.org. Accessed October 2, 2005.

[25a] Wikipedia. Available at: http://en.wikipedia.org.

[25b] NOAA. Available at: www.noaa.gov.

[26] The tsunami story. Available at: http://www.tsunami.noaa.gov/tsunami_story.html. Accessed October 2, 2005.

[27] Stein S, Okal E. Seismology: speed and size of the Sumatra earthquake. Nature 2005;434: 581–2.

[28] Lay T, Kanamori H, Ammon CJ, et al. The great Sumatra-Andaman earthquake. Science 2005;308:1127–33.

[28a] Life of a tsunami. Available at: www.usgs.gov.

[29] US Department of the Interior. Earthquake hazard program. Available at: http://earthquake.usgs.gov/docs/020204mag_policy.html. Accessed September 18, 2005.

[30] National oceanic and atmospheric administration. Tsunami. Available at: www.tsunami.noaa.gov. Accessed October 2, 2005.

[31] Taylor PRP, Emonson DL, Schlimmer JE. Operation Shaddock—the Australian Defense Force response to the tsunami disaster in Papua New Guinea. Med J Aust 1998;169:602–6.

[32] Holian A, Keith P. Orthopedic surgery after the Aitape Tsunami. Med J Aust 1998;169: 606–9.

[33] Maegele M, Gregor S, Steinhausen E, et al. The long-distance tertiary air transfer and care of tsunami victims: Injury pattern and microbiological and psychological aspects. Crit Care Med 2005;33(5):1136–40.

[34] Masur H, Murray P. Tsunami disaster and infection: beware what pathogens the transport delivers to your intensive care unit. Crit Care Med 2005;33(5):1179–80.

[35] Allworth A. Tsunami lung: a necrotizing pneumonia in survivors of the Asian Tsunami. Med J Aust 2005;182(7):364.

[36] Athan E, Allworth AM, Engler C, et al. Melioidosis in tsunami survivors [letter]. Emerging Infectious Diseases [serial on the Internet] 2005;11(10). Available at: www.cdc.gov/eid.

[37] Chierakul W, Winothai W, Wattanawaitunechai C, et al. Melioidosis in 6 Tsunami survivors in southern Thailand. Clin Infect Dis 2005;41:982–90.

[38] Kao AY, Munander R, Ferrara SL, et al. Case 19–2005: a 17-year-old girl with respiratory distress and hemiparesis after surviving a tsunami. N Engl J Med 2005;353:2628–36.

[39] Andersen D, Donaldson A, Choo L, et al. Multifocal cutaneous mucormycosis complicating polymicrobial wound infections in a tsunami survivor from Sri Lanka. Lancet 2005;365: 876–8.

[40] Morgan O, Ahern M, Cairncross S. Revisiting the tsunami: health consequences of flooding. Public Library of Science 2005;2(6):e184.

[41] Guha-sapir D, van Panhuis W. The Andaman Nicobar earthquake and tsunami 2004: impact on disease in Indonesia. July 2005 Centre for research on the epidemiology of disasters (CRED). EM-DAT: the OFDA/CRED International disaster database. Available at: www.em-dat.net.

[42] Bartlett JG. Tetanus. In: Goldman L, Ausiello D, editors. Cecil textbook of medicine. 22nd edition. Philadelphia: W.B. Saunders Company; 2004.

[43] Lim JH, Yoon D, Jung G, et al. Medical needs of tsunami disaster refugee camps: experience in Southern Sri Lanka. Fam Med 2005;37(6):422–8.

[44] Sondorp E, Bornemisza O. Public health, emergencies and the humanitarian impulse. Bull World Health Organ 2005;83(3):163–4.

[45] Noji E. Public health issues in disasters. Crit Care Med 2005;33(1):S29–33.

[46] Available at: http://www.bt.cdc.gov/disasters/tsunamis/healtheff.asp.

[47] De Jong K, Prosser S, Ford N. Addressing psychological needs in the aftermath of the tsunami. PLoS Med 2005;2(6):e179.

[48] Ursano RJ, Fullerton CS, Norwood AE. Psychiatric dimensions of disaster: patient care, community consultation, and preventive medicine. Harv Rev Psychiatry 1995;3:196–209.

ELSEVIER
SAUNDERS

SURGICAL
CLINICS OF
NORTH AMERICA

Surg Clin N Am 86 (2006) 579–600

Civilian Preparedness and Counter-terrorism: Conventional Weapons

COL Edward B. Lucci, MD

*Emergency and Operational Medicine, Building 2, Room 1B09, Walter Reed
Army Medical Center, 6900 Georgia Avenue, Washington, DC 20307, USA*

Everything should be made as simple as possible, but not simpler.

Albert Einstein (1879–1955)

The modern era of terrorism began in the late 1960s and is the most destructive in history [1]. This global crisis has resulted in unexpected mass-casualty incidents descending on civilian medical systems. Experience demonstrates that a hospital's proximity to a terrorist bombing, rather than its trauma designation, is the best predictor of casualty load delivered to its doors. The victims of these bombings suffer a combination of blast, penetrating, and thermal injuries whose management falls outside the routine experience of most physicians. Because of these circumstances, it is imperative that all surgeons and emergency physicians be familiar with triage and treatment to optimize survival. Specifically, they should be familiar with the principles and application of the concepts of minimal acceptable care, damage control surgery, and managing complex wounding patterns [2]. A successful strategy should not be interpreted as streamlining care for a large group of casualties with varying severities of injury but rather as providing consistently high-quality trauma care to the small group of critical but salvageable patients from the larger mix [3].

Most terrorist attacks involve explosive devices, and the frequency of bombings directed at civilians is increasing [1,4–6] There are nearly five illegal bombing incidents in the United States per day [7]. Between 1992 and 2002 more Americans were injured and killed from bombings within the

---

The opinions or assertions contained herein are the private views of the author and are not to be construed as official or representing the position of the Department of the Army or the Department of Defense.

E-mail address: edward.lucci@na.amedd.army.mil

surgical.theclinics.com

United States than overseas [7]. Nonetheless, most American health care providers continue to consider terrorism and bombings an international rather than a domestic problem, and few have experience caring for victims of a true mass-casualty event. Therefore it is necessary to learn from others' experiences [8]. Although individuals may be the target of conventional weapons, such as knives and guns, most medical literature has focused on planning and response to mass-casualty incidents from conventional explosive devices of various degrees of sophistication [5]. Of the 93 terrorist attacks reported worldwide between 1991 and 2000 involving more than 30 casualties, most resulted from conventional bombings [3,9]. For these reasons all hospitals must be prepared to deal with trauma mass casualties.

Ambulances commonly are diverted from their usual destinations in the United States because of emergency department (ED) overcrowding, reflecting limited surge capacity in the event of a multiple- or mass-casualty event in their communities [10]. Terrorist bombings produce mass casualties that have the potential to overwhelm even the best-prepared emergency medical systems and hospitals. A rational approach to civilian preparedness for conventional weapons terrorism suggests that lessons learned from previous terrorist attacks be incorporated into the current response posture. Two recent surveys of preparedness for mass-casualty events confirm that hospitals in the United States are poorly prepared at multiple levels to care for large numbers of severely injured patients [11,12]. This article examines current thinking regarding civilian preparedness for a conventional weapon terrorist attack, emphasizing hospital planning and surgical response.

Bombing characteristics and injury frequency

Most terrorist attacks employ conventional explosive weapons. These devices are of various levels of sophistication and power with diverse characteristics regarding the location of the explosion, the time of day it occurs, the exposed population, and the distance from hospitals [5]. A recent study by Arnold and colleagues [9] that analyzed large bombings with more than 30 casualties worldwide during the period from 1991 to 2000 found that the number of victims and their injuries were related to multiple factors including the magnitude and setting of the explosion and the number of potential casualties at risk [9]. Specifically, one in four victims died immediately in bombings where structural collapse occurred, 1 in 12 died immediately in confined-space bombings (often buses), and 1 in 25 died immediately in open-air bombings [9].

In terrorist bombings, most deaths are immediate, with few deaths occurring early or late afterwards. The relatively low early and late mortality rates are consistent with other studies in this area [9,13]. The low early mortality rates, as the authors suggest, suggest that EDs probably will not be confronted with many simultaneously dying patients, and physicians involved in resuscitation rarely will face the difficult choice of withholding medical care from a nonsalvageable expectant patient in the resuscitation bay [9]. A biphasic distribution of mortality rates is seen in large terrorist bombings; that is, there is a high immediate mortality rate followed by low early and late mortality rates. This pattern contrasts with the triphasic distribution of deaths typically associated with conventional blunt and penetrating trauma [5,9,14,15]. Other reports confirm higher fatality rates, increased Injury Severity Scores, increased rate of blast injury, and more extensive burns associated with confined-space bombings. No differences regarding penetrating injuries or traumatic amputations were reported [5].

A study comparing 43 mass-casualty terrorist bombings found ED use and hospital admission rates varied greatly by event, and immediate mortality rates depended most on whether building collapse occurred [14]. This study suggested that median values for mortality, ED use, and hospitalization might be useful as predictors of what to expect in future events. Although the use rates for EDs after bombings are complex, in simple terms, the lower the immediate mortality, the higher the ED use rate becomes, because bombings that kill fewer victims generate more ED patients [14]. Available data may not reflect patients who have minor injuries and seek care in venues other than the ED; also, in overwhelmed Eds, documentation may have been poor [14].

Prehospital care

Most patients, particularly most urgent patients, are brought to the nearest hospital (Fig. 1). A critical task for the emergency medical services (EMS) leader at the scene is to assume control of the entire scene to the maximum extent possible. Protection of critically injured and assurance that the most seriously injured are evacuated first are primary objectives. As patients are evacuated, they should be taken from the scene based on their level of criticality, and each patient leaving the scene should be the next most urgent, in sequential order. Finally, EMS must ensure that no casualties are overlooked.

The initial search and rescue in a terrorist bombing are conducted by untrained survivors, and most casualties arrive at hospitals by a variety of non-ambulance vehicles, having received little or no treatment in the field. The local EMS system is likely to have limited control over subsequent casualty care activities such as triage, first aid, decontamination, field resuscitation, stabilization and transport, patient regulation, and hospital notification. These facts have a significant effect on required hospital preparedness and response.

Traditionally, patients are not distributed evenly to local trauma centers (Fig. 2) [16,17]. Patients who can bypass field triage and decontamination sites do so. Hospital personnel must be prepared to carry out triage and decontamination at the hospital entrance, while recognizing that the least

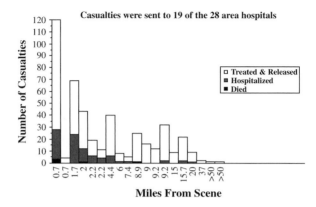

Fig. 1. Distribution of casualties among area hospitals after the bombing of the Murrah Federal Building, Oklahoma City, 1994. (*From* Auf der Heide E. Common misconceptions in disasters: panic, the "disaster syndrome," and looting. In: O'Leary M, editor. The first 72 hours: a community approach to disaster preparedness. Lincoln (NE): iUniverse Publishing; 2004. p. 366.)

injured are likely to arrive first, with little notification. Furthermore, communication between the event site and the receiving hospital can be expected to be poor or nonexistent [16]. Auf der Heide [16] suggests ways to influence inefficient prehospital casualty distribution by EMS, such as sending ambulances to outlying hospitals and thus avoiding the hospitals closest to the disaster site. In Washington, DC, for example, mass-casualty situation mutual aid agreements with surrounding jurisdictions send trauma patients who are stable for transport back to the jurisdiction hospitals corresponding with the ambulances that responded (Capt. Henry Lyles, Chief, Special Events Unit, DC Fire and EMS, Washington, DC, personal communication, 2005).

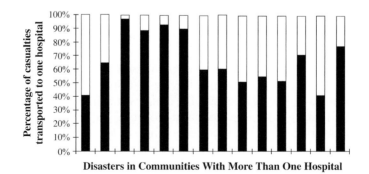

Fig. 2. The Disaster Research Center study: the percentage of casualties transported to one hospital. Of the 29 disasters in the study, 14 are included on this chart; the 15 communities with only one hospital were excluded. (*From* Auf der Heide E. The importance of evidence-based disaster planning. Ann Emerg Med 2006;47:42; with permission.)

It is difficult to distinguish between casualties requiring immediate and delayed treatment by a rapid examination in the field, particularly when there is no organization or crowd control on site [17]. For this reason, the tendency of EMS in mass-casualty settings is a "scoop and run" approach, with minimal medical intervention at the site and rapid evacuation to the nearest medical facility [3,17]. Few differences exist between the initial requirements for prehospital care of the victim of a bombing and a regular trauma patient. Quick evacuation increases the chance of survival for critically injured patients in either circumstance; therefore, transport to the closest medical facility is prudent. Stein [5] recommends the following basic field medical care guidelines:

1. Victims with amputated body parts and no signs of life are dead.
2. Victims without breathing or pulse and with dilated pupils are dead.
3. Cardiopulmonary resuscitation is not indicated at the scene [18].
4. Airway management with cervical spine control is indicated.
5. Improve oxygenation with supplemental O_2 or needle decompression, as needed.
6. Control hemorrhage by tourniquet or direct pressure.
7. Align fractures, splint limb-to-limb, and cover open wounds.

Based on 33 Israeli civilian mass-casualty experiences between 2000 and 2002, Einav and colleagues [17] propose the following on-scene management sequence for a terrorist bombing in the civilian setting:

1. Rapid on scene triage with minimal medical intervention
2. Immediate evacuation of the severely injured to the nearest hospital for primary resuscitation and stabilization (Israeli evacuation hospital concept)
3. Evacuation of all other casualties to other hospitals in the region to avoid exhausting the capacity of any one hospital

The Israeli evacuation hospital concept has emerged from the experience of the Israeli Defense Force medical corps [17]. The mission of the evacuation (front-line) hospital is to perform primary triage and resuscitation, limited to life- or limb-saving surgery, and to evacuate patients promptly to civilian medical centers. Einav and colleagues [17] suggest that every hospital should be prepared to act as an evacuation hospital should a mass-casualty event occur in its proximity; therefore an appropriate degree of surgical expertise and trauma management capability should be maintained.

Prehospital triage

The primary goal of triage is to identify salvageable surviving victims who have life-threatening injuries. Rapid identification of immediate needs in the field and at the hospital entrance is critical. It is reasonable to plan for a rough distribution of 80% nonurgent and 20% immediate/urgent [2]. Over-triage is expected and necessary because the blast mechanism makes it difficult to assess the extent of a patient's injuries accurately; however, inundation of the system with casualties inaccurately assessed as critical can jeopardize the survival of critical patients. Furthermore, victims of blast injury frequently have significant hearing compromise that may impact their rescue [5].

A prehospital protocol proposed by Almogy and colleagues [19] based on lessons learned in Israel recommends that burns over more than 10% of the body surface area, skull fractures, or penetrating wounds to the head or torso be considered markers of proximity to the center of the blast and be used to identify patients at high risk for blast lung injury, thus warranting early evacuation to a level one trauma center. Additionally, they suggest a patient who has traumatic amputations, open fractures, or burns and who has no signs of life should be triaged for secondary evacuation or pronounced dead [19].

Hospital planning and response

The emphasis in hospital emergency planning and response needs to shift from "not just where to go, but how to think when disaster strikes" [3]. Knowledge of the type of bombing, proximity of the bombing to the hospital, and the likely distribution of victims to local hospitals will help a hospital make an initial estimate of its need for ED and hospital bed capacity and for the hospital resources that are likely to be required [14]. An explosion with structural collapse is likely to produce many casualties requiring wound and orthopedic care but relatively fewer patients who have pulmonary injury requiring chest tubes or endotracheal intubation than an explosion in a confined space where the structure remains intact. In addition, higher immediate mortality rates tend to be associated with a reduced demand for ED care [14].

Immediately upon learning about an event, the hospitals in the vicinity should perform a preliminary needs assessment [20] to identify key information from local EMS, police sources, or perhaps patients already arriving at the hospital [16]. Because the ED is probably the place in the hospital where the news is first received, an ED staff member should be assigned this task. Essential information to be collected includes

1. Identification of the bombing site, which suggests the number of potential victims at risk, the proximity to the hospital, and the potential distribution of casualties through EMS [20]
2. Further information about the bombing characteristics, including use of a vehicle delivery system, explosion setting, and explosion sequelae, which helps identify the resources that should be mobilized (Table 1) [20]

Table 1
Bombing characteristics and anticipated impact on hospitals

Bombing characteristic	Implication	Anticipated impact		
		Number of injured survivors seeking emergency care[a]	Injury frequency	Injury severity
Blast site close to hospital	↑ number of injured survivors will arrive at ED outside EMS ↓ EMS transport time to hospital	↑ at nearby hospital	↑ primary blast injuries, traumatic amputations, and many minor injuries	Variable – more minor and more serious injuries
Vehicle delivery system	↑ explosive magnitude Structural collapse possible ↑ immediate deaths close to detonation point or inside collapse	↑ May produce 100s to 1000s of injured survivors	Variable	↑
Pre explosion or precollapse evacuation	↑ distance between potential victims and detonation point ↓ number at risk	↓	↓ primary blast injury, traumatic amputations, flash bums	↓
Open-air setting	Blast energy dissipated, but spread over greater area Structural collapse unlikely ↓ number of immediate deaths	↑ May produce up to 200 injured survivors	↑ secondary blast injury	↓ - more injuries minor
Confined-space setting	Blast energy potentiated, but contained in lesser area ↑ number of immediate deaths inside space ↑ number of injured exposed to blast effects ↑ effects in smaller space (bus >> public room)	↓ Usually produces <100 injured survivors	↑ primary blast injury, amputations, burns	↑↑

(*continued on next page*)

Table 1 (*continued*)

Bombing characteristic	Implication	Anticipated impact		
		Number of injured survivors seeking emergency care[a]	Injury frequency	Injury severity
Structural collapse result	↑ explosive magnitude Collateral damage outside structure possible ↑ number of immediate deaths inside collapse ↑ effects with taller building	Variable ↓ number from inside structural collapse ↑ number from outside structural collapse May produce 100s to 1000s of injured survivors	↑ inhalation injury, crush injury	↑
Structural fire result	↑ number of victims inside structure exposed to smoke and fire ↑ effects with taller building ↑ evacuation time in high-rise fire	↑ number from inside structure	↑ bums, inhalation injury ↑ inhalation injury in high rise fire	Variable

Abbreviations: ED, emergency department; EMS, emergency medical services; ↑, increased; ↓, decreased.

[a] Relative to population at risk.

From Halpern P, Tsai MC, Amold J, et al. Mass-casualty, terrorist bombings: implications for emergency department and hospital emergency response (part II). Prehosp Disast Med 2003; 18:236; with permission.

Ideally, before patients start arriving, the ED should accomplish several key tasks:

1. Activate the hospital mass-casualty plan. Activate the Hospital Emergency Incident Command System (HEICS) [21], if previously established at the hospital. The HEICS is becoming a national standard management tool based on the Incident Command System. The system is a product of a cooperative interagency effort by fire and EMS in California to develop a common organizational structure to use when responding to incidents. The HEICS employs a logical management structure, shared common nomenclature, and clear reporting channels with a goal of promoting interoperability between health care organizations and community-wide emergency response agencies. The HEICS is designed to function independently of the availability of key individuals. The system identifies key positions that must be filled and provides accompanying job action sheets and an initial list of priority tasks. The HEICS is intended to help clarify roles and responsibilities in a hospital's

disaster response plan. A recent report by Zane and colleagues [22] addressing HEICS implementation at their institution noted that the training process itself exposed many critical institution-specific weaknesses, such as the need to create redundancy in their system [21–23].

2. Simultaneously activate plans to clear the ED rapidly in anticipation of incoming patients and to expand hospital capacity. In Israel, routine ED patients are sent to the internal medicine wards for further management, and the EDs are required to prepare for a patient casualty load equaling 15% to 20% of their total number of beds [20]. Because occupancy of critical care beds tends to be high, patients in ICUs should be evaluated for transfer out or for step-down to ward beds [20,24]. All routine procedures and surgeries should be postponed.

3. Mobilize additional personnel and equipment. Initially physicians trained in rapid assessment and general trauma care (emergency physicians and trauma surgeons) are needed, and extra resuscitation bays should be designated. All specialties routinely involved in caring for seriously injured trauma patients should be included in the initial response [20].

4. Control access to the ED [18].

5. Establish an ED command and control post with dual command (because the volume of information is likely to be too great for one person) [25]. One command physician (emergency physician) is responsible for the overall medical and administrative operation of the ED. A second command physician (trauma surgeon/surgeon in charge) supervises the delivery of trauma care, including assigning priorities for surgery and supervising trauma teams [25].

Several authors have recommended the following guidelines in a mass-casualty setting when patient influx continues and the estimated number of casualties arriving to the hospital is unknown [5,18,20,26]:

1. Perform plain radiographs only when the results will have an immediate impact on management.

2. Advanced trauma life support should be practiced in the resuscitation/shock rooms.

3. There is no role for ED thoracotomy.

4. Salvageable hemodynamically unstable patients go to the operating room (OR).

5. A focused abdominal sonography for trauma examination is an acceptable method for detecting abdominal bleeding.

6. CT scans are reserved for patients who have head injury.

7. The use of blood is restricted, with predetermined limits for individual cases.

8. Secondary distribution is practiced: for example, orthopedic fixations and débridement are transferred out to the surrounding community.

9. Organizational flexibility that allows frequent re-evaluation and retriage of survivors is critical to screen for commonly associated occult injuries

such as pulmonary and intestinal blast injury, compartment syndrome, ophthalmologic injuries, and delayed vascular compromise.

10. Blast wounds receive extensive irrigation, débridement, and delayed primary closure [27].
11. Casualty flow is unidirectional [5,20,25,27].
12. Patient disposition is made by a senior trauma surgeon to ensure appropriate OR and ICU use. Stein and colleagues [5] suggest dividing surgical care into two phases: minimal acceptable surgical care (damage-control surgery) while casualties are still arriving and definitive optimal surgery when new arrivals have ceased [5,19,20,25,27]. The following priority for OR disposition is recommended [5]:
    a. Hemodynamically unstable patients requiring hemorrhage control
    b. Hemodynamically stable patients with life-threatening torso injuries
    c. Closed head injury with expanding hemorrhage and without extensive brain injury
    d. Vascular and orthopedic injuries
    e. Wounds requiring extensive irrigation and débridement

Virtually all injury types occurred in all bombing categories; therefore hospital physicians need to be prepared to treat all types of blast injuries, regardless of the specific bombing mechanism [9,14]. Some patterns of injury distribution emerge, however (Table 2).

Inhalational injury was associated only with bombings where structural fire or structural collapse occurred. The highest rate of inhalation injury reported was 93% in the 1993 World Trade Center (WTC) bombing where structural fire occurred and delayed evacuation led to prolonged smoke exposure [28]. Fifty-two percent of immediate survivors of the 2001 WTC bombing sought emergency care for inhalation injury because of structural fire or dust from structural collapse [14].

Crush injury and fractures are associated with structural collapse. Crush injury is particularly associated with structural collapse [9,20,28].

Pulmonary blast injuries (blast lung syndrome, pneumothorax) and tympanic membrane rupture are associated with confined-space bombings [20,29,30]. The highest rate of blast lung injury reported in large casualty bombings is 44% in two bus bombings in Israel in 1996. In addition, patients involved in confined-space bombings have a higher rate of burns, inhalation injury, and hepatic and splenic trauma [9,13,14,20].

The highest rate of penetrating soft tissue trauma caused by fragments in an explosion is associated with open-air bombings. These injuries typically are minor. The rate of penetrating soft tissue injuries seen at the Olympic Park bombing in Atlanta in 1996 was 100% [31].

When OR resources are thin, the hospital emergency response plan must account for relief of medical teams and for secondary distribution, that is, possible evacuation of stable patients who require lengthy procedures (eg, orthopedic stabilization, wound débridement, plastic surgery, nerve

Table 2
Injury-frequency data for six subgroups of victims who presented to the emergency department compiled from 43 mass-casualty terrorist bombings

Median (IQR)

Subgroup	Pulmonary contusion (%)	Pneumothorax (%)	Blast lung syndrome (%)	TM rupture (%)	Intestinal perforation (%)	Penetrating soft tissue (%)	Eye (%)	Penetrating eye (%)	Penetrating abdomen (%)	Penetrating vascular (%)	Fracture (%)	Open fracture (%)	Amputation (%)	Intracranial (%)	Liver of spleen (%)	Burn (%)	Inhalation (%)	Crush (%)
Vehicle delivery	1 (0–2)	1 (0–2)	2 (1–4)	3 (2–3)	0 (0–1)	56 (61–72)	8 (3–14)	0 (0–1)	1 (1–2)	3 (2–3)	6 (2–11)	11 (10–11)	0 (0–1)	6 (2–6)	1 (0–1)	3 (2–4)	2 (0–40)	1 (0–1)
Terrorist suicide	-	11 (3–19)	25 (5–44)	4*	2 (0–4)	17*	19*	-	-	-	6*	-	-	12*	6 (1–10)	6*	52*	1*
Confined-space	3 (2–4)	13 (5–19)	11 (1–38)	32 (20–53)	4 (4–4)	54 (34–55)	2 (2–7)	2 (2–3)	2 (2–3)	3 (2–3)	14 (11–25)	6*	3 (3–5)	3 (2–4)	7 (3–10)	23 (20–27)	-	-
Open-air	0 (0–0)	2 (0–3)	3 (0–5)	2 (0–5)	0 (0–0)	91 (72–100)	3 (3–3)	0 (0–2)	2 (1–3)	2 (1–3)	2 (2–6)	3 (2–22)	0 (0–4)	1 (1–2)	1 (1–1)	0 (0–0)	0 (0–0)	0 (0–0)
Structural collapse	2 (0–2)	2 (1–2)	2 (1–2)	2 (1–2)	0 (0–1)	42 (29–54)	8 (3–14)	1 (0–1)	1 (1–2)	3 (2–3)	12 (9–13)	9 (7–11)	1 (0–1)	5 (3–6)	1 (0–1)	3 (3–5)	2 (1–15)	1 (1–2)
Structural fire	-	-	7*	-	-	17*	19*	-	-	-	6*	-	-	-	-	50 (28–72)	73 (62–83)	1*
All	1 (0–2)	2 (0–4)	2 (0–6)	7 (2–23)	0 (0–3)	64 (54–88)	3 (2–12)	1 (0–3)	1 (1–3)	3 (2–4)	9 (6–14)	7 (5–10)	1 (0–3)	4 (2–6)	1 (0–1)	5 (0–21)	1 (0–15)	1 (0–1)

Abbreviations: IQR, interquartile range; TM, tympanic membrane.

* Data from one bombing only.

From Arnold J, Tsai MC, Halpern P, et al. Mass casualty, terrorist bombings: epidemiological outcomes, resource utilization, and time course of emergency needs (part 1). Prehosp Disast Med 2003;18:227; with permission.

reconstruction) and burn casualties [5,20,25,27]. It is recommended that hospitals establish and exercise mutual aid memoranda of understanding in their regions that address emergency support such as accepting transfer patients, assistance with hospital evacuation, and the loan of medical personnel, pharmaceuticals, supplies, and equipment.

Most injuries seen in the ED from a mass-casualty bombing event are minor [5,9,32]. Responders must understand the focus of management should be on identifying and treating the small number of critically injured patients within the larger group of injured victims. The 2004 bombing in Madrid, Spain, is a reasonable model for planning purposes [33]. In that attack, 10 terrorist bombs simultaneously exploded in four commuter trains, instantly killing 177 people and injuring more than 2000. The closest hospital received 312 patients within approximately 3 hours of the explosions, with a 30% admission rate, 12% of which were admitted to critical care areas. In addition, over the next 9 hours they performed 34 surgical interventions (Table 3). Of the critical patients admitted, more than half had both severe head injury and blast lung injury [34].

In general, victims who are not incapacitated or entrapped bypass the prehospital EMS system and go rapidly by any means available to the nearest hospital. In some cases, these victims arrive within 5 minutes of the event. Their arrival represents the first-wave phenomenon [5,14,35]. They arrive without warning, and usually the least injured arrive first. The initial response to the first-wave capacity depends on in-house resources, and the normal workload of the hospital continues [34]. A part of the success of the medical community's response to the Madrid bombing and the September 11, 2001, response in the United States was the result of the time of day that these attacks occurred, because an abundance of medical and nursing staff was available immediately [24,34].

Hospital surge capacity

The term "surge capacity," a hospital's ability to accommodate an influx of patients above its routine daily volume, is difficult to quantify. Trauma

Table 3
Types and number of surgical interventions performed on 34 victims during the first 24 hours of the Madrid, Spain, bombing 2004

Types of intervention	No (%) (N = 37)
Orthopedic	15 (40.5)
Abdominal	7 (18.9)
Neurosurgical	6 (16.2)
Maxillofacial	5 (13.5)
Plastic	3 (8.1)
Ophthalmic	1 (2.7)

From Gutierrez de Ceballos JP, Turegano Fuentes F, Petez Diaz D, et al. Casulties treated at the closest hospital in the Madrid, March 11 terrorist bombings. Crit Care Med 2005;33 (Suppl):S109; with permission.

centers define the term as the number of critical casualties arriving per unit of time that can be managed without compromising care (ie, patients receive the same level of care given to similar patients under normal circumstances) [36]. The Israelis routinely use an arbitrary number of 20% of a hospital's bed capacity as its required "surge capacity" for determining the amount of supplies and equipment required to be kept on hand at for immediate use [26]. Hirshberg and colleagues [36] define the "surge capacity" of a level one trauma center in the United States by using computer modeling to analyze the impact of a mass-casualty bombing event on trauma assets. They suggest that surge capacity is a rate, not a number of casualties or number of beds, and they found it varies with the assets on hand and the level of care one is willing to designate as approximating the "normal daily level of trauma care." The level of trauma care depends on the availability of trauma teams, CT, ORs, and other key resources. Their surge capacity is a rate that corresponds with their hospital's ability to provide 90% of the optimal care given to a single trauma patient during normal operations (Fig. 3). They looked at two scenarios: one using only immediately available staff and one allowing the recruitment of off-site staff [36]. They determined the hospital's "critical casualty load" as a sigmoid-shaped curve and defined "multiple-casualty incident," "mass-casualty incident," and "major medical disaster" as corresponding to regions on the curve [36]. They suggest that the sigmoid shape of the curve reflects a fundamental characteristic of any hospital confronting a trauma mass casualty, and they propose ways to shift the curve to the right, that is, to increase the hospital's casualty capacity [36].

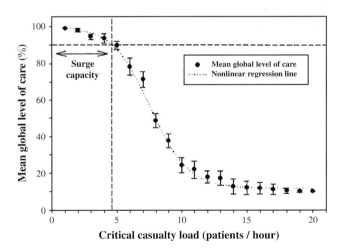

Fig. 3. Model prediction of the effect of critical casualty load on global level of trauma care (mean ± 95% confidence interval). The surge capacity of the hospital's trauma assets is the critical casualty load, corresponding to a 90% level of care on the fitted curve. (*From* Hirshberg A, Bradford S, Granchi T, et al. How does casualty load affect trauma care in urban bombing incidents? a quantitative analysis. J Trauma 2005;58:690; with permission.)

Auf der Heide [35] has introduced the concept of a first-wave protocol in which hospitals predetermine the number of patients in each triage category they can receive comfortably in a disaster occurring under minimum staffing (eg, at 2 AM on a weekend) [35]. This information is maintained by local EMS and is used as a guide for initial casualty distribution during a disaster.

Victims who have injuries requiring hospitalization are likely to arrive in a second wave through EMS [18]. Peak arrival time to the ED is reported to occur 30 to 60 minutes after the event; but there has been great variability. In the 1993 WTC bombing, only 50% of injured had been transported to EDs within 3.5 hours, and injured personnel were still arriving at EDs 24 hours later [14,28,37]. Most injured survivors extricate themselves or are extricated by bystanders. Early extrication is critical, and the likelihood of survival after a few hours is very low. In Oklahoma City, only three victims were extricated after the first 5 hours. After structure collapse occurred at the 2001 WTC bombing, only five victims were extricated, the last being rescued at 32 hours [14,38].

In the United States, as in Israel, every hospital employee should have a modified role in the emergency plan, ideally similar to the employee's routine role and practiced regularly in disaster drills. Every employee should be dedicated to the institutional effort [3,19].

Communication

Historically, communication has been a problem at multiple levels in every significant terrorist bombing event and will continue to be a problem at future disasters. Telephone and cellular circuits are likely to be overloaded. The 2002 state-by-state assessment of public health preparedness for a mass-casualty event in the United States by Mann and colleagues [12] found that communications across states were fragmented and that few states have an operating communications system linking health and medical resources [24,39]. The Arlington County Fire Department (Incident Command at the Pentagon on September 11, 2001) reported in their After-Action Report that almost all aspects of communication were problematic, from the initial notification of the incident through all levels of tactical operations [40]. Cellular telephones were of little value in the first few hours, and emergency responders were not given priority access to cellular service. Radio channels were oversaturated, and interoperability problems between jurisdictions and agencies persisted. Pagers and Nextel two-way devices were the most reliable form of notification [24,41].

In a successful effort to circumvent the expected communications problems associated with a major terrorist event, the District of Columbia Hospital Association has funded a private radio-frequency system, the hospital mutual aid radio system (known as H-MARS) to provide a direct ED–ED link among hospitals in the area. Recently recognized by the RAND

Corporation (Santa Monica, CA) as an "exemplary practice in public health preparedness," the system, a privately licensed radio frequency, uses existing infrastructure to facilitate reliable communications during an emergency, enabling health care providers to coordinate easily without telephones or cell phones. Daily communications checks and monthly ED "critical capacity" reports are conducted also. The system has proven effective in several emergencies by allowing prompt dissemination of information and interhospital coordination, including management of surge capacity. It is the communications foundation for implementing the Hospital Mutual Aid Memorandum of Agreement, facilitating the sharing of personnel, equipment, and bed capacity during a crisis. It provided invaluable interhospital communications during the September 11, 2001, attack on the Pentagon and the subsequent anthrax incident in October 2001 [41].

Patient tracking/information sharing

Health insurance portability and accountability act (HIPPA) constraints, interhospital communication problems, and poorly integrated local public health and medical communities in many areas guarantee that patient tracking and critical information sharing between hospitals in a disaster will continue to be a challenge. Multiple Web-based products designed to share information are available, but payment, maintenance, interoperability, patient privacy, and security issues are barriers to widespread implementation. Furthermore, many hospitals do not yet have the technologic infrastructure to operate and support such systems adequately. One of the hallmarks of a functioning trauma system is its ability to move injured patients safely and in a timely fashion to the appropriate level of care at a certified facility that has the appropriate resources and expertise needed to care for the injured. States with functioning statewide trauma systems were more likely to possess functioning key disaster-readiness components. Statewide trauma systems may provide the framework for building future disaster readiness capacity [11,12].

Hospital medical care

The approach to medical care in a mass-casualty bombing cannot be managed on the basis of "business as usual, just more of it" [42]. The goal is to recognize and provide critically injured patients with a level of care comparable to that given to injured patients under normal circumstances [25,36]. To do so requires a system in place that quickly and reliably identifies and treats the small group of critical but salvageable patients, rather than a system designed to streamline care for a large group of mostly noncritical patients [2,3,25,36]. The high number of potentially urgent patients requires that the initial assessment be rapid and that only minimally acceptable care be given until casualties stop arriving [17,19,25,43]. Noncritical casualties must queue for care [36]. Critically injured patients should be handled by dedicated trauma teams in a suitable resuscitation bay [25,36]. The ED should avoid providing care to patients categorized as "expectant survivors" [2,19,25,27]. Performing resuscitation efforts such as ED thoracotomy on unsalvageable victims (eg, those without signs of life) may compromise the delivery of care to salvageable patients [5,19]. In the initial phases of a response, hospitals must consider restricting the use of imaging and blood supplies and consider treating the moderately injured before the severely injured while casualty influx is occurring.

The realistic admitting capacity of a hospital is determined by the available surgical resources, that is, the number of trauma teams available. Approximately 10 trauma teams are required for 100 to 150 patients [25]. Hirshberg and colleagues' [36] computer modeling of an urban terrorist bombing, based on Israeli data, predicted that the admitting capacity of a hospital depends primarily on the number of available surgeons and that the major bottlenecks to patient flow are the limited number of ED resuscitation beds and the CT scanner, not the operating rooms. In their model, there was a direct relationship between the number of surgeons available and the number of patients who could be treated. In fact, increasing the number of surgeons from eight to nine doubled the admitting capacity of the hospital (Table 4) [36]. The study also suggested that the effects of overtriage can be mitigated by adding improvised resuscitation bays in the ED [25,36,44].

The importance of repeat evaluations in these patients cannot be overemphasized [19]. Hospital care must include a plan for reassessing stable casualties for occult life-threatening injuries. Missing subclinical blast injury has been reported and can be a fatal error [5].

Casualty flow through the facility will depend on a core group of critical decision-makers prepared to improvise unconventional solutions to difficult situations, such as using an OR suite as an ICU bed [3,19]. The critical mortality rate (ie, the death rate in critically injured survivors) more accurately reflects the magnitude of the medical disaster and the effectiveness of medical response and should be used when evaluating outcome as a more

Table 4
Effect of number of surgeons on institutional capacity

No. of surgeons	Time of zero surgeons	No. of patients treated
6	59 ± 3	20 ± 1
7	95 ± 6	31 ± 2
8	122 ± 7	39 ± 2
9	238 ± 11	77 ± 3

From Hirshberg A, Stein M, Walden R. Surgical resource utilization in urban terrorist bombing: a computer simulation. J Trauma 1999;47:547; with permission.

meaningful indication of the quality of care provided than is the overall mortality rate [2,27,34]. Deaths that occur among noncritical survivors should be analyzed to assess the quality of medical management [45].

New recommendations

Based on recent experience with bombing victims, Almogy and colleagues [46] have recommended a modification to the concept of damage control surgery in the unstable trauma patient that includes packing of multiple entry sites before abbreviated laparotomy and the use of recombinant factor VIIA. All victims who have multiple fragment wounds receive total-body CT imaging when possible, and unexplained sepsis or hemodynamic instability results in aggressive evaluation of the abdomen as the possible source [47]. Also, findings of "human remains" fragments in victims of penetrating blast injuries has resulted in a guideline mandating hepatitis B immunization for all bombing victims who have dermal penetration [47].

Blast injury

The standard approach to blast injury and clinical manifestations of blast lung injury have been well described in the literature [4,29,48–52]. The hallmark of blast injury involves the respiratory system. The distribution of primary blast injuries suggests that barotrauma affects the tympanic membrane, lungs, and intestinal tract in order of decreasing susceptibility [4,9,14]. The highest rate of primary blast lung syndrome reported is 44%, associated with confined-space bombings [14]. A recent review by Avidan and colleagues [53] of all ICU admissions at their hospital from terrorist bombings in Israel between 1983 and 2004 revealed 29 ICU admissions for blast lung injury. All patients presented with progressive hypoxemia and respiratory distress. Most had some degree of hemoptysis, and all had pulmonary infiltrates on chest radiograph. Although 76% required mechanical ventilation, short- and long-term prognosis was good [53].

An interesting finding in one open-air market bombing was that 30% of hospitalized victims developed candidemia after associated pulmonary blast injury. Subsequent air sampling detected a significant concentration of airborne Candida species in the blast area [47].

The experience in Israel has demonstrated that victims of terror bombings have a higher requirement for intensive care, more prolonged hospital course, and higher mortality than other trauma victims [47].

Gaps

Recent surveys suggest the level of preparation for domestic terrorism and mass-casualty events is inadequate. Gaps in emergency response exist at multiple levels in training and education, communications, planning guidelines for triage and resource allocation, and trauma systems coverage, to name a few areas of concern [11,12,34,54–56].

Federal funding

In the Washington, DC, region, efforts have been underway to build hospital surge capacity for all patients. Several initiatives are underway to include use of federal funds through the Urban Area Security Initiative (UASI) provided by the Department of Homeland Security to high-risk urban areas. Individual hospitals received limited flexibility in how they applied the UASI funding and used it toward various projects tied to surge capacity such as increasing ICU and negative pressure/isolation capacity and for other necessary infrastructure upgrades. Future funding is earmarked for improving burn capacity (eg, by procuring hospital burn packs). Mobile surge facilities also have been evaluated (Dr. J.A. Elting, Medical Director, District of Columbia Hospital Association, Washington, DC, personal correspondence, 2006.).

Training requirements

There is broad agreement that a wide range of provider training is needed to ensure an effective health and medical response to a mass-casualty terrorist event [56]. Most would agree that some training is better than none. It is safe to predict that in a mass-casualty, disaster response, people will do best what they have been trained to do daily [57]. The Joint Council on Accreditation of Healthcare Organizations mandates hospital-level disaster drills and encourages community-wide participation. The secret to hospital readiness is having simple, straightforward plans that everyone knows and will automatically carry out [57]. In many cases mandatory individual training is being tied to hospital privileges and credentials, state licensure, and specialty board certification and renewal. Some disaster and mass-casualty training should be incorporated into residency and medical school curricula. Through its Military Unique Curricula, the Uniformed Services University provides guidance to graduate medical education training programs in military-relevant topics such as blast injuries [58].

Strategic National Stockpile

The Centers for Disease Control and Prevention currently maintains 12 Strategic National Stockpile push packages of pharmaceuticals and equipment to treat or provide prophylaxis for a large population against a wide range of health threats. Push packages can be sent to states within 12 hours of a request. The program is designed to support states facing public health emergencies. Although the stockpiles are focused toward response to chemical, biologic, or radiologic terrorism, the supplies contained within them (eg, chest tubes, airway equipment, burn packs, and portable ventilators) have obvious utility in a major trauma event. States and local public health agencies are tasked with storing and distributing these supplies in the event of a disaster. These packages also can be prestaged before high-visibility special events. In Washington, DC, before the fifty-fifth Presidential inauguration in 2005, this program was used to stage caches of portable ventilators at local hospitals (Dr. J.A. Elting, Medical Director, District of Columbia Hospital Association, Washington, DC, personal correspondence, 2006.) [59,60].

Summary

In the United States medical personnel have limited experience with bombings and mass-casualty events, and blast injuries are rarely encountered in civilian institutions [2,3,5].

Despite increased awareness, significant deficiencies persist in community emergency preparedness and response. Civilian emergency preparedness is not thoroughly ingrained in this culture for an appropriate level of emergency response, but considerable progress is being made in many areas [3].

Between 1983 and 2002, 36,110 illegal bombing incidents occurred in the United States [7]. During this same period, there have been only two biologic terrorism incidents in the United States, and, fortunately, there have been no chemical or nuclear events [7]. The current focus on weapons of mass destruction may be misguided given past experience with terrorism and the resulting trauma. Trauma centers, however, must continue to compete for limited resources with expensive technologies aimed at weapons of mass destruction. Similarly, regional and state coordinators must ensure that funding is distributed equitably to maintain and expand the existing infrastructure appropriately [54,55]. Perhaps funding priorities should be re-examined.

On the local level, hospitals must maintain a trained cadre of personnel who are prepared to deal effectively with the multidimensional injuries of bombing victims [61]. They also must continue to establish reasonable emergency management plans and galvanize those plans, with a focus on ensuring that critical casualties are not left to compete with noncritical casualties for limited trauma resources. Moreover, surgical leadership is required to ensure that critical hospital resources are conserved and applied appropriately to patient care. A critical challenge to surgeons is balancing their roles as key leaders in the hospital mass-casualty response against their roles in the OR. If the expectations placed upon general surgeons are unrealistic, perhaps it is time to consider seriously other alternative approaches [62].

Communication and interoperability must be improved between hospitals and partners in the response community. An even distribution of patients by a centrally acting EMS system should ensure the best treatment for all patients. Finally, communities should consider adopting an all-hazards approach to certain aspects of preparedness when it is the efficient and right thing to do and should continue to incorporate lessons learned into the basis for future planning and preparedness.

Acknowledgments

The author is extremely grateful to Robert Kurlantzick, MD, John Schlesser, MD, Valerie Waldorff, RN, JD, and Margaret Lazzerini, JD, for their assistance in researching and editing and the encouragement they provided.

References

[1] US Department of Justice. Federal Bureau of Investigation. Terrorism in the United States 1999: counterterrorism threat assessment and warning unit. Washington (DC): US Department of Justice, Counterterrorism Division; 1999. p. 1–62.

[2] Frykberg E. Principles of mass casualty management following terrorist disasters. Ann Surg 2004;239:319–21.

[3] Hirshberg A. Multiple casualty incidents: lessons from the front line. Ann Surg 2004;239: 322–4.

[4] DePalma R, Burris D, Champion H, et al. Blast injuries. N Engl J Med 2005;352:1335–42.

[5] Stein M, Hirshberg A. Medical consequences of terrorism: the conventional weapon threat. Surg Clin North Am 1999;79:1537–52.

[6] Tavenise S, Myers SL. Toll in Russia climbs to 41 in bombing at a hospital. The New York Times. August 3, 2003. Available at: http//www.sullivan-county.com/bush/41_russia.htm om. Accessed February 9, 2006.

[7] Kapur GB, Hutson RH, Davis MA, et al. The United States twenty-year experience with bombing incidents: implications for terrorism preparedness and medical response. J Trauma 2005;59:1436–44.

[8] Slater M, Trunkey D. Terrorism in America: an evolving threat. Arch Surg 1997;132:1059–66.

[9] Arnold J, Halpern P, Tsai MC, et al. Mass casualty terrorist bombings: a comparison of outcomes by bombing type. Ann Emerg Med 2004;43:263–73.

[10] Stobbe M. One ambulance per minute diverted in us, study finds: overcrowded emergency rooms send arriving patients to other hospitals, elderly most affected. The Washington Post. National News. February 7, 2006. p. A8.

[11] Ciraulo D, Frykberg E, Feliciano D, et al. A survey assessment of the level of preparedness for domestic terrorism and mass casualty incidents among Eastern Association for the Surgery of Trauma members. J Trauma 2004;56:1033–41.

[12] Mann NC, MacKenzie E, Anderson C. Public health preparedness for mass-casualty events: a 2002 state-by-state assessment. Prehosp Disast Med 2004;19:245–55.

[13] Leibovici D, Gofrit O, Stein M, et al. Blast injuries: bus versus open-air bombings—a comparative study of injuries in survivors of open-air versus confined-space explosions. J Trauma 1996;41:1030–5.

[14] Arnold J, Tsai MC, Halpern P, et al. Mass casualty, terrorist bombings: epidemiological outcomes, resource utilization, and time course of emergency needs (part I). Prehosp Disast Med 2003;18:220–34.

[15] Subcommittee on Advanced Trauma Life Support for the American College of Surgeons Committee on Trauma. Advanced trauma life support course for physicians. 5th edition. Chicago: American College of Surgeons; 1995.

[16] Auf der Heide E. The importance of evidence-based disaster planning. Ann Emerg Med 2006;47:34–49.

[17] Einav S, Feigenberg Z, Weissman C. Evacuation priorities in mass casualty terror-related events: implications for contingency planning. Ann Surg 2004;239:304–10.

[18] Hogan DE, Waeckerle JF, Dire DJ, et al. Emergency department impact of the Oklahoma City terrorist bombing. Ann Emerg Med 1999;34:160–7.

[19] Almogy G, Luria T, Richter E, et al. Can external signs of trauma guide management? Lessons learned from suicide bombing attacks in Israel. Arch Surg 2005;140:390–3.

[20] Halpern P, Tsai MC, Arnold J, et al. Mass-casualty, terrorist bombings: implications for emergency department and hospital emergency response (part II). Prehosp Disast Med 2003;18:235–41.

[21] Hospital emergency incident command system, version 3, vol. I. Redwood City (CA): San Mateo County Health Services Agency Emergency Medical Services; 1998.

[22] Zane RD, Prestipino AL. Implementing the Hospital Emergency Incident Command System: an integrated delivery system's experience. Prehosp Disast Med 2004;19(4):311–7.

[23] Firescope. Available at: www.firescope.org. Accessed February 6, 2006.

[24] Wang D, Sava J, Sample G, et al. The Pentagon and 9/11. Crit Care Med 2005;33(Suppl): S42–7.

[25] Hirshberg A, Holcomb J, Mattox K. Hospital trauma care in multiple-casualty incidents: a critical view. Ann Emerg Med 2001;37:647–52.

[26] Levi L, Michaelson M, Admi H, et al. National strategy for mass casualty situations and its effects on the hospital. Prehosp Disast Med 2002;17:12–6.

[27] Frykberg E, Tepas J. Terrorist bombings: lessons learned from Belfast to Beirut. Ann Surg 1988;208:569–76.

[28] Quenemoen LE, Davis YM, Malilay J, et al. The World Trade Center bombing: injury prevention strategies for high-rise building fires. Disasters 1996;20:125–32.

[29] Wightman J, Gladish S. Explosions and blast injuries. Ann Emerg Med 2001;37:664–78.

[30] Leibovici D, Gofrit ON, Shapira SC. Eardrum perforation in explosion survivors: is it a marker of pulmonary blast injury? Ann Emerg Med 1999;34:168–72.

[31] Feliciano DV, Anderson GV, Rozycki GS, et al. Management of casualties from the bombing at the centennial Olympics. Am J Surg 1998;176:538–43.

[32] Adler J, Golan E, Golan J, et al. Terrorist bombing experience during 1975–79. Casualties admitted to the Shaare Zedek Medical Center. Isr J Med Sci 1983;19(2):189–93.

[33] Carlton PK. Training together—first responders and first receivers playing the same game. Presented at the Georgetown University conference: Hospitals on the frontline: adapting to a new global reality. Washington, DC, January 19–20, 2006.

[34] Gutierrez de Ceballos JP, Turegano Fuentes F, et al. Casualties treated at the closest hospital in the Madrid, March 11 terrorist bombings. Crit Care Med 2005;33(Suppl.):S107–12.

[35] Auf der Heide E. Disaster response. Principles of preparation and coordination. St. Louis (MO): CV Mosby; 1989.

[36] Hirshberg A, Bradford S, Granchi T, et al. How does casualty load affect trauma care in urban bombing incidents? A quantitative analysis. J Trauma 2005;58:686–95.

[37] Centers for Disease Control. Rapid assessment of injuries among survivors of the terrorist attack on the World Trade Center—New York City, September 2001. MMWR Morb Mortal Wkly Rpt 2002;51:1–5.

[38] Asaeda G. The day that the START triage system came to a stop: observations from the World Trade Center disaster. Acad Emerg Med 2002;9:255–6.

[39] Auf der Heide E. Principles of hospital disaster planning. In: Hogan D, Burstein JL, editors. Disaster medicine. Philadelphia: Lippincott Williams & Wilkins; 2002. p. 57–89.

[40] Arlington County Fire Department. After action report on the response to the September 11 terrorist attack on the Pentagon. Available at: http://www.mipt.org/pdf/pentagonafteractionreport.pdf.2002. Accessed January 20, 2006.

[41] Tanielian T, Ricci K, Stoto M, et al. Exemplary practices in public health preparedness. Technical report. RAND Center for Domestic and International Health Security. Santa Monica (CA): RAND Corporation; 2005.

[42] Hawkins M. Surgical resource utilization in urban terrorist bombing: A computer simulation (Editorial comment). J Trauma 1999;47:550.

[43] Peleg K, Aharonson-Daniel L, Stein M, et al. Gunshot and explosion injuries: characteristics, outcomes, and implications for care of terror-related injuries in Israel. Ann Surg 2004;239:311–8.

[44] Hirshberg A, Stein M, Walden R. Surgical resource utilization in urban terrorist bombing: a computer simulation. J Trauma 1999;47:545–50.

[45] Frykberg E. Medical management of disasters and mass casualties from terrorist bombings: how can we cope? J Trauma 2002;53:201–12.

[46] Almogy G, Belzberg H, Mintz Y. Suicide bombing attacks: update and modifications to the protocol. Ann Surg 2004;239:295–303.

[47] Singer P, Cohen J, Stein M. Conventional terrorism and critical care. Crit Care Med 2005; 33(Suppl):S61–5.

[48] Argyros G. Management of primary blast injury. Toxicology 1997;121:105–15.

[49] Katz E, Ofek B, Adler J, et al. Primary blast injury after a bomb explosion in a civilian bus. Ann Surg 1989;209:484–8.

[50] Mellor SG. The pathogenesis of blast injury and its management. Br J Hosp Med 1988;39: 536–9.

[51] Hadden WA, Rutherford WH, Merrett JD. The injuries of terrorist bombing. A study of 1532 consecutive patients. Br J Surg 1978;65:525.

[52] Stuhmiller J, Phillips Y, Richmond D, et al. The physics and mechanisms of primary blast injury. In: Zajtchuk R, Jenkins D, Bellamy R, editors. Conventional warfare: ballistics, blast, and burn injuries. Textbook of military medicine, part I. Washington (DC): Office of the Surgeon General. Washington, DC: Borden Institute; 1991. p. 241–70.

[53] Avidan V, Hersch M, Armon Y, et al. Blast lung injury: clinical manifestations, treatment, and outcome. Am J Surg 2005;190:927–31.

[54] MacKenzie E, Hoyt D, Sacra J, et al. National inventory of hospital trauma centers. JAMA 2003;289:1515–22.

[55] Trunkey D. Trauma centers and trauma systems. JAMA 2003;289:1566–7.

[56] Altered standards of care in mass casualty events. Prepared by Health Systems Research, Inc. under contract No. 290–04–0010. AHRQ Publication # 05–0043. Rockville (MD): Agency for Healthcare Research and Quality; 2005.

[57] Burstein JL. The myths of disaster education. Ann Emerg Med 2006;47:50–2.

[58] Boyer M. Surgical education in the new millennium: the military perspective. Surg Clin North Am 2004;84:1453–70.

[59] Centers for Disease Control and Prevention. Receiving, distributing, and dispensing the national pharmaceutical stockpile: a guide for planners. Version 9. Atlanta (GA): Centers for Disease Control and Prevention; 2002.

[60] Interstate planning for the strategic national stockpile. Experiences in five regions. Association of State and Territorial Health Officials (ASTHO) Report 2005. Available at: www.ASTHO.org. Accessed February 6, 2006.

[61] Kluger Y, Peleg K, Daniel-Aharonson L, et al. The special injury pattern in terrorist bombings. J Am Coll Surg 2004;199:875–9.

[62] Trunkey D. In search of solutions. J Trauma 2002;53:1189–91.

ELSEVIER
SAUNDERS

SURGICAL
CLINICS OF
NORTH AMERICA

Surg Clin N Am 86 (2006) 601–636

Nuclear Terrorism: Triage and Medical Management of Radiation and Combined-Injury Casualties

COL Daniel F. Flynn, MD[a,b,c,*],
Ronald E. Goans, MD, PhD[b,d,e]

[a]US Army Reserves Medical Corps, Office of the Command Surgeon,
94th Regional Readiness Command,
11 Saratoga Boulevard, Devens, MA 01434, USA
[b]Radiation Emergency Assistance Center and Training Site, Oak Ridge Institute for Science
and Education, P.O. Box 117, MS 39, Oak Ridge, TN 37831, USA
[c]New England Radiation Therapy Associates, Radiation Oncology Department,
Holy Family Hospital, 70 East Street, Methuen, MA 01844, USA
[d]MJW Corporation, University Park, 1900 Sweet Home Road, Amherst, NY 14228, USA
[e]Center for Applied Environmental Public Health, Tulane University School of Public Health
and Tropical Medicine, 1440 Canal Street, New Orleans, LA 70112, USA

Intentional radiation incidents, such as terrorist attacks, have a wide range of possible scenarios—from a dirty bomb to a nuclear bomb detonation. Medical preparedness for nuclear terrorism also means preparedness for treating casualties resulting from unintentional causes, ranging from transportation accidents that involve an airplane or truck carrying radioactive material, an industrial accident, a fire in a hospital, to a nuclear power reactor "meltdown." Treatment, regardless of cause, involves the medical management of patients who have conventional mechanical trauma or burns and who also have been exposed to radiation or are contaminated by radioactive material. Today, nuclear war between major powers is considered unlikely. Nuclear terrorism is now the major threat.

Thermonuclear weapon detonation

In 1945, the two nuclear bombs that exploded in Japan were both in the 10- to 20-kiloton range, equivalent to 20,000–40,000 pounds of trinitrotoluene (TNT). The Hiroshima and Nagasaki bombs, which were low-altitude air

---

* Corresponding author. N.E.R.T.A., Department of Radiation Oncology, Holy Family Hospital, 70 East Street, Methuen, MA 01844.
  E-mail address: daniel_f_flynn_md@cchcs.org (D.F. Flynn).

0039-6109/06/$ - see front matter © 2006 Elsevier Inc. All rights reserved.
doi:10.1016/j.suc.2006.03.005   surgical.theclinics.com

bursts, were detonated at approximately 2000 feet altitude. At Hiroshima, within 20 days of the detonation, the fatality rate was 86% up to 0.6 miles from the detonation, 27% at 0.6 to 1.6 miles, and 2% at 1.6 to 3.1 miles [1,2]. People who were in reinforced concrete buildings had a 50% chance of survival at only 0.2 miles from the detonation, whereas those who were in the open and unshielded from the explosion had a 50% chance of survival at 1.3 miles. The affected area of Hiroshima contained 328,081 inhabitants. The total number of deaths in this population was 122,338 (118,661 accounted for and 3,677 missing persons), of which approximately 68,000 deaths occurred in the first 20 days. Among the survivors there were 79,130 persons injured and 118,613 uninjured. The majority of the doctors and nurses in the area were killed or injured, and most of the hospitals were totally destroyed or severely damaged. Approximately 82,000 survivors have been part of a cohort established to study long-term effects. Results of the study indicate that the incidence of thyroid cancer was increased in those less than 20 years old at the time of exposure; in the 60-year period since the detonation, about 500 persons developed cancers (leukemias and solid tumors) attributable to radiation exposure.

A full nuclear exchange between powers at war probably would involve weapons that have yields in megatons of TNT. The predominant cause of fallout is actual contact of the fireball with the ground, which usually happens with either low-altitude, or surface-level detonations. Massive amounts of contamination are injected into the lower atmosphere, producing a downwind radioactive plume containing radioactive dust and particles. Prolonged contact with fallout on the skin can result in serious skin damage plus increased whole-body dose. Therefore, the public response should be "shelter and shower." Sheltering (particularly at home) is prudent early in a radiologic event, because families congregate at home and showers, clean clothing, food, and water are available. Sheltering also provides authorities time to assess the situation more completely. Evacuation might be indicated later for people in some locations, depending on the specific situation and the extended dose estimates. In other locations, remaining sheltered may result in lower radiation exposure.

Medical effects of nuclear weapon detonation

The medical effects of nuclear weapon detonation include blast, thermal, and radiation effects, all of which cause significant casualties [1]. Casualties generally are caused by a combination of effects; immediate deaths result from blast and thermal injuries. Among those who experienced significant clinical effects at Hiroshima, an estimated 90% had burns, 83% had mechanical trauma, and 37% had radiation injuries.

Blast injury

Two types of blast forces occur simultaneously in the shock front of a nuclear detonation: direct blast wave peak overpressure, which is measured by the magnitude of sudden pressure rise over ambient pressure, and indirect blast wind drag forces, which are measured by wind velocities. Both blast forces decrease with increasing distance from the detonation site.

Direct blast wave peak

Overpressure refers to sudden pressure changes above the stable ambient pressure. Ambient pressure at sea level is 14.7 pounds per square inch (psi). Sudden peak overpressures may cause windows to shatter at 1 psi or some brick houses to collapse at 5 psi. Rapid compression and decompression with transmission of pressure waves through tissues results in damage at junctions between tissues of different densities. This damage is noted particularly at air–tissue interfaces, including eardrums and lungs. Rupture of the tympanic membrane may cause tinnitus, pain, and hearing loss, and there may be otoscopic evidence of perforation and blood in the external canal. The threshold pressure for eardrum rupture is 5 psi. Nearly all eardrums rupture at 20 psi, which is the threshold for lung injury. Severe lung injury occurs between 30 and 40 psi. Thus, the finding of ruptured eardrums signals that lung injury may be present, because pressure levels high enough to cause serious injury to the lung invariably rupture the eardrums.

Injury to the lungs is the major cause of morbidity and mortality in direct blast injuries [3,4]. Clinically diffuse pulmonary contusions become apparent as local or diffuse infiltrates on radiographs over the course of hours. Symptoms may include chest tightness, pain, tachypnea, and hemoptysis. At the interface between soft tissue and air in the lung, the direct blast pressure wave results in local tensions that cause microscopic tears; hemorrhage and edema then develop. An alveolar–pulmonary venous communication can be the source of air emboli, which can be immediately life threatening. Pneumothorax, hemothorax, and mediastinal extravasation of air are all possible manifestations of severe direct blast injury.

Indirect blast wind drag force

Winds of much greater than hurricane force cause flying debris (missiles) to strike people or project people into the air to impact other objects. Traumatic injuries, including penetrating trauma (eg, caused by glass at high velocity) or blunt trauma, are much more common than direct blast effects. Crush injuries may result because blast winds cause the collapse or fragmentation and displacement of buildings or large objects such as vehicles. There is a relationship between the peak overpressure and the maximum wind velocity at the blast shock front (Table 1). As noted in Table 1, both the blast wind velocity and the direct blast peak overpressure decline with increasing distance from the detonation. The actual distance is not listed in the table, because it would depend on the magnitude of the nuclear detonation yield. For example, for a 20-kiloton nuclear detonation, the blast wind velocity is 180 mph at 0.8 miles. For a 1-megaton nuclear detonation, the estimated velocity of the blast wind is 400 mph at 1.1 mile, 180 mph at 3.0 miles, and 40 mph at 9 miles.

Table 1
Indirect blast effects: maximum wind velocity of shock front and associated blast peak overpressure

Indirect blast maximum wind velocity (mph)	Direct blast peak overpressure (psi)
2078	200
1415	100
934	50
294	10
163	5
70	2

Data from Glasstone S, Dolan PJ. The effects of nuclear weapons. 3rd edition. Washington (DC): US Department of Defense; 1977. p. 22.

Thermal radiation injury

The intense heat of the expanding fireball and thermal infrared radiation cause thermal injury consisting of flash burns, flame burns, flash blindness (resulting from temporary depletion of photopigment from the retinal receptors), and retinal burns (relatively rarely). Thermal effects also decrease with increasing distance from the detonation. In a 10-kiloton detonation, second-degree burns on exposed skin are seen on people located up to 1.4 miles from the site, and first-degree burns are seen on those within 2 miles of the site. In a 1-megaton detonation, second-degree burns are seen on people at distances up to 10 miles, and first-degree burns are seen on those within 15 miles.

Flash burns

Flash burns are caused by thermal infrared radiation that travels in a straight line. Exposed skin absorbs the infrared radiation, and the victim is burned on the side of the body facing the explosion (profile burns). At a sufficient distance from the detonation, objects covering the skin, including clothing, may shield against this injury. A little closer to the detonation, where thermal energy is higher, radiation can cause flash burns through clothing, even at temperatures below those required to cause ignition. Depending on its thermal conduction properties and whether the clothing is in actual contact with the skin, light-colored clothing reflects the infrared and dark colors absorb it, resulting in pattern burns. Still closer to the detonation, the higher thermal energy ignites clothing and causes third-degree burns. This effect, however, is considered a flame burn rather than a flash burn.

Flame burns

Flame burns are caused by ignition of clothing relatively close to the detonation or by the secondary effect of fires. Firestorms cause many burn injuries and deaths as damaged buildings burn with people trapped inside. Severe thermal injuries include respiratory injuries from hot gases. Close to the fireball of the explosion, everything is totally incinerated, with immediate 100% lethality.

Nuclear radiation injury

Two types of radiation injury occur. Prompt radiation injury is caused by the exposure to radiation released immediately upon the detonation. Residual radiation injury is caused by the delayed exposure to radioactive contamination or fallout. Most acute radiation casualties result from prompt radiation. As with blast and thermal effects, the radiation effects decrease with increasing distance from the detonation. In a 10-kiloton detonation, an absorbed radiation dose of 4.5 Gy would be noted at a distance of 0.7 miles from the detonation site, whereas this dose would be seen at a distance of 1.6 miles from the site of a 1-megaton detonation.

The effects of whole-body irradiation increase with higher doses of radiation. The published literature and information on Websites may use different units to express radiation measurements. Radiation dose is often expressed in Gy or Sv. The older units are R (roentgen), rad, and rem, respectively, whereby 1 Gy = 100 cGy = 100 rad = approximately 100 R, and 1 Sv = 100 rem = 100,000 mrem. The primary clinical effects observed within hours of sufficient whole-body irradiation are nausea and vomiting; the primary early hematologic effect is reduced lymphocyte count, which is seen in less than 48 hours. Reduced neutrophil and reduced platelet counts are seen at approximately 2 to 6 weeks. For an acute whole-body exposure, the lethal dose (LD) that will kill 50% of an exposed group in 60 days is expressed as $LD_{50}(60)$. For untreated humans, the $LD_{50}(60)$ is about 3.5 Gy (350 cGy). With aggressive treatment, as is possible when casualties are limited, the $LD_{50}(60)$ might be doubled. The clinical dose–effect relationships for acute whole-body exposure are given in Table 2, in which, for the purpose of the data presented, 1 Gy = 1 Sv. These doses can be compared with doses that do not cause symptoms or acute injury (Box 1):

Table 2
Whole-body radiation dose-effect relationship

Dose	Effect
0.2 Gy	No observable symptoms; threshold for minor chromosome changes in circulating blood lymphocytes
0.5 Gy	Threshold for minor lymphocyte depression
1 Gy	Threshold for nausea and vomiting; mild lymphocyte depression at 48 hr; no deaths from acute effects of radiation
2 Gy	Nausea and vomiting within hours commonly seen; moderate lymphocyte depression at 48 hr; few, if any, deaths provided no combined injuries are present
3.5 Gy	Probable nausea and vomiting within hours; significant lymphocyte depression at 48 hr; 50% lethal within 60 days (if untreated); more lethal if combined injuries are present
6 Gy	100% nausea and vomiting within 1 hr; severe lymphocyte depression at 48 hr; 100% lethal within 60 days (if untreated); 100% lethal even with treatment if significant combined injuries are present

Adapted from Radiation Emergency Assistance Center/Training Site (REAC/TS), Training Material, Oak Ridge (TN), March 2006.

Box 1. Noninjurious radiation doses

Overseas roundtrip flight or a chest radiograph (posteroanterior
  and lateral): 10 mrem (0.01 cGy or 0.1 mSv)
Average annual background absorbed dose (United States):
  360 mrem (0.36 cGy or 3.6 mSv)
Diagnostic radiology CT scan of chest or abdomen: 500 mrem
  (0.5 cGy or 5 mSv)
Maximum annual dose allowed radiation worker
  (United States): 5000 mrem (0.05 Gy or 5 cGy or 50 mSv)

Acute clinical effects of whole-body or significant ($>60\%$) partial-body radiation are characterized as acute radiation syndrome [5]. In addition to nausea and vomiting, other clinical effects (sometimes delayed) may be noted, including erythema, fever, headache, diarrhea, hair loss, delayed radiation skin burns (as distinguished from prompt thermal burns), and fatigue. Table 3 outlines the three classic acute-radiation syndromes: hematopoietic, gastrointestinal, and cardiovascular/central nervous system. Whole-body exposures between 0 and 1 Gy generally are asymptomatic. Potentially survivable exposures generally are in the range for hematopoietic syndrome (1–8 Gy). Even with aggressive treatment, no one with a total body dose in excess of about 12 Gy will survive for more than 6 months. Death results not only from the severe hematologic and gastrointestinal effects but also from the intolerance of the lungs for high single doses. For the very few who survive the combined bone marrow and gastrointestinal effects within the first 60 days, death from radiation pneumonitis is likely within the next 60 days (ie, about 2–4 months after exposure). Other organ systems, such as the heart, kidney, and liver, are also likely to suffer potentially lethal damage.

Assessment of radiation dose

Clinical assessment of radiation dose

Once the immediate medical needs of a trauma and burn patient have been met, radiation decontamination and estimation of radiation dose should begin. Assessment of the radiation dose is important for modifying patient triage. The radiation dose can be estimated by the time to first emesis. Goans has demonstrated that the time to first emesis decreases with increasing radiation dose in a predictable pattern [5]. The original work was performed by Ricks and Lushbaugh [6] at Oak Ridge Associated Universities and involved 502 patients who had undergone therapeutic or accidental radiation between 1964 and 1975. With low-to-moderate dose rates (0.8–90 R/hr), the estimated dose resulting in emesis in 50% of the patients was 2.4 Gy. When a dose is absorbed over a short period of time (ie, at

Table 3
Classic acute radiation syndromes

Dose	Clinical status	Description
1–8 Gy	Hematopoietic syndrome	Clinical effects may include nausea, vomiting, and, occasionally, skin erythema, fever, mucositis, and diarrhea. Laboratory analysis in cases with acute whole-body exposure >1 or 2 Gy can show lymphocytopenia (8–48 hr), neutropenia, and thrombocytopenia (20–30 d). Other common effects in the weeks after exposure include impaired wound healing, anemia, bleeding (frequent gingival bleeding, petechiae, and/or ecchymoses of skin or mucous membranes), increased infectious complications, and death. Death from hematopoietic syndrome may occur about 3 to 8 weeks after exposure.
8–30 Gy	Gastrointestinal syndrome	Clinical effects include onset of severe nausea and vomiting, from minutes up to 1 hour after exposure, diarrhea (hours later), fever, headache, and fatigue. Death from gastrointestinal syndrome (added to severe hematopoietic syndrome) usually occurs 1 to 2 weeks after exposure.
>30 Gy	Cardiovascular/central nervous syndrome	Clinical effects within minutes after exposure include vomiting, burning sensation, and prostration. Neurologic signs include dizziness, ataxia, and confusion. Hypotension, high fever, and explosive diarrhea are seen. Death is inevitable within 24 to 48 hours.

Adapted from Medical preparedness and response subgroup of the Homeland Security Department Working Group on Radiological Dispersal Devices (RDD) and Preparedness (p. 15), December 9, 2003 update. Available at: www1.va.gov/emshg/docs/Radiological_Medical_Countermeasures_Indexed-Final.pdf. Accessed January 12, 2006.

a high dose rate), the dose resulting in emesis in 50% of the patients is expected to be significantly lower, as consistent with clinical experience in radiation oncology treatment where the dose is delivered in a few minutes. Although a relatively small percentage of patients acutely exposed to a dose of 1 Gy vomit, most vomit when the dose is higher than 2 Gy, provided the dose is absorbed over a short time rather than over many hours or days. As a guide for rapid clinical radiologic triage in a mass casualty situation, it has been proposed, based on Goans' REAC/TS data, that persons who vomit within 4 hours of exposure be referred for hospital evaluation and possible hospital admission [7]. Persons who do not vomit within 4 hours can be referred for delayed evaluation (24–72 hours). If they have no concurrent injury, outpatient care probably is appropriate.

A summary of Goans' analysis of the Radiation Emergency Assistance Center/Training Site (REAC/TS) International Accident Registry data is presented in Table 4 [7]. Worldwide accident data are recorded and

Table 4
Radiation Emergency Assistance Center/Training Site estimates of time to vomiting after exposure in relation to whole-body radiation dose

Percentile of dose	Radiation dose	
	<4 hr to vomiting	>4 hr to vomiting
25th percentile	2.5 Gy	0.5 Gy
Median dose	3.6 Gy	0.9 Gy
75th percentile	6.0 Gy	1.7 Gy

Data from Goans RE, REAC/TS, and the Medical Preparedness and Response Subgroup of the Homeland Security Department Working Group on Radiological Dispersal Devices (RDD) and Preparedness (p. 23), December 9, 2003 update. Available at: www1.va.gov/emshg/docs/Radiological_Medical_Countermeasures_Indexed-Final.pdf. Accessed January 12, 2006.

maintained at the REAC/TS in Oak Ridge, Tennessee. The International Atomic Energy Agency also has published dose estimates relative to the time to first emesis after a single acute-radiation exposure (Table 5) [8]. If no vomiting occurs during the first 4 hours after an acute exposure, one may assume that severe clinical effects are unlikely unless there are significant conventional injuries. If there is insufficient laboratory support in a mass-casualty situation, triage of casualties according to radiation dose will depend on the length of time to initial vomiting. More recently, Goans [9] reported that if the time to emesis is less than 2 hours after exposure, the effective whole-body dose is at least 3 Gy. Patients who have radiation-induced emesis within 1 hour have received a whole-body dose that probably exceeds 4 Gy. The median radiation dose for patients vomiting in less than 1 hour after exposure is 6.5 Gy, with an interquartile range (25%–75%) of approximately 5 to 11 Gy [7].

Laboratory assessment of radiation dose by depression of lymphocyte count

Peripheral blood lymphocyte counts are known to follow a predictable radiation dose–dependent exponential decline in the first few days after a significant, but often unknown, whole-body dose. The classic nomogram

Table 5
International Atomic Energy Agency estimates of whole-body radiation dose in relation to time to onset of vomiting after a single acute exposure

Time to vomiting	Estimated dose
<10 min	>8 Gy
10–30 min	6–8 Gy
30 min–1 hr	4–6 Gy
1–2 hr	2–4 Gy
>2 hr	<2 Gy

Data from Diagnosis and treatment of radiation injuries. International Atomic Energy Agency safety report series # 2. Vienna (Austria): International Atomic Energy Agency; 1998. table VIII. p. 7.

developed by Andrews [10] has been used to predict the prognosis roughly based on the degree of lymphocyte depression. For example, at 24 hours after exposure, if the lymphocyte count is less than 10% of a normal count, the exposure is lethal even with treatment. If it is 90% or more of a normal count, survival is likely even without treatment. If it is about 50% of a normal count, the corresponding dose is in the mid-hematopoietic syndrome range (about 5 Gy). In that case, aggressive treatment should be started before the end of the first week to decrease the risk of death in the following weeks. As a quantitative enhancement of the classical Andrews model, Goans and colleagues [11,12] developed a predictive algorithm to estimate the effective whole-body dose soon after an accident. The method uses the measured lymphocyte depletion rate from serial complete blood cell counts performed within the first 8 to 12 hours after exposure. This algorithm was developed to provide both the physician and the health physicist with an early approximation of the dose, so that cytokine therapy, if indicated, could be begun early. A rough estimate of the whole-body dose may be obtained by using Goans' data and taking the absolute lymphocyte count at approximately 8 to 12 hours after exposure (Table 6). The dose estimate is independent of the preirradiation lymphocyte count, which often is unknown. This technique is designed to be a radiation triage mechanism applied early in the postexposure period and should be considered along with the time to radiation-induced emesis. Between 12 and 48 hours after exposure, the lymphocyte count continues to drop exponentially. The lymphocyte counts of patients receiving different radiation doses will differ more at 48 hours than at 12 hours. This is because the counts of different patients are decreasing at different dose-dependent depletion rates. Therefore, at the 48-hour point, a better estimate of dose and prognosis can be made (Table 7). Algorithms from the Armed Forces Radiobiology Research Institute's Biodosimetry Assessment Tool [13] combine various factors, including time to emesis and lymphocyte depletion rate, to estimate the radiation dose and help guide therapy. These algorithms can be downloaded from www.afrri.usuhs.mil.

Table 6
Whole-body estimated dose based on early lymphocyte count depression

Absolute lymphocyte count 8–12 hr after exposure[a]	Absorbed dose (rough estimate)
1700–2500/mm^3	1–5 Gy
1200–1700/mm^3	5–9 Gy
<1000/mm^3	>10 Gy

[a] A whole body dose of 1 Gy or less should not noticeably depress the lymphocyte count below the normal range taken as 1500–3500/mm^3.

Data from Goans RE, REAC/TS, and Medical Preparedness and Response Subgroup of Homeland Security Department Working Group on Radiological Dispersal Devices (RDD) and Preparedness. (p. 23), December 9, 2003 update. Available at: www1.va.gov/emshg/docs/Radiological_Medical_Countermeasures_Indexed-Final.pdf. Accessed January 12, 2006.

Table 7
Prognosis based on lymphocyte count depression after acute whole-body exposure

Absolute lymphocyte count 48 hr after exposure	Absorbed dose (estimate)	Prognosis
1000–1500/mm^3	1–2 Gy	Moderate injury, probably nonlethal; good prognosis
500–1000/mm^3	2–4 Gy	Severe injury; fair prognosis
100–500/mm^3	4–8 Gy	Very severe injury; poor prognosis
<100/mm^3	>8 Gy	High incidence of death even with treatment

Adapted from Koenig KL, Goans RE, Hatchett RJ, et al. Medical treatment of radiological casualties and current concepts. Ann Emer Med 2005;45:646.

Laboratory assessment of radiation dose by cytogenetic studies

A second laboratory method for assessing radiation dose involves chromosome-aberration bioassay in cultured peripheral blood lymphocytes [5]. Blood samples need to be drawn in heparinized tubes and refrigerated (not frozen). Chromosome dicentrics are interchanges between two chromosomes that form a distorted chromosome with two centromeres. The frequency of chromosome dicentrics correlates better with the absorbed dose than does lymphocyte count depression and changes can be detected as low as 0.2 Gy dose. The technique is very labor intensive, however, and results cannot be obtained rapidly: even in ideal situations, the delay in obtaining results typically is up to 1 week after exposure. Thus, the method has limited usefulness in a mass-casualty situation. Nevertheless, when there are relatively few casualties, cytogenetics can guide therapy in selected cases. The current cytogenetic laboratory capability in the United States is at the Armed Forces Radiobiological Research Institute in Bethesda, Maryland. The REAC/TS in Oak Ridge, Tennessee, is presently reestablishing its cytogenetics laboratory.

Triage and emergency medical treatment of mass casualties

Conventional injury triage

Initial primary triage is based on conventional injuries (mechanical trauma and burns), not on radiation dose. In the first few hours after a nuclear terrorism event with mass casualties, trauma will be the primary life-threatening problem to address [14–18]. A patient presenting with hypotension must be presumed to be hypovolemic as a result of trauma and not as a result of a massive radiation dose. Therefore, hypotensive patients must be evaluated quickly to determine if their hypotension has a surgically correctable cause (eg, hemorrhage).

Triage categories identical to those used in the military for conventional injuries (trauma and burns) [19–23] should be adopted to prioritize care when the number of victims overwhelms available medical resources (Box 2).

Box 2. Triage categories used by the military

Immediate (red)—Patients require immediate treatment to save
life, limb, or sight (highest triage priority)

Delayed (yellow)—Patients require less urgent treatment than
those in the immediate category

Minimal (green)—Patients require outpatient treatment and are
often returned to duty

Expectant (black)—Patients require extensive treatment
and resources and usually have a very poor prognosis, even
with treatment (lowest triage priority)

This conventional-injury triage system is the first approach. Patients in the immediate-treatment category and many patients in the delayed-treatment category require surgical intervention for blunt or penetrating trauma or burns. Many patients in the immediate-treatment category may be unstable because of localized, surgically correctable conditions. It is likely that there will be many more patients in the immediate-treatment category than the operating room has the capacity to handle. Given two equally compelling immediate-category patients requiring emergency surgery, the one estimated to require less operating room table time should be taken first. Surgeons will need to prioritize on whom they will operate. The remaining patients in the immediate- and delayed-treatment categories will be stabilized as much as possible while awaiting surgery. Patients in the expectant-treatment category are given comfort care only. After a period of time, which might range from hours to several days—once all the patients in the immediate- and delayed-treatment categories have been cleared—available resources will address the few expectant patients still alive and the patients in the minimal-treatment category still requiring care. This conventional military triage system is based on mechanical trauma and burn assessment.

Combined injury is defined as concurrent trauma (mechanical or thermal) and radiation injury. The prognosis is much worse for victims who have serious combined injuries than for those with the same degree of conventional injury without radiation. Historical experiments demonstrated that animals that have received a dose of radiation plus an experimental thermal burn have greatly reduced survival as compared with animals receiving the same dose of radiation alone or the same thermal burn alone. Studies also have demonstrated that for the same radiation dose, adding an experimental wound significantly reduces survival. Early wound closure has been shown to reverse this effect. In a mass-casualty situation after a nuclear detonation, many will die from the effects of combined injuries. Unfortunately, there are no modern data regarding combined-injury survival with modern medical and surgical techniques. A theoretical combined-injury military triage guide that tries to factor in radiation dose would be difficult to implement because of the uncertainty of the radiation dose during initial triage. The "golden hour" for trauma patients is actually the first 1 to 2 hours following the trauma. In a mass-casualty situation with patients needing immediate life-saving surgery, there would be no opportunity to accurately estimate the absorbed dose within the first 2 hours. Nevertheless, if it is judged (later in the first day or in the second day) that an immediate or delayed trauma victim has also received a radiation dose in the mid-hematopoietic syndrome range (about 3.5 Gy) or higher, the triage category for this victim might have to be changed to expectant, because survival is probably unlikely even with aggressive treatment. A patient in the minimal-treatment category who has received a dose of 3.5 Gy might be switched to the delayed-treatment category or kept in the minimal-treatment category, because the treatment for the presumed minor conventional injury plus significant radiation injury could be delayed for a few days before appropriate therapy for an absorbed dose in the mid-hematopoietic syndrome range is instituted.

Radiation injury triage

On the basis of the severity of radiation exposure, the REAC/TS uses four basic treatment categories that are listed as hospital care groups (Table 8). The four categories are mild (<2 Gy), moderate (2–5 Gy), severe (5–10 Gy), and lethal (>10 Gy) exposure. The assumption is that these patients do not have significant conventional injuries (trauma or burns) but are primarily radiation-alone patients. If the patients are numerous enough to require triage, the four REAC/TS hospital groups are somewhat parallel to the military triage categories. Those who have received a mild radiation dose might be considered in the minimal-treatment category, in that they are expected to survive with no immediate treatment; those who have received a lethal radiation dose would obviously be considered expectant and would be given comfort care. Clinical resources would be prioritized to treat the victims in the moderate (2–5 Gy) and severe (5–10 Gy) groups, similar to trauma and burn patients in the delayed-treatment and immediate-treatment categories, respectively, on the assumption that there are no patients who have mechanical trauma or burns. Patients in the immediate-treatment category, by strict definition, are those requiring immediate lifesaving intervention. Neither the moderate nor the severe radiation-alone category is immediately life threatening. Any patients who have trauma that falls in the immediate- or delayed-treatment categories will certainly take priority over all categories of radiation-alone patients.

In combined-injury cases, lymphocyte count may be an unreliable indicator in some patients, because severe burns or trauma to more than one system may result in lymphopenia. If there were major conventional injuries (trauma or burns), all patients in Group III (Table 8, 5–10 Gy) would clearly

Table 8
Hospital care groups

Group I mild (<2 Gy)	Group II moderate (2–5 Gy)[a]	Group III severe (5–10 Gy)[a]	Group IV lethal (>10 Gy)
Triage by symptoms, lymphocyte count	Hospitalization	Hospitalization	Symptomatic and supportive care only. If there are no mass casualties, or if resources become adequate, some of these patients can be treated as if in Group III
Close observation and complete blood cell with differential count	Reverse isolation	Reverse isolation	
Outpatient management appropriate if no significant mechanical trauma or burns	Consider early growth factor (cytokine) therapy	Early growth factor (cytokine) therapy	
	Consider selective gut decontamination (oral antibiotics)	Selective gut decontamination	
	Viral prophylaxis	Viral prophylaxis	
	Consider early antifungal therapy	Early antifungal therapy	
	Antibiotics for febrile neutropenia	Early antibiotics for anticipated severe neutropenia	

[a] Patients in Groups II and III require assistance of a hematologist knowledgeable in treatment of severe pancytopenia and experimental growth factor and assistance of an infectious disease expert knowledgeable in treatment of resistant opportunistic infections with anticipation of profound febrile neutropenia. If resources become depleted, some patients in Group III may be considered Group IV.

Modified from MacVittie TJ, Weiss JF, Browne D. Advances in the treatment of radiation injuries. Elsevier Press; 1996. p. 327.

be considered expectant, because their combined injuries would indicate an expected lethality, even with aggressive use of resources. A major difference between conventional injuries and radiation injuries is the time line. Thermal burns and mechanical trauma result in many deaths within hours. Survivable injuries caused by radiation alone do not cause death in the first week. A death caused by radiation alone within the first week indicates a dose so high that it would have been nonsurvivable regardless of treatment (ie, a dose high in the gastrointestinal syndrome [24] or in the cardiovascular/central nervous system syndrome range). For this reason, initial care in a combined-injury scenario always focuses first on serious mechanical trauma and burns.

The cutaneous syndrome caused by radiation (Table 9) may occur with any of the three classic syndromes previously described. Occasionally, an early, very transient skin erythema is seen. The principal effects, however, are not noted until several weeks after exposure. They include a brisk erythema, with blistering and wet desquamation at higher doses. At still higher doses, ulcerations with necrosis may evolve. Burns appearing within 48 hours of exposure are thermal burns, because radiation burns take up to several weeks to manifest.

Virtually all survivors at Hiroshima had estimated whole-body doses of less than 3 Gy [25], which may approximate the $LD_{95}(60)$, the dose that kills 95% of victims ("virtually all") within 60 days. The $LD_{50}(60)$ is known now to be about 3.5 Gy, which implies that the $LD_{95}(60)$ for untreated individuals is probably closer to 5 to 5.5 Gy. Therefore one may speculate that the combined-injury effect of trauma or burns with whole-body radiation injury at Hiroshima probably resulted in a rough decrease of 2 Gy in both the $LD_{95}(60)$ and the $LD_{50}(60)$.

Emergency treatment of combined injuries

During the first 72 hours the initial phase of treatment will be directed toward treatment of trauma and burns, external decontamination, and very early initiation of potassium iodide, where appropriate. After detonation of a nuclear weapon, most casualties will be combined-injury patients. Emergency surgical care involves resuscitation, control of hemorrhage, and minimization of sepsis with débridement techniques. Traditionally, combat or traumatic wounds are left open, but wounds left open by secondary intention in the irradiated patient (who has received a dose in the hematopoietic syndrome range) will serve as a nidus of infection. Therefore, wounds in the combined-injury patient should be débrided thoroughly and closed at a second-look operation within 36 to 48 hours. Emergency nonsurgical care includes administration of fluids and electrolytes, transfusions, covering of wounds and burns, and pain control. External radiation decontamination is

Table 9
Radiation dose thresholds for cutaneous effects (single acute exposure)

Dose	Cutaneous effects
3 Gy	Epilation (threshold) beginning several weeks after exposure
> 10 Gy	Dry desquamation 2–3 weeks after exposure
> 20 Gy	Wet desquamation 2–3 weeks after exposure
> 50 Gy	Radionecrosis and deep ulceration

Data from Goans RE. Critical care of the radiation-accident patient: patient presentation, assessment and initial diagnosis. In: Ricks RC, Berger ME, O'Hara FM, editors. The medical basis of radiation-accident preparedness: the clinical care of victims. Boca Raton (FL): Parthenon Publishing Group, CRC Press; 2002. p. 14.

started and performed so that it does not interfere with continuing emergency care. Traumatic wounds are handled somewhat similarly to burns. Major surgical procedures are prioritized for unstable but salvageable patients. Ideally, if surgical correction of major injuries is required, it should be performed as soon as possible. Otherwise, major surgical procedures should be postponed, if possible, until late in the convalescent period (45–60 days) following hematopoietic recovery. Obviously, patients requiring lifesaving surgery during the first 2 months will receive it even if the time is not optimal. Topical antibiotics with nonadherent dressings are essential, with systemic antibiotics added if necessary. For vomiting, treatment includes drugs such as prochlorperazine, granisetron, and ondansetron. Vomiting usually abates within 48 hours, ameliorating the need for prolonged antiemetic therapy. For diarrhea, treatment includes drugs such as loperamide and diphenoxylate hydrochloride with atropine sulfate. Radiation oncologists and medical oncologists frequently use these drugs. Patients who have serious trauma or burns without serious radiation injury should be stabilized and referred to trauma or burn centers. Patients who have severe radiation injury should be referred later to oncology centers equipped to treat opportunistic infectious complications of bone marrow failure. Patients who have mild, uncomplicated injuries may be kept in community hospitals.

Definitive treatment of radiation casualties

During the first 72 hours of the emergency treatment phase, while clinical and laboratory assessments of whole-body dose are being made, potentially salvageable patients should be identified who are destined to develop radiation-induced bone marrow aplasia of the hematopoietic syndrome. Early in the definitive treatment phase of casualties, the initiation of cytokines (such as granulocyte colony-stimulating factor [G-CSF]) and probably antimicrobials will improve the chances of survival for these patients [26–29].

Treatment of hematopoietic injury

Both in the immediate posttraumatic period and later during the manifestation of hematopoietic radiation injury, aggressive use of transfused blood products should be considered when indicated. In the 2- to 4-week period after radiation exposure, further transfusions may be needed if the delayed myelosuppressive effects of radiation are seen. If possible, blood products should be irradiated (25 Gy) to decrease the risk of transfusion-associated graft-versus-host disease in the immunosuppressed patient. If necessary, nonirradiated blood may be used [30].

Growth factors or cytokines (colony-stimulating factors [CSFs]) are endogenous glycoproteins that induce bone marrow stem cells to proliferate and differentiate into specific mature blood cell types. For those who receive radiation doses in the hematopoietic syndrome range (1–8 Gy), successful treatment depends upon maintaining a surviving fraction of stem cells capable of spontaneous regeneration, assuming that any nonhematopoietic injuries present are survivable. The Food and Drug Administration approved CSFs more than 10 years ago for use in neutropenic patients receiving myelosuppressive chemotherapy. Such drugs currently approved in oncology practice include filgrastim (G-CSF), pegfilgrastim (pegG-CSF), and sargramostim (granulocyte-macrophage colony-stimulating factor [GM-CSF]). These, along with newer growth factors under development, are potent stimulators of the bone marrow for hematopoiesis. Data indicate that CSFs may both ameliorate radiation-induced neutropenia and also shorten its duration, suggesting a survival advantage. Unfortunately, no data showing increased survival in higher animals or humans using this regimen are currently available. In the REAC/TS registry, however, 25 of 28 patients treated with G-CSF or GM-CSF after radiation accidents seemed to have a faster neutrophil recovery. Although the optimal interval between radiation exposure and initiation of CSF therapy is unknown, the results of animal experiments and several radiation accidents suggest that CSFs should be initiated prophylactically early in patients who have been exposed to a potentially survivable whole-body dose of radiation and are at risk for the hematopoietic syndrome. For patients who were not offered early G-CSF and who become profoundly neutropenic (ie, an absolute neutrophil count [ANC] <500/μL), a CSF should be employed when severe neutropenia develops. Although radiation-induced neutropenia is a main issue to be addressed early in the hematopoietic syndrome, anemia may need to be addressed later in some patients, particularly to decrease the need for transfusion of packed red blood cells. Erythropoietin is a glycoprotein hormone that is a CSF for red blood cell precursors in the bone marrow. Synthetic forms include epoetin alpha and darbepoetin alpha. Although the benefits of epoetin and darbepoetin have not been established in radiologic events, these agents may be considered in patients who have significant radiation-induced anemia.

Transfusion of peripheral blood or of cord/placenta blood progenitor cells is controversial but may be considered in highly selected cases, when there are a limited number of casualties who received high doses of radiation (>8 Gy but clearly <12 Gy) and who are without serious burns or trauma. In a nuclear detonation, most casualties whose dose exceeds 6 to 8 Gy also may have significant blast and thermal injuries that preclude survival, regardless of treatment. Bone marrow transplantation (BMT) cannot salvage anyone who has received a whole-body dose of about 12 Gy, because serious radiation injury to the lungs and other vital organs would result in nonsurvivable conditions. The outcomes of patients undergoing BMT after radiation accidents have been poor. BMT would have no role in mass casualties, given the presence of current alternative therapies (such as cytokine therapy), the probability of combined injuries, uncertainties about radiation dose, and non-uniform exposure of radiation victims. The patient's physical environment often affords partial shielding, resulting in variability in the absorbed dose. Because the absorbed radiation dose is non-uniform, there may be unexpected reservoirs of viable hematopoietic stem cells that received a lower dose than the average whole-body dose. Both spared and radiation-resistant stem cells are capable of promoting hematologic reconstitution. This ability seems to be augmented with CSF therapy.

Treatment of infectious complications

Controlling infection during the critical neutropenic phase is a major factor for producing a successful outcome in patients who have absorbed radiation doses in the hematopoietic syndrome range [31–33]. Infections are a major cause of mortality in the irradiated host because of immunosuppressive effects that result from declining lymphohematopoietic elements secondary to radiation-induced bone marrow aplasia (reversible or irreversible). After wounds or burns have been débrided, topical antibiotics should be used, and the wound should be covered with nonadherent dressings. Life-threatening gram-negative bacterial infections are universal among neutropenic patients. The goal of antibiotic therapy is to suppress potentially pathogenic aerobic bacteria while preserving anaerobic bacteria, which act as a protective barrier against colonization by pathogenic bacteria. Prophylactic selective gut decontamination with oral fluoroquinolones (FQ) may be used electively in severely neutropenic patients. The management of established or suspected infection (neutropenic and febrile) in irradiated patients is similar to that used for febrile neutropenic patients undergoing chemotherapy. For those who have significant neutropenia (ANC < 500/µL), broad-spectrum prophylactic antimicrobials should be used, because the duration of neutropenia is likely to be prolonged. Treatment might include a FQ with streptococcal coverage (with penicillin or amoxicillin, if the streptococci are not inherently covered by the FQ), an oral antiviral agent such as acyclovir, and an oral antifungal agent such as fluconazole. Acyclovir is effective against herpesvirus, which has a high risk of reactivation during periods of immunosuppression. Fluconazole has been shown to reduce fungal infections and mortality in immunosuppressed patients undergoing allogeneic bone marrow transplantation. Other antifungals, such as voriconazole (oral or intravenous) or amphotericin B (intravenous), could be used for infections that do not respond to fluconazole, such as those from Aspergillus molds or resistant Candida species. Other antivirals, such as foscarnet, are useful for the treatment of acyclovir-resistant Herpes simplex and Cytomegalovirus infections. Ganciclovir also can be used for Cytomegalovirus infections, but blood counts must be monitored when using ganciclovir because of possible adverse effects of neutropenia and thrombocytopenia.

Antimicrobial agents should be continued until the treatment fails or the patient has a neutropenic fever or shows evidence of neutrophil recovery (ANC rising and > 500/µL). Any foci of infection that develop during the neutropenic period will require a full course of antibiotic therapy. For patients who have fever while receiving FQ, the FQ should be stopped.

Suspicion of the presence of FQ-resistant gram-negative bacteria, in particular *Pseudomonas aeruginosa*, calls for the urgent administration of parenteral therapy, because gram-negative infections may be rapidly fatal. Vancomycin should be added if a resistant gram-positive infection is suspected. The prevalence of life-threatening gram-positive bacterial infections varies greatly among hospitals, and therefore antimicrobial therapy should be matched against hospital susceptibility patterns. Infectious disease experts will be the center of the decision-making process regarding opportunistic, drug-resistant infections in patients who have altered immunity or burns.

The specific hematopoietic and antimicrobial treatment described is one idealized approach to the treatment of victims who have radiation doses in the hematopoietic syndrome range. Hematologists and infectious disease physicians would determine the actual treatment. A truly overwhelming mass-casualty situation would, to some degree, preclude the strict use of any idealized approach. For example, oral antimicrobials might be used primarily if inadequate staffing and hospital resources limited the capability for intravenous therapy, or weekly injections of a specific cytokine might be given instead of daily injections. Because some drug supplies would run short in a mass-casualty scenario, alternative available second-choice drugs could be used on the basis of ongoing expert guidance.

Treatment of cutaneous syndrome

Skin decontamination needs to be done early because reducing the time radioisotopes remain in direct contact with the skin lessens the severity of the radiation burn that develops later [5,16]. In contrast to thermal burns, which appear almost immediately, the development of radiation burns takes weeks to evolve fully. In certain circumstances a burn could be a combination of thermal and radiation burns.

The two main approaches to managing radiation skin injury are conservative and surgical treatment. Sometimes both approaches are necessary in managing cutaneous syndrome. Conservative treatment is the initial approach. Treatment should consist of gentle flushing, early excision, and débridement of potentially septic tissue. Steroid ointment should be used for relatively intact skin, a topical antibiotic with dressings for the blistering phase, and silver sulfadiazine cream with nonadherent dressings for the moist desquamation phase. Depending on the specific case, systemic antibiotics may be added. Decisions regarding surgical treatment may be impossible at an early stage, because it takes several weeks or more for the radiation burn to evolve fully. Once indications for surgery appear—radiation ulcers and localized necrosis without signs of regeneration, and severe, intractable pain—surgical intervention should not be delayed, because the patient's immune system may deteriorate further. The resection of tissues must be performed in a zone around the exposed skin that was not exposed or at least was only slightly exposed, and a whole block of injured dead tissue must be removed to provide an effective graft. The type of grafting should be decided for each individual case.

Therefore, the cutaneous syndrome can be managed as follows: conservative nonsurgical treatment initially, especially for superficial lesions; surgical excision for painful, deep, or necrotic ulcers, followed by wound covering (grafting); amputation for necrotic extremity. Cutaneous injuries in some individuals may be quite protracted and require the expertise of reconstructive surgeons and other specialists.

Nuclear terrorism

The goals of nuclear terrorism include (1) creating fear, social disruption, and widespread psychologic damage; (2) causing major lasting economic effects; (3) undermining authority and demonstrating the vulnerability of the targeted government; and (4) sending a political message to the targeted population [34,35].

After the detonation of a terrorist nuclear device, the Federal Bureau of Investigation (FBI) will be the lead federal agency for crisis management. The detonation site will be treated as a crime scene. The FBI will balance law-enforcement interests, including the prevention of further detonations, with public health concerns, including emergency medical treatment of casualties. Once the major security issues have been dealt with, the FBI will shift authority to the Department of Homeland Security (DHS). State and local authorities will also assume greater involvement with DHS oversight. Available medical emergency response should be integrated efficiently with the designated lead federal agency. Nuclear terrorist events have a range of possible scenarios. Medical planning requires flexible, incident-specific approaches that are proportional to the size and complexity of the incident.

Classes of radiologic and nuclear devices for terrorism

Simple radiologic device

A simple radiologic device consists of a nondispersible radioactive source that could be left in a highly populated area or a heavily used public place, such as a subway station, tourist site, or sports facility. In 1995, Chechen separatists left a cesium-137 source in a Moscow park and later notified a news service. There were no known injuries. Such devices have limited value to terrorists, because the radiation is confined, and hence they do not produce contamination problems. A knowledgeable terrorist would want to cause prolonged contamination that would instill fear in the public and have lasting psychologic, economic, and political effects.

Radiologic dispersal device such as a dirty bomb

A dirty bomb employs a conventional explosive to disperse radioactive materials. Detonated in a public place, the conventional explosive produces acute casualties, but significant radiation injuries are unlikely because of dispersal (dilution) of the limited radioactive material. The dispersed radioactive contamination would have lasting psychologic and economic effects, even without producing a single radiation casualty. Contamination of the local environment would typically involve a number of city blocks and might take months or longer to remove.

Reactor core damage

The probability of nuclear reactor sabotage is low because of high security, reactor safety systems, and sound construction of the reactors. Significant amounts of explosives would be required to breach the reactor core to cause a loss of coolant, resulting in a nuclear emergency. Security measures would prevent terrorists from bringing significant amounts of explosives inside the plant. It is not clear whether even a large commercial airplane crashing into a reactor could breach the coolant system. If serious reactor core damage occurred, and a radioactive plume was generated, radioactive iodine in the population downwind would be a significant problem, as would large-area contamination.

Improvised nuclear device

An improvised nuclear device (IND) might be developed by terrorists who had a high level of technical support. Such a device could be a modification of an existing nuclear bomb or could be fabricated in a completely improvised manner. Acquiring plutonium or highly enriched uranium would be extremely difficult, however. Success would hinge on obtaining enough material to form a supercritical mass to permit a chain reaction. In addition, the technology and triggering mechanism conditions must be met. If the stringent requirements were not met, the terrorist would end up with a device that would produce a partial nuclear yield or no yield at all. If there were no yield, the conventional explosive component of the device would detonate and blow the device apart, dispersing weapons-grade radioactive material such as plutonium and uranium. In that case, the IND would be a type of dirty bomb, because no actual nuclear detonation would have taken place. Next to an IND with full nuclear yield, however, an IND with a partial yield would produce the most casualties and contamination.

Nuclear weapon

Military weapons, such as those used at Hiroshima and Nagasaki, are designed to be detonated as a low-altitude air burst to maximize destructive power. Conversely, a terrorist nuclear weapon would probably be of a lower yield, and most likely would be a surface burst, so the destructive power would be reduced. A full-yield nuclear device is considered the least likely device to be used as a terrorist weapon because of high security and technical issues involved in detonation. Nevertheless, disaster planning must include this worst-case scenario.

A dirty bomb is the most likely choice for terrorists because it would be relatively easy to make and could be highly effective. All or nearly all casualties from a dirty bomb are likely to be the result of the conventional explosion. The conventional explosion could be as large as that in the Oklahoma City bombing. The explosives generate a pulse of heat that may vaporize or aerosolize some of the radioactive material and propel it across an area. Stolen solid radioactive material wrapped around a stick of dynamite would constitute a clumsy weapon capable primarily of scattering large chunks of the radioactive material over a limited area, making cleanup and recovery relatively easy. Nevertheless, there would have to be monitoring for localized highly radioactive shrapnel. A dirty bomb cannot produce overwhelming mass casualties from radiation. A nuclear weapon detonation would produce thousands of times more casualties, with widespread heavy contamination and fallout. The infrastructure would be severely affected by consequent physical damage and damage from its electromagnetic pulse, including the loss of electrical power and damage to transportation systems, evacuation routes such as bridges, and communications. These weapons would damage medical care facilities, and many health care workers would be among the casualties. None of these effects would result from the use of a dirty bomb (Table 10).

A dirty bomb could be preset to explode at a fixed location or delivered by a mobile system, probably by using a common vehicle, such as an automobile, truck, train, or airplane. Delivery by truck might be the most likely means, because a truck can carry more explosives than an automobile, and the use of a truck would avoid the security measures involved in boarding a train or entering an airport. A truck could be loaded and prepared in a private garage out of sight. To access potential sources of radioactive materials, terrorists probably would use someone with knowledge of the characteristics of the ideal radiation source used for terrorism. Such characteristics would include availability, high activity, and long half-life. The security for nuclear weapon sites and nuclear power plants is such that these areas probably will not receive serious consideration by terrorists. Plutonium-239 and highly enriched uranium therefore would be unlikely sources. Sources used in diagnostic nuclear medicine and in many research laboratories have weak activity and short half-lives and would make an ineffective dirty bomb.

Table 10
Effects of detonation of a dirty bomb and a nuclear weapon

Effect	Dirty bomb	Nuclear weapon
Major damage to infrastructure	No	Yes
Expected casualty range	10–1000	50,000–1,000,000
Range of significant contamination	A few city blocks	Hundreds of square miles (or more with fallout)

High-activity sources of certain isotopes such as cesium-l37, iridium-192, cobalt-60, radium-226, strontium-90, and americium-241 would be the target isotopes to be stolen from hospitals, laboratories, or industrial irradiators (Table 11). Terrorists are known to be interested in acquiring chemical warfare agents classified as persistent agents that remain effective for a prolonged time. Nuclear agents (radioisotopes) selected by a terrorist probably also would be persistent, meaning they would have decay properties (half-lives) of many years. Cesium-137 has a 30-year half-life and in the form of cesium chloride is a highly water-soluble powder that could be disseminated readily. Terrorists probably would choose an internationally known site with high symbolic value, preferably in a highly populated, major transportation center or prominent daily-use public site. Terrorists would want to create a scenario in which there would be mandatory evacuation, and millions of people might be prevented from using or entering the area for a significant period of time. An example of a site meeting all these criteria would be Times Square in New York City.

Medical lessons from major radiologic events at Chernobyl and Goiania

Two major accidents have provided valuable lessons in the medical management of radiation casualties [2]. The first was the 1986 accident at the nuclear power reactor in Chernobyl, Ukraine. This was the worst-case scenario of any possible nuclear power reactor incident [36,37]. Bypassing safety systems resulted in loss of reactor coolant, followed by two chemical explosions, fires, the meltdown of the reactor core in a reactor designed without a containment facility, and a delay in instituting community emergency procedures. The overall findings from the accident were the following:

- Cesium-137 was the radionuclide that contributed most to the total-body dose, both of the emergency workers and later of the general population.
- Iodine-131 contributed to thyroid dose in a significant number of the general population (especially children). Because of the lack of initial public health countermeasures, many children ingested milk

Table 11
Potential sources of radioactive materials for terrorism

Material	Source
Cesium-137	Industry, food irradiators, and medical therapy
Iridium-192	Industry and medical therapy
Cobalt-60	Industry, food irradiators, and medical therapy
Radium-226	Medical therapy
Strontium-90	Industrial heating devices
Americium-241	Exploratory oil drilling and density gauges
Iodine-131	Medical therapy and nuclear reactors
Plutonium-239	Nuclear weapons programs and reactors
Highly enriched uranium	Nuclear weapons programs

contaminated with iodine-131 and did not receive timely potassium iodide therapy.

- Approximately 116,000 persons living in a 30-km zone around the plant were evacuated; none was seen to have acute radiation effects during the evacuation period.
- Three hundred of the approximately 600 workers who were on site during the night of the accident were hospitalized within 2 days.
- Fifty-eight firemen and workers, unaware they had intense external contamination for a day or more, failed to shower or change clothes and later developed extensive cutaneous radiation burns that contributed to the death of 19 of them.
- Thirteen patients received bone marrow transplants, with subsequent poor results.
- Two workers who had severe combined injuries (trauma, thermal, and radiation) died soon after the initial explosion at the plant, primarily from the effects of the blast.
- One hundred thirty-four persons had eventually confirmed acute radiation syndrome, having received the following estimated doses: 0.8 to 2.1 Gy, 41 persons; 2.2 to 4.1 Gy, 50 persons; 4.2 to 6.4 Gy, 22 persons; 6.5 to 16 Gy, 21 persons [2,38].
- Twenty-eight of the 134 persons with acute radiation syndrome, primarily firemen, died within 60 days from radiation effects, with estimated doses: 0.8 to 2.1 Gy, no deaths; 2.2 to 4.1 Gy, 1 person (2%); 4.2 to 6.4 Gy, 7 persons (32%); 6.5 to 16 Gy, 20 persons (95%).
- When workers who were in the reactor area at the time of the accident were later decontaminated, the medical staff at the site wore protective clothing, used proper technique, and themselves received very low radiation doses (less than 0.01 Gy = 0.01 Sv = 1 rem).
- There was substantial regional radioactive contamination with short-lived iodine and long-lived cesium.
- Although some late effects (such as thyroid cancer in children) have been observed, most adults and children in the exposed population did not experience any effects attributable to radiation.

In addition to the acute effects, the long-term effects of the Chernobyl accident, such as thyroid cancer in children but not adults, have been well documented and support the Hiroshima data. As has been done in the mature Hiroshima studies, other long-term effects of Chernobyl currently are being quantified. A large cohort population is being followed that includes people living in the affected area at the time of the accident and the tens of thousands of cleanup workers who subsequently worked in the contaminated areas. Comprehensive outpatient medical checkups, including a battery of diagnostic tests, are being performed periodically on each patient. Hospital admissions are reserved for inpatient treatment. The work is being conducted at the Ukrainian Research Center for Radiation Medicine in Kiev.

Medical lessons learned from Chernobyl include the value of using the time to emesis during the first day and lymphocyte depression within the first 2 days for triage, the importance of monitoring initial responders for the radiation dose-rate environment in which they will work and for radioactive contamination they may subsequently receive, the importance of early decontamination for protection of the skin, the recognition of a life-threatening cutaneous syndrome, the need for early potassium iodide prophylaxis to protect the thyroid, the ability of medical personnel to limit their own exposure by using good technique in caring for highly contaminated patients, the failure of bone marrow transplantation, and the effectiveness of aggressive conventional treatment (such as antimicrobial therapy).

The Chernobyl reactor accident was not a terrorist event, but the aftermath is comparable, as a worst-case scenario, to that of severe reactor core damage caused by a terrorist using high explosives or crashing a large commercial airplane to breach the cooling system. Therefore, the medical and contamination management issues of the Chernobyl accident serve as lessons learned in planning for the worst-case scenario for this class of nuclear terrorism.

The second incident was the 1987 accident that occurred in Goiania, Brazil [39]. A mishandled 1375-curie cesium-137 radiation therapy source was stolen, and the shielding was breached. Intensely radioactive cesium chloride powder was spread by hand from person to person within the community. The accident went undetected for 16 days, until residents turned up at hospitals with unexplained symptoms (nausea and vomiting) and unexplained burns on the hands. The overall findings of the accident were the following:

- Cesium-137 was the only radionuclide involved.
- Approximately 125,000 persons eventually were surveyed for contamination.
- Two hundred forty-nine persons were contaminated.
- One hundred twenty persons were externally contaminated (primarily on the clothing or shoes).
- One hundred twenty-nine persons were both externally and internally contaminated.
- Forty-six persons received ferric ferrocyanide (Prussian blue) therapy for internal contamination with cesium-137.
- Twenty persons were hospitalized.
- Fourteen persons eventually had confirmed acute radiation syndrome.
- Eight persons received cytokine therapy (GM-CSF).
- Four persons died within 30 days of hospital admission from radiation effects.

Medical lessons learned from Goiania include the value of Prussian blue in reducing internal contamination with cesium-137 and undoubtedly reducing the number of deaths, the usefulness of cytogenetic dose estimates in selected cases, the value of cytokine therapy together with conventional treatment, and the difficulties with delayed treatment when early medical intervention is not possible. An additional lesson learned was the value of using designated sites (such as a soccer stadium) away from the hospital to deal with the tens of thousands of uninjured anxious persons demanding to be checked for contamination.

Prussian blue has a high affinity for cesium, whose metabolism follows an enterohepatic cycle. Ingested cesium is absorbed into the blood, extracted by the liver, secreted by the bile into the gut, reabsorbed again into the blood, and so forth. Prussian blue given orally traps cesium in the gut and thereby increases fecal excretion. The 46 Goiania patients who had cesium-137 internal contamination were treated with Prussian blue in daily divided doses of 3 to 20 g. Because of augmented fecal excretion, the average effective biologic half-life of cesium-137 was reduced from 39 to 16 days, with consequent reduction in radiation dose from the internal contamination.

The Goiania accident, if it had been intentional, would have been an example of terrorists' use of a simple radiologic device employing radioactive material left in a public place. If the source material had been attached to an explosive, it would have been classified as a dirty bomb. In that case, the blast could cause injuries and death, but there would have been no deaths from the radiation, for two reasons. First, the source would have been widely dispersed (diluted) rather than passed from person to person in an intensely concentrated form. Second, the explosion would have triggered an immediate medical response, in contrast to the weeks of delay that followed the Goiania accident. Once the radiation contamination was detected, any required therapy would have been initiated much sooner, including external decontamination, internal decontamination techniques such as Prussian blue and growth-factor (cytokine) therapy.

Planning for emergency medical care after a nuclear terrorist attack

Emergency medical care of injured, irradiated, and radioactively contaminated patients begins at the site of the incident and continues in a local hospital emergency room [40–42]. Transport of the severely injured to the hospital should not be delayed in cases of suspected or confirmed radiologic contamination. Lives will be lost if critically injured patients are held at the explosion site with delayed transport to the hospital because of exaggerated fears concerning contamination.

Site of the incident

The first responders to the site of an incident with enormous radioactive contamination—such as that resulting from the detonation of a nuclear device or an IND or from a serious nuclear reactor breach—may knowingly expose themselves to high levels of radiation to save lives. The maximum-dose guideline for first responders who are trying to rescue people who would otherwise die is 500 mSv (= 0.5 Sv = 50 rem = approximately

50 cGy). Any vomiting would be an indicator that an individual rescuer should be removed from the site. Initial emergency responders should have appropriate dose-rate meters, such as Geiger-Mueller (GM) counters, to evaluate the radioactive levels. Different locations within and around the incident site may have different radiation dose-rate levels: "cold zones" are those with less than 10 mR/hr, "warm zones" are those with 10 mR/hr to 10 R/hr, and "hot zones" are those with more than 10 R/hr. The time of exposure and the accumulated dose for these rescuers would be monitored continuously. It is highly unlikely that the dose would be at acutely harmful levels, especially if established protocols were followed. Amifostine is a "radioprotector" administered just before radiation treatment for some oncology patients. It cannot be administered orally, is effective for only a short time, and has risk of significant side effects of hypotension, nausea, and vomiting. For these reasons, amifostine is not recommended for emergency responders who must engage in physically demanding activities and must sometimes wear respirators. The National Council on Radiation Protection and Measurements currently is completing a report entitled *Preparing, Protecting and Equipping Emergency Responders for Nuclear and Radiological Terrorism*, which should be available later in 2006.

For the typical dirty bomb, there would not be enormous radioactive contamination, there would be no expected hot-zone levels anywhere around the incident site, and emergency responders would not receive symptomatic radiation doses. For example, following the dispersal of radiation after a dirty bomb detonation, assume the radiation levels are 40 mR/hr over an area of a few city blocks. A first responder who spends 5 hours working in that area receives a total accumulated exposure of 200 mR (200 mR = 0.2 R), which is roughly equivalent to 0.2 Gy or 0.2 Sv absorbed dose. This dose is roughly equal to the average annual dose all United States citizens receive from natural background radiation, is less than the additional annual dose (over natural background) a commercial airplane pilot receives from flying at high altitudes, and is only about half the dose received by a patient who has a diagnostic radiology chest or abdominal CT scan. It is critical that emergency responders and health care providers not be fearful of exposure to relatively low radiation levels. Emergency responders and hospital staff who do not have a clear understanding of the risks posed by radiation or of how to protect themselves may experience irrational fear resulting in absenteeism and dereliction of duty.

The following measures should be taken at the site of a radiologic incident in a mass casualty situation:

- Establish control and safe perimeters.
- Medically stabilize the injured and preferably perform initial decontamination. The presence of radiologic contamination must not interfere with rapid triage and removal of medically unstable trauma victims from the scene.

- Transport to the hospital injured patients needing medical care, including those who have no apparent injuries but who have nausea or vomiting or otherwise appear ill. Contaminated patients may be wrapped to minimize contamination of the ambulance.
- Transport uninjured persons who require further decontamination to a site other than the hospital by means other than an ambulance. Large numbers of contaminated, uninjured persons arriving at a hospital emergency department will threaten to disrupt care of the injured, divert personnel away from patients needing medical attention, and contaminate the emergency department. Decontamination of the uninjured should be performed at a site with extensive shower facilities (eg, school gymnasium, YMCA, indoor arena). Those who are ambulatory can shower themselves. When total-body showering is not possible, simply removing the outer layer of clothing and washing the hands, face, head, and exposed areas with wet washcloths or paper towels will provide a large measure of protection. The site should have supplies such as replacement clothing, surgical scrub suits and blankets, and individually bottled water. Nutrition could be provided by the Meals-Ready-to-Eat system widely used by the military or by an equivalent nonperishable, time-durable food supply that requires neither cooking nor refrigeration.

Prior notification to emergency department

Ideally, the radiation accident response plan will be activated at the same time that the rescuers begin their work at the site. If possible, the following information should be obtained from the bomb site before the arrival of victims at the hospital: the number and nature of the injuries, the estimated time of arrival of the patients, whether a radiologic survey has been performed at the bomb site, whether the patients have only been exposed to radiation or are radioactively contaminated, and which radioisotopes are involved. Often it will not be possible to get all this information before the patients arrive.

Radiation response team notification

Key health care professionals from the hospital staff or in the community should be notified, including radiation oncologists, radiation physicists, and nuclear medicine staff, together with emergency physicians, trauma surgeons, and medical support staff. Within a day or two of a major event, infectious disease and hematology experts would assume key roles. It is to be hoped that a priority list with telephone numbers already will have been established as part of the hospital's existing disaster plan. Additional staff who should be added to the on-site emergency department team and the on-call surgeons and trauma specialists would include

- Emergency department physicians
- Triage nurses

- Radiation safety officer and health physicist and associated staff with their GM counters
- Radiation oncologists and radiation physicist and associated staff with their GM counters
- Nuclear medicine technologists who can serve as radiation safety physics technicians with their GM counters
- Security personnel

The decontamination-treatment area

The decontamination-treatment area for those injured needs to be delineated and, if possible, established in an area away from the main flow of emergency department activity, near a separate emergency department entrance. It should be appropriate for both emergency medical care and decontamination, with access to water. Ideally, the floor should be covered and with taped-down nonskid plastic sheets (however, butcher's paper or other appropriate covering may be substituted). The covering should extend from the ambulance entrance to the decontamination area. The decontamination rooms should be emptied of any unnecessary supplies or equipment, and fixed equipment not in use should be covered to minimize possible contamination.

Equipment and supplies

Ideally, the emergency department will have a dedicated decontamination supply cabinet. If so, the case, the cabinet must be locked (with a quick-break lock), and the contents must be checked periodically for the presence of key items such as

- Radiation-detection devices, particularly a GM counter and film thermoluminescent dosimetry badges or pocket dosimeters; extra batteries
- Operating room attire for staff involved in patient treatment or decontamination
- Floor covering for treatment area; 2-inch-wide masking tape
- Radiologic sample-taking equipment
- Radiologic decontamination supplies
- Waste containers (barrels) for water and many hundreds of large plastic bags for decontamination waste and clothing
- Forceps to remove any metal fragments or shrapnel from patients and a means to place them in a shielded container or area away from the patients and staff. Radiation oncology or nuclear medicine staff may supply such shielded containers

Decontamination team dress

Caregivers should follow strict isolation-type procedures (universal precautions). Barrier clothing is worn, including cap, mask, eye protection, gown, gloves, and shoe covers. All seams and cuffs should be secured with masking tape. Ideally, a dosimeter should be worn at the collar level. A complete surgical scrub suit ideally would include a plastic apron or water-proof gown for use when washing contaminated patients and double gloves, with the inner gloves taped to the scrub suit, to prevent cross contamination, because glove changes may be necessary.

Hospital site: emergency department procedure

Ideally, emergency responders and medical personnel will monitor and perform initial decontamination of patients at the scene. Because decontamination at the scene sometimes will not be possible, evaluation of contamination levels and decontamination procedures must be part of hospital disaster plans. Military training for nuclear, biologic, and chemical (NBC) attack is now termed "chemical, biologic, radiologic, nuclear" (CBRN). Under military CBRN policy, decontamination of persons exposed to chemical and biologic agents takes place before admission to a deployed medical facility (such as a Combat Support Hospital), because of the potential risks from even small amounts of some chemical or biologic agents. Persons with radiologic contamination, however, pose no significant medical risk to health care personnel using proper decontamination techniques. In addition, unlike biologic and chemical contamination, the level of radiation contamination can be monitored easily by hand-held instruments such as the commercially available GM counter or the military RADIAC meter [17,43–46].

The patient's history is obtained, including the time of onset and severity of the symptoms following a radiologic incident. A complete blood cell count with differential should be performed several times on the first day, then daily as indicated. Emergency surgical procedures involve resuscitation (including intravenous fluids), control of hemorrhage, and early débridement of wounds to prevent sepsis. A portable radiograph machine should be brought to the emergency department. Security personnel should be present in the emergency room for several reasons, including control of access and physical protection of emergency caregivers. Remember that the terrorists themselves may be injured or irradiated and may be among those brought to the hospital. Casualties from an explosion caused by unexplained circumstances should raise the possibility that radioactive material is involved, and an appropriate radiologic survey should be done [47]. Definitive care follows emergency care and decontamination.

Contamination control at the hospital

Upon arrival of the patients, the combined decontamination-treatment area needs to be controlled strictly. Ideally, the ambulance crew and patient are met and monitored outside the emergency department. Access to the medical decontamination-treatment area is roped off and monitored by security and radiation safety personnel located in the clean zone at the edge of the control line. A control line is established at the entrance to the decontamination room to mark clearly the boundary between the clean zone and the dirty zone in which the patient receives medical stabilization plus decontamination. Radiation safety personnel check everyone (and all equipment) for contamination before allowing them to proceed from the dirty zone to the clean zone. Security personnel also help control access. Care is taken to minimize contamination as much as practicable upon leaving the room. Contamination can be minimized by unrolling a clean paper floor covering into the room, followed by a clean litter for patient transfer. Universal precautions are taken when removing patients from the dirty zone and discharging them home, admitting them to the hospital, or transferring them to the operating room for surgery. Performing surgery on a patient who has acceptable residual radiation contamination is no different from performing surgery on a patient who has diagnostic or therapeutic radioisotopes or a patient undergoing radiation oncology brachytherapy, such as a patient receiving a prostate radioactive seed implant. Lives will be lost if patients who require emergency surgery but who have some radioactive contamination are not transported to the operating room without delay. In the emergency department, hospital personnel also should be monitored for contamination before leaving the dirty zone area. Their barrier clothing should be removed, considered contaminated, and remain with the other waste. All contaminated waste is collected in barrels and plastic trash bags, and all waste stays in the dirty zone for later cleanup.

External decontamination techniques

A health physicist, medical radiation physicist, or radiation safety physics technician will help supervise and interpret contamination measurements and advise the medical staff on the contamination levels. In doing so, the physicist will answer questions and provide guidance and reassurance [48–51]. This supervision would include the evaluation and handling of any radioactive metal fragments (shrapnel) in patients. Without interfering with initial emergency care, specimens may be collected (if needed) by taking nasal swabs (individual swabs for each nostril) and wound swabs and by collecting urine and feces. Strongly positive nasal swabs may indicate inhalation of radioactive particles. As part of medical resuscitation, clothing should have been removed. Clothing should be placed in plastic trash bags and labeled with the patient's name. Evidence must be labeled and preserved both at the scene and at the hospital to provide for isotope analysis later or to assist law enforcement. For seriously injured victims, the skin is decontaminated in the emergency department to decrease the dose of radiation to the skin, decrease the risk of internal contamination, and limit contamination of medical personnel and the hospital.

A GM counter will guide external decontamination. Removing clothing alone can decrease external radioactive contamination by 90%. Washing with soap and lukewarm or room-temperature water is effective and removes another 90% of contamination (about 99% of the total is removed after both steps have been performed). Soap emulsifies and dissolves most contaminants. Wounds and body orifices usually are decontaminated first. Wounds should be rinsed with saline. To prevent cross-contamination, wounds and burns should be covered with waterproof dressings before the skin is decontaminated. Abrasions and lacerations usually are relatively easy to decontaminate. Stubborn contamination may be excised from lacerations. Puncture wounds, most often on the hands, are sometimes difficult because of poor access to the contaminants and difficulty in determining the degree and depth of contamination. Irrigation with standard water picks may be successful. Burns should be rinsed gently with water and cleared of debris. In patients whose burns cannot be completely decontaminated, most of the contamination will remain in the burn eschar when it sloughs. Some patients may have imbedded metal fragments (shrapnel). When metallic shrapnel is removed, it should be evaluated for radioactivity and either shielded or placed in a safe location. Potentially radioactive fragments should be handled with forceps, not with gloved hands. Contaminated wastewater can be released into sewers without restriction. For intact skin, a wet washcloth and basin (with or without a low-velocity, low-volume water spray) may be used to remove a significant amount of superficial contamination. Gentle brushing may help remove contamination from the skin, but care should be taken not to damage the skin, because some contamination could be absorbed through injured skin. Experience has shown that shampoo can be effective for skin decontamination in addition to soap, if soap alone is inadequate. On some occasions, povidone-iodine can be used as an antiseptic-germicide on the intact skin. It has the added benefit of nonradioactive iodine absorption through intact skin to block the thyroid partially when there is internal contamination from radioactive iodine-131. Hair can be decontaminated with any commercial shampoo. Cutting or clipping the hair, if appropriate, can remove contaminants, but cutting the eyebrows should be avoided, because they may not grow back. Fingernails and toenails should be checked and cut if necessary.

After each skin and wound decontamination, the patient should undergo another check of the contamination level with a GM counter to determine the effectiveness of the decontamination. The goal, which is not always reached, is to decontaminate down to two or three times the background radiation count rate. An alternate goal is to stop if subsequent decontamination attempts are ineffective at reducing the count rate by no more than 10% of the prior count rate.

Internal decontamination techniques

Once the patient has been stabilized medically and decontaminated externally, attention should focus on minimizing internal contamination. Samples may have been collected from the patient previously. Internal contamination is minimized by reducing absorption, increasing excretion, or both. Organ doses from internal contamination are rarely high enough to cause acute radiation syndrome. Therefore, clinical judgment needs to be exercised so that the steps undertaken to decontaminate internally do not carry greater risk than the contamination itself [52]. Techniques to be applied might include

- Oral/nasopharyngeal suction
- Stomach lavage
- Laxatives (cathartics) such as a biscodyl or phosphate soda enema or magnesium sulfate to decrease gastrointestinal transit time
- Antacids, particularly aluminum hydroxide, to reduce absorption
- Intravenous hydration and/or diuretics
- Emetics to induce vomiting in highly selected cases
- Therapeutic agents: blocking or diluting agents (such as potassium iodide for radioactive iodine); mobilizing agents (such as ammonium chloride for radiostrontium); chelating agents (such as calcium or zinc diethylenetriaminepentaacetic acid [DTPA]) for plutonium, americium, and curium; other specific agents such as ferric ferrocyanide (Prussian blue), which has proven useful for cesium and thallium internal contamination; and sodium bicarbonate, which is used to prevent kidney toxicity from uranium

The use of iodine-131 is not ideal for terrorists because it has a relatively short half-life of 8 days. The quantities in any one hospital would be limited, so that a dirty bomb made with iodine-131 stolen from a hospital would be widely dispersed (and diluted) and would not give a clinically significant dose. The primary threat from radioactive iodine would occur after breach of a nuclear reactor or a nuclear detonation. These events would release large amounts of airborne radioactive iodine over the surrounding area. Therapy is effective if administered early. Potassium iodide is a blocking agent that prevents uptake of radioiodine by the thyroid, which is the target organ, thus allowing the radioactive iodine to be excreted in the urine. The treatment is especially important for children and for pregnant or lactating women. One must remember that a dirty bomb does not create radioactive iodine. The recommended daily doses [53] of potassium iodide are 130 mg for adults (including pregnant or lactating women), 65 mg for children 4 to 17 years old, 32 mg for children 1 month to 3 years old, and 16 mg for infants less than 1 month old.

Detailed information on a range of radioisotopes is available from the National Council on Radiation Protection and Measurements in their Report No. 65, *Medical Management of Radiation Accidents* [52]. A major project to update this publication is currently in progress and should be completed later in 2006.

Psychologic effects of nuclear terrorism

Terrorists believe they can achieve their goals by inducing widespread fear among the general population. There no doubt will be a range of psychologic effects, both for victims and their loved ones and for those not directly affected, termed "the worried well." Among those at highest risk are pregnant women, mothers of young children, and children. In the case of a large radiologic incident, there would be a potential for people wanting to be checked for contamination to flood emergency rooms or to tie up communications. Reactions to this kind of psychologic trauma will produce symptoms ranging from insomnia and impaired concentration to social withdrawal, anxiety, and irrational and perhaps aggressive behavior. Some psychosomatic symptoms that mimic symptoms of high-radiation exposure (nausea, vomiting, rashes) may be seen in patients who were not exposed. Victims who have real physical injuries or who received a significant radiation dose also may experience acute psychologic effects, as might some of the emergency responders, hospital personnel, and cleanup workers. The appropriate response will be to establish firm command and control. In a mass-casualty situation, persons seeking medical care could be checked at roadblocks leading to medical facilities, with clearance required to proceed. The noninjured requiring only radiation checks and the noninjured who have only external contamination would be diverted to appropriate nonmedical facilities. These facilities will be staffed with decontamination teams or Red Cross personnel, plus a few medical personnel to evaluate and handle first aid or deal with medical problems that might arise. Extra police and security personnel will be needed at triage sites, at hospital sites, and along roads leading to hospitals. There must be no doubt as to who is in charge of the situation. A single, unified federal command must be maintained over numerous federal, state, and local entities. The public will respond to strong, effective leadership. People need to believe that decisions made are rational and, when possible, include their input. At the same time, there must be good communication and openness to restore trust by the general population after such a tragedy. Communication to affected populations on the verge of panic must provide reassurance that the leadership is concerned about radiation effects, will monitor radiation exposure levels, and will treat injuries found. Communication, when appropriate, should relate that the overall expectation is that most exposed persons will remain asymptomatic and will not suffer adverse health effects, based upon the experience gained from accidents such as Chernobyl and Goiania. The general public needs accurate information and reassurance when it is possible to give such reassurance. In the months that follow the radiation event, those who suffer from posttraumatic stress disorder should receive treatment.

Acknowledgments

David G. Jarrett, MD, FACEP, Director, Armed Forces Radiobiology Research Institute (AFRRI)

William E. Dickerson, MD, Colonel, USAF, Medical Corps, Director, Military Medical Operations, AFRRI

Daniel C. Garner, MD, Radiation Oncologist, Stonecrest Medical Center, Smyrna, TN (Formerly AFRRI, USAF Medical Corps [ret.])

Jamie K. Waselenko, MD, Hematologist-Oncologist, Sarah Cannon Research Institute, Nashville, TN (Formerly AFFRI, USA Medical Corps [ret.])

Albert L. Wiley, Jr., MD, PhD, Director, Radiation Emergency Assistance Center/Training Site (REAC/TS)

Patrick C. Lowry, MD, MPH, Medical Section Leader, REAC/TS

Mary Ellen Berger, PhD, REAC/TS Consultant

References

[1] Glasstone S, Dolan PJ. The effects of nuclear weapons. 3rd edition. Washington (DC): US Department of Defense; 1977.

[2] Gonzalez AJ. Lauriston S. Taylor lecture: radiation protection in the aftermath of a terrorist attack involving exposure to ionizing radition. Health Phys 2005;89(5):418–46.

[3] Stein M, Hirsberg A. Medical consequences of terrorism. Surg Clin North Am 1999;79(6): 1537–52.

[4] Emergency war surgery. 3rd revision. Washington (DC): US Department of Defense; 2004. Available at: www.bordeninstitute.army.mil/index.htm?/borden.htm. Accessed January 12, 2006.

[5] Ricks RC, Berger MC, Ohara FM. The medical basis for radiation accident preparedness: clinical care of victims. Boca Raton (FL): CRC Press; 2002.

[6] Ricks RC, Lushbaugh CC. Studies related to the radiosensitivity of man: based on retrospective evaluations of therapeutic and accidental total-body irradiation. Washington: ORAU/ NASA-CR 1444439; Oak Ridge Associated Universities, Oak Ridge, TN; 1975.

[7] Medical preparedness and response subgroup of the Department of Homeland Security: Working Group on Radiological Dispersal Sevices (RDD) and Preparedness. Dec 9, 2003 update. Available at: www1.va.gov/emshg/docs/Radiological_Medical_Countermeasures_ Indexed-Final.pdf.

[8] Diagnosis and treatment of radiation injuries. International Atomic Energy Agency (IAEA) safety reports series #2. Vienna (Austria): International Atomic Energy Agency; 1998.

[9] Goans RE, Waselenko JK. Medical management of radiological casualties. Health Phys 2005;89(5):505–12.

[10] Andrews GA. Medical management of accidental total-body irradiation. In: Hubner K, Fry S, editors. Medical basis for radiation accident preparedness. New York: Elsevier Press; 1980.

[11] Goans RE, Holloway EC, Berger ME, et al. Early dose assessment following severe radiation accidents. Health Phys 1997;72(4):513–8.

[12] Goans RE, Holloway EC, Berger ME, et al. Early dose assessment in criticality accidents. Health Phys 2001;81(4):446–9.

[13] Blakely WF, Salter CA, Prasanna P. Early-response biological dosimetry—recommended countermeasure enhancements for mass-casualty radiological incidents and terrorism. Health Phys 2005;89(5):494–504.

[14] Browne D, Weiss JF, MacVittie TJ, et al. Treatment of radiation injuries. New York: Plenum Press; 1990.

[15] Ricks R, Fry S. Medical basis for radiation accident preparedness II. New York: Elsevier Press; 1990.

[16] MacVittie TJ, Weiss JF, Browne D. Advances in treatment of radiation injuries. New York: Elsevier Press; 1996.

[17] Gusev IA, Guskova AK, Mettler FA. Medical management of radiation accidents. 2nd edition. Boca Raton (FL): CRC Press; 2001.
[18] Leikin JB, McFee RB, Walter FG, et al. A primer for nuclear terrorism. Dis Mon 2003;49: 479–516.
[19] Medical management of radiological casualties handbook. 2nd edition. Bethesda (MD): Armed Forces Radiobiological Research Insttitue; 2003. Available at: www.afrri. usuhs.mil.
[20] NATO handbook on medical aspects of NBC defensive operations. AMED P-6(B). Washington (DC): US Departments of the Army, Navy, and Air Force; 1995.
[21] Treatment of nuclear and radiological casualties. Army FM 4–20.83. Washington (DC): US Headquarters: Departments of the Army, Navy, Air Force and the Commandant Marine Corps; 2001.
[22] Bland SA. Mass casualty management for radiological and nuclear incidents. J R Army Med Corps 2004;150:27–34.
[23] Yehezkelli Y, Dushnitsky T, Hourvitz A. Radiation terrorism—the medical challenge. Isr Med Assoc J 2002;4(7):530–4.
[24] Flynn DF, Mihalakis I, Mauceri T, et al. Gastrointestinal syndrome after accidental overexposure during radiotherapy. In: Dubois A, editor. Radiation and the GI tract. Boca Raton (FL): CRC Press; 1994.
[25] Schull WJ. Effects of atomic radiation: a half-century of studies from Hiroshima and Nagasaki. New York: J. Wiley; 1996.
[26] Mettler FA, Voelz GL. Major radiation exposure—what to expect and how to respond. N Engl J Med 2002;346:1554–61.
[27] Waselenko J, MacVittie TJ, Blakely WF, et al. Medical management of acute radiation syndrome: recommendations of the strategic national stockpile radiation working group. Ann Intern Med 2004;140:1037–51.
[28] Koenig KL, Goans RE, Hatchett RJ, et al. Medical treatment of radiological casualties: current concepts. Ann Emerg Med 2005;45:643–52.
[29] Jarret DG, Sedlak RG, Dickerson WE. Current status of treatment of radiation injury in the United States. In: Proceedings of the Human Factors and Medicine (HFM) Panel Research Task Group (RTG) 099 meeting, Radiation Bioeffects and Countermeasures. Bethesda, MD, June 21–23, 2005. Available at: www.afrri.usuhs.mil.
[30] Dainak N, Waselenko JK, Armitage JO, et al. The hematologist and radiation casualties. Hematology 2003;473–96.
[31] Pizzo PA. Fever in immunocompromised patients. N Engl J Med 1999;341(12):893–9.
[32] Hamza NS, Ghannoum MA. Choices aplenty: antifungal prophylaxis in hematopoietic skin cell transplant recipients. Bone Marrow Transpl 2004;34:377–89.
[33] Dalal S, Zhukovsky D. Pathophysiology and management of fever. J Support Oncol 2006;4: 9–16.
[34] Management of terrorist events involving radioactive material. NCRP report #138. Betheseda (MD): National Council on Radiation Protection and Measurement; 2001.
[35] Levi MA, Kelly HC. Weapons of mass disruption. Sci Am 2002;287(5):76–81.
[36] Summary report on the post-accident review meeting in the Chernobyl accident. Vienna (Austria): International Atomic Energy Agency; 1986.
[37] Baranov A, Gale P, Guskova A, et al. Bone marrow transplantation after the Chernobyl nuclear accident. N Engl J Med 1989;321:205–12.
[38] Savkin MN, Ilyin LA, Guskova AK. First measures applied immediately after Chernobyl accident. Proceedings from the World Health Organization (WHO, Geneva, Switzerland) Radiation Emergency Preparedness and Assistance Network (REMPLAN) Meeting. Kiev, Ukraine, April 2006.
[39] The radiological accident in Goiania. Vienna (Austria): International Atomic Energy Agency; 1988.

[40] Berger ME, Leonard RB, Ricks RC, et al. Hospital triage in the first 24 hours after a nuclear or radiological disaster. Radiation Emergency Assistance Center/Training Site (REAC/TS) 2004 Update. Available at: www.orau.gov/reacts/triage.pdf.

[41] Turai I, Katalin V, Gunalp B, et al. Medical response to radiation incidents and radionuclear threats. BMJ 2004;328:568–72.

[42] Mettler FA Jr. Medical resources and requirements for responding to radiological terrorism. Health Phys 2005;89(5):488–93.

[43] Kilpatrick J. Nuclear attacks. RN 2002;65(5):46–51.

[44] Willis D, Coleman E. The dirty bomb: management of victims of radiological weapons. Medsurg Nurs 2003;12(6):397–401.

[45] Hogan DE, Meadows SM, Kellison T. Nuclear and radiological emergencies. J Okla State Med Assoc 2003;96(10):499–503.

[46] McFee DO, Leikin JB. Radiation terrorism. JEMS 2005:78–96.

[47] Koenig KL, Hatchett RJ, Mettler FA, et al. Use high awareness to screen emergency department patients for radiation exposure. Ann Emerg Med 2006;47(1):120–1.

[48] Miller K, Erdman M. Health physics considerations in medical radiation emergencies. Health Phys 2004;87(Suppl 1):S19–24.

[49] Smith JM. Hospital management of mass radiological casualties: reassessing exposures from contaminated victims of an exploded radiological dispersal device. Health Phys 2005;89(5): 513–20.

[50] Miller K, Groff L, Erdman M, et al. Lessons learned in preparing to receive large numbers of contaminated individuals. Health Phys 2005;89(Suppl 2):S42–7.

[51] Ring JP. Radiation risks and dirty bombs. Health Phys 2005;86(Suppl 1):S42–7.

[52] Management of persons accidentally contaminated with radionuclides. NCRP Report #65. Washington (DC): National Council on Radiation Protection and Measurement; 1980.

[53] Balk SK and the American Academy of Pediatrics Committee on Environmental Health. Policy statement on radiation disasters and children. Pediatrics 2003;111(6):1455–64.

SURGICAL
CLINICS OF
NORTH AMERICA

ELSEVIER
SAUNDERS

Surg Clin N Am 86 (2006) 637–647

Chemical Threats

Donald E. Fry, MD*

*Department of Surgery, MSC10 5610, 1 University of New Mexico,
Albuquerque, NM 87131, USA*

The use of chemical agents as military weapons has been recognized for many centuries but reached the most feared and publicized level during World War I. Considerable political effort has been exercised in the twentieth century to restrict military strategies with chemicals. However, considerable concern currently exists that chemical weapons may be used as agents in civilian terrorism. The distribution of acetaminophen tablets contaminated with potassium cyanide [1] and the release of sarin in the Tokyo subway system [2–4] show that larger-scale deployment of chemical agents can be a reality. This reality makes it necessary for civilian disaster-planning strategies to incorporate an understanding of chemical agents, their effects, and the necessary treatment.

Cyanide

Cyanide is an easily produced chemical that can be manufactured as a vapor or a sodium or potassium salt. The vapor can be inhaled with rapid absorption and physiologic effects, and transcutaneous absorption can occur with cutaneous contact. The vapors may either be hydrogen cyanide, which has a bitter almond odor, or cyanogen chloride, which has a pungent biting odor. The salt preparations could be used for contamination of food or water.

Cyanide ion is rapidly distributed by the circulation and binds to iron within the oxidative phosphorylation process of the mitochondria to produce its physiologic effect. The binding of the cyanide ion to cytochrome A_3 results in inhibition of electron transport and the cessation of oxidative energy production within the cell [5]. Although binding to the iron moiety in the mitochondria is not irreversible, a critical level of exposure results in

---

* Michael Pine & Associates, 5020 South Lake Shore Drive, Suite 304N, Chicago, IL 60615.

E-mail address: dfry@mpine-inc.com

death if an effective antidote is not promptly administered. Oxygen is abundant in the cell but cannot be used for oxidative purposes.

The diagnosis of cyanide poisoning requires a higher index of suspicion among casualties where exposure to the vapor may have occurred. Vapor exposure will occur in confined spaces and not outside because rapid dispersal negates the toxic effects. Exposures that are not quickly lethal result in acute fatigue, dyspnea, nausea, vomiting, headache, and confusion (Table 1) [6]. Acutely poisoned individuals will have a red appearance, reflecting 100% hemoglobin saturation with oxygen. Metabolic acidosis will be present. Severe exposure results in rapid progression to seizures, coma, apnea, and cardiac arrest.

The opportunity for therapeutic intervention is very brief. Individuals must undergo rapid intravenous administration of sodium nitrite and sodium thiosulfate [7]. The sodium nitrite is given as 10 mL of the standard 30-mg/mL solution over 5 to 15 minutes. This aggregate dose of 300 mg of sodium nitrite should convert approximately 20% of the patient's hemoglobin to methemoglobin. The ferric ion of methemoglobin has a greater affinity for the cyanide anion than does the ferrous ion in the cytochrome pathway of oxidative phosphorylation. In severe cases a second 5 mL of the standard sodium nitrite solution is given, but excessive methemoglobin formation must be avoided. Blood pressure and vital signs are carefully monitored during the sodium nitrite administration. The sodium nitrite is then followed by the intravenous administration of 50 mL of a 25-mg/mL (12.5 g) solution of sodium thiosulfate. The thiosulfate reacts with the cyanmethemoglobin complex, resulting in thiocyanite and sulfite salts that are eliminated in the urine [8]. In severe cases, 50% of the thiosulfate dose may be administered as a second dose. The combined sodium nitrite and sodium thiosulfate preparation is available as the Lilly Cyanide Antidote Kit (Eli Lilly, Indianapolis, Indiana).

Table 1
Organ-specific observations seen in patients poisoned with cyanide

Organ system	Clinical finding
Eye	Mydriasis
	Blurred vision
Cardiac	Arrhythmias
	Reduced force of contraction
Vascular	Increased blood pressure
Pulmonary	Tachypnea
	Deep breathing pattern
Gastrointestinal	Vomiting
	Defecation
Urinary tract	Incontinence
Metabolic	Metabolic acidosis
Central nervous system	Coma
	Seizure activity

Alternative antidotes to sodium nitrite and sodium thiosulfate have been used. Dicobalt edetate, the cobalt salt of ethylenediaminetetraacetic acid [9], directly binds the cyanide ion. It is available in Europe but not in the United States. However, it has been associated with angina and ventricular arrhythmias. Hydroxocobalamin (vitamin B_{12a}) is another agent that directly binds the cyanide ion [10]. It is potentially useful in patients who have anemia where significant methemoglobinemia may not be tolerated with sodium nitrite, but is a very expensive therapy.

Immediate administration of the antidote is critical, but patient decontamination is also necessary. Vapor in the clothing and on the skin subject the patient to ongoing absorption of the chemical. Vapor-contaminated clothing is also a potential risk for health personnel. Skin decontamination using soap and water is desirable, but all clothing should first be removed for complete decontamination. If oral ingestion is suspected, gavage and charcoal administration may prevent further absorption, but health care workers must be careful to avoid an aspiration event. Ventilation and cardiac support may be necessary, and monitoring blood gas for metabolic acidosis will show the effectiveness of therapy [11].

Nerve agents

Nerve agents are organophosphates and are commonly used as insecticides [12]. The five agents developed as chemical weapons include sarin, tabun, soman, GF, and VX (GF and VX have no common names). Although chemically these compounds have unique properties and chemical structures, they all bind to cholinesterase enzymes in general and to acetylcholinesterase specifically [13]. They are all liquids at room temperature and generally have been applied in vapor form when used as chemical weapons.

The cholinergic nervous system must be understood to appreciate the toxic mechanism of action of nerve agents. Acetylcholine is the neurotransmitter for the preganglionic nerves of the autonomic nervous system, the postganglionic nerves of the parasympathetic nervous system, and the neurons to skeletal muscle. Postganglionic parasympathetic nerves are muscarinic sites and include salivary glands, smooth muscle of the respiratory and gastrointestinal tracts, and the cranial nerves. Skeletal muscle and the autonomic ganglia are nicotinic sites.

The neuron's propagated action potential arriving at the presynaptic area causes axonal vesicles to release presynthesized acetylcholine. The neurotransmitter is released into the synaptic space where diffusion causes acetylcholine to bind to specific binding sites on the postsynaptic membrane. Binding results in depolarization and continued propagation of the nerve impulse. In nicotinic sites, the postsynaptic transmission causes skeletal muscle contraction. In muscarinic sites, the transmitted impulse causes glandular secretions. The released acetylcholine that transmits the impulse across the synapse is then hydrolyzed by the enzyme acetylcholinesterase.

Enzymatic degradation of acetylcholine is necessary so that each release of the neurotransmitter has only a single postsynaptic response and the post-synaptic site responds to the next discrete signal.

The acetylcholinesterase activity that regulates synaptic transmission of the cholinergic nervous system is tissue-bound. Circulating cholinesterase enzyme can be found free in the plasma and within red blood cells (RBCs). A physiologic role for these circulating cholinesterases have not been defined, but these blood cholinesterases may play a protective role or serve as a buffer for the tissue-bound enzyme. Transcutaneous absorption or inhalation of vapor results in dissemination of the organophosphate chemical, resulting in the dramatic loss of cholinesterase activity from RBCs before any systemic symptoms are identified. This buffering effect of circulating cholinesterase activity seems to be more significant with RBCs than with the free plasma enzyme. The plasma enzyme is produced by the liver and requires 50 days for recovery after depletion. RBC cholinesterase requires bone marrow to produce new RBCs and 120 days for complete replacement of depleted activity.

Nerve agents are very potent inhibitors of acetylcholinesterase. They inhibit the enzyme by binding it in an efficient and irreversible manner that completely neutralizes enzyme activity. Consequently, a rapidly increasing concentration of neurotransmitter accumulates in the synaptic space. This accumulation results in sustained and unrelenting cholinergic stimulation that causes a serious array of pathophysiologic consequences.

Certain signs and symptoms reflect the cholinergic crisis (Table 2) [14]. Cardiac response may be either tachycardia or bradycardia even though the hypertension from increased vascular resistance would seemingly predict a slow heart rate from increased afterload. Extremity weakness followed by fasciculations and flaccid paralysis are characteristic with large exposures. Large exposure events result in unconsciousness, apnea, and seizure activity. Sweating, rhinorrhea, and salivation rapidly evolve, and miosis, ocular pain, and blurred vision occur. Bronchospasm with wheezing; bronchorrhea; and chest tightness develop rapidly after the vapor is inhaled. Cramping abdominal pain, nausea, vomiting, and diarrhea are symptoms affecting the gastrointestinal tract [15].

The rapidity of onset and severity of symptoms from nerve agents depend on the total dose of exposure. Inhalation of the vapor results in rapid uptake of large amounts of the organophosphate. Although absorption of the exposure dose can occur through intact skin, this is usually less efficient compared with absorption through the lung. Because nerve agents are vapors, condensation can occur on the skin and within the clothing, which can result in sustained uptake of the chemical if not recognized and managed. Exposure to nerve agents shares some common features with cyanide poisoning and botulinum toxin, and the clinical syndrome associated with each requires differentiation (Table 3).

After exposure to a nerve agent, treatment of the casualty begins with decontamination. The individual should be rapidly removed from the exposure

Table 2
Effects of nerve agents on exposed individuals

Organ system	Pathophysiologic effects
Nicotinic effects	
Cardiac	Tachycardia or bradycardia
	Acute arrhythmias
	Atrial-ventricular heart block
Vascular	Hypertension
Muscular	Weakness, flaccid paralysis
	Fasciculations
Muscarinic effects	
Skin	Sweating
Nose	Rhinorrhea
Mouth	Salivation
Eye	Miosis
	Ocular pain
	Conjunctival injection
Lungs	Bronchospasm, wheezing
	Bronchorrhea
	Shortness of breath
Gastrointestinal tract	Cramping abdominal pain
	Nausea and vomiting
	Diarrhea
Central nervous system	Coma
	Apnea
	Seizures

environment and all clothing removed because this is the most effective initial form of decontamination. Because the nerve agent can be absorbed transdermally, recovery personnel must be appropriately protected, and removed clothing should be placed in sealed bags or containers for subsequent evaluation and incineration. Skin decontamination is performed using tepid water. Hot water may cause cutaneous vasodilation and increased uptake of the chemical and has no advantage over a room-temperature rinse.

Decontamination should ideally be performed before the casualty arrives at the hospital. However, incidents involving many casualties, such as the

Table 3
Comparison and contrast of botulinum toxin, nerve agents- (eg, sarin), and cyanide poisoning

Comparisons	Cyanide	Botulinum toxin	Nerve agent
Physical property	Gas (almonds)	Fine powder	Vapor (odorless)
Mechanism of action	Inhibits oxidative phosphorylation	Inhibition of acetylcholine release	Inhibition of cholinesterase
Eye effects	Pupil dilation	Pupil dilation	Miosis
Mouth/throat	No changes	Salivation/dysphagia	Salivation/dysphagia
Chest	No changes	Congestion	Bronchospasm
Muscles	Weakness, coma	Fasciculations and paralysis	Flaccid paralysis
Neurologic	Seizures	No seizures	Seizures

one in the Tokyo subway system, cause logistical problems for at-the-scene decontamination. Furthermore, casualties will likely be transported to the hospital by private transportation and will not be decontaminated before arrival. Designated facilities should be identified in the community disaster plan for victims of biologic and chemical terrorism so that trategies for hospital-based decontamination can be executed.

Current definitive treatment of nerve agent casualties is with a combination of atropine and pralidoxime chloride to manage the cholinergic crisis [12,16]. Atropine competes with the accumulated acetylcholine in the synaptic space for the receptor site and diminishes the cholinergic effects. The amount of atropine administered must be adjusted or titrated to the severity of exposure. An initial dose of 2 mg of atropine is administered intravenously or intramuscularly. The military has used intramuscular injection of the atropine and pralidoxime in premade kits for self-administration on the battlefield, and this route may be considered in a mass exposure situation. Physiologic effects of the treatment are best achieved through intravenous delivery. The 2-mg dose is repeated every 10 to 15 minutes until hypersecretion and shortness of breath resolve. A 6-mg initial dose has been recommended for casualties who are unconscious at presentation. A dose of atropine has physiologic effects for about 4 to 6 hours, so redosing may be necessary. The patient's response determines whether repeated doses are necessary.

Pralidoxime chloride is from the oxime group of drugs and is the only oxime approved by the Food and Drug Administration for the treatment of nerve agent exposure. The oxime drugs dissociate the bound nerve agent from the cholinesterase and regenerate enzyme activity. The oxime–organophosphate complex is then excreted in the urine. The dose of pralidoxime is 15 to 25 mg/kg and is also given either intravenously or intramuscularly. Intravenous administration should occur over 20 to 30 minutes. The atropine and pralidoxime should be given simultaneously. The effects of the pralidoxime are principally for the paralysis (nicotinic effects), whereas atropine therapy is most useful in managing the hypersecretory symptoms (muscarinic effects).

Timing in administering pralidoxime is very important. The complex formed between the organophosphate and the cholinesterase enzyme undergoes an aging process; that is, the capacity to dissociate the organophosphate from the enzyme gradually diminishes depending on the nerve agent. For sarin, an estimated 50% of the bound organophosphate ages by 5 hours and cannot be regenerated [17]. Nevertheless, any regenerated cholinesterase activity is beneficial and treatment should not be avoided because of a delay. Some spontaneous regeneration of cholinesterase activity occurs from synthesis of new enzyme.

Supportive care of the nerve agent casualty is also important. Ventilation support to maintain oxygenation is commonly necessary and some volume resuscitation may be required. Support of airway, breathing, and circulation allows full resynthesis of the acetylcholinesterase. Administration of diazepam, which is used to manage seizures, has been recommended for sedation and anticonvulsive effects in exposed casualties even before the onset of seizure activity.

Lung toxicants

Lung toxicants are the general class of gases that are toxic to the alveolar–capillary membrane of the human lung when inhaled [18]. The toxic inhalation results in a severe inflammatory response that leads to pulmonary edema, reduced pulmonary compliance, and altered gas exchange. Hydrolysis of the inhaled gas produces hydrochloric acid that may mediate some of the severe local toxicity to pulmonary tissue. Death is caused by fulminate respiratory failure, hypoxemia, and noncardiac pulmonary edema. Chlorine gas was the first lung toxicant used as a weapon in World War I, but was replaced later in the war by phosgene gas, which is currently the agent of greatest concern.

Phosgene is chemically carbonic dichloride ($COCl_2$), a synthetic chemical that does not occur naturally in our environment [19]. It is produced and used commercially to manufacture plastics and pesticides, is a gas at room temperature, and has a pungent and offensive odor at high concentrations, although at lower concentrations smells of newly mowed hay or freshly cut corn. This gas is heavier than air and would settle into low-lying areas.

Phosgene would be used as a gas for delivery in a terrorism situation. Some condensation occurs at temperatures less than 47°F and it may cause skin or direct eye irritation, but pulmonary contact with the gas is the source of injury. It could be swallowed as a contaminant in food or water, but toxicity through the alimentary tract is unknown.

Symptoms usually occur within 30 minutes after inhalation [20]. Burning of the throat and eyes, lacrimation, and blurred vision are followed shortly by cough, shortness of breath, and bronchospasm. Nausea and vomiting may follow. Depending on the degree of exposure, extreme cases may have rapid-onset pulmonary edema within 2 hours. Phosgene generally shows a dose–effect relationship, with large exposures associated with more severe lung injury.

Paradoxically, some individuals may undergo significant exposure but experience only minimal symptoms initially. However, at 48 hours the individual may experience rapid onset of potentially life-threatening pulmonary edema. The delay in onset of the typical lung failure indicates that patients who experience suspected or proven exposure must be observed for 48-hours before discharge.

Managing the exposed person begins with decontamination. Clothing is removed and placed in sealed containers to avoid secondary exposures of health care personnel. Surfaces are decontaminated with soap and water. Local irrigation for eye exposure may be necessary.

Care is supportive for casualties exposed to phosgene [21]. No specific antidote or neutralizing agent is currently recognized. Care for the disease becomes the management of severe pulmonary chemical inflammation. Ventilatory support is usually required to maintain oxygenation, and volume resuscitation and cardiac support may be necessary. Predisposing lung disease or tobacco use is a risk factor for a poor outcome. Steroids are not considered helpful. Long-term ventilator support will commonly be needed, and early tracheostomy is advisable for patients who have clearly sustained severe exposure. Systemic absorption of phosgene is not considered a hazard and complications of system toxicity are generally not considered a problem.

Secondary ventilator-associated pneumonia is a major concern in patients who have a severely injured lung and are undergoing long-term ventilator management. Pressure-controlled (<30 mm Hg) and appropriate tidal volume (<6–7 mL/kg) strategies are used to avoid barotrauma. Positive end-expiratory pressure will probably be needed. Preventive antibiotics are not indicated and will only result in microbial selection and the emergence of resistant nosocomial pathogens.

The long-term consequences of phosgene exposure are likely related to the severity of the initial event. Experts believe that most patients will experience a full recovery, but some degree of lung fibrosis and pulmonary restriction can be anticipated in severe cases.

Vesicants

The vesicant group of chemicals consists of agents that cause severe blistering on contact with human skin. Vesicants disable the target and only infrequently cause death. Incapacitation and anguish are the objectives. The psychologic consequences of the vesicant compounds are significant. A large civilian attack would saturate the health care infrastructure with large numbers of casualties requiring extensive care.

Sulfur mustard was the vesicant used as a chemical weapon in World War I [22]. It is a yellow, oily liquid that is aerosolized when used as a weapon. It is easily manufactured and numerous countries have accumulated stockpiles of this agent.

Topical exposure to sulfur mustard results in blistering and sloughing of the epidermal layers of the skin from 2 to 12 hours after contact, depending on the exposure dose. Sulfur mustard is an alkylating agent, but no consensus exists as to how it actually works [23]. One theory is that the agent directly damages cellular DNA, which then activates a repair enzyme system that depletes nicotine adenine dinucleotide (NAD+) within the cell. The NAD+ depletion causes stimulation of the hexose monophosphate shunt and activation of cellular proteases [24,25]. Cellular proteases are indicted as responsible for separation of the epidermal cells from the basement membrane. An alternative theory about sulfur mustard action is that it depletes the cell of glutathione, which causes the loss of protection against reactive oxygen intermediates that then leads to lipid peroxidation of cellular membranes and cell death [26]. The inability to satisfactorily explain the mechanism of action of sulfur mustard has made development of an antidote difficult. Regardless of mechanism, topical contact with human skin causes a response that is analogous to a second-degree scald wound, toxic epidermal necrolysis, or Stevens-Johnson syndrome.

Symptoms after skin exposure begin with cutaneous erythema and itching, which lead to large blisters that rupture and produce a weeping surface with shaggy sloughing skin. Pain from the wounds is analogous to second-degree burns. Eye contact from the sulfur mustard vapor results in pain, swelling, and tearing. Photophobia and temporary blindness may follow. Unusually large exposures can lead to permanent corneal damage. Inhalation may result in rhinorrhea, dysphonia, epistaxis, cough, and dyspnea. Respiratory distress may be seen with severe inhalational injury. Nausea, vomiting, diarrhea, and abdominal pain may accompany significant gastrointestinal ingestion. Sulfur mustard exposure has overall mortality rates of 2% to 5%.

Systemic uptake of sulfur mustard through the skin, lung, or gastrointestinal tract can lead to hematopoietic, immunologic, and central nervous system effects. Monitoring white blood cells and platelets is appropriate after an exposure event. In severe cases, vigilance for increased susceptibility to infection is appropriate.

Management requires decontamination and wound management. The exposed individual should be removed from the exposure environment because the vapor lingers in the environment where it was released. In a suspected terrorist incident involving a vesicant, the health personnel who are evacuating casualties must have appropriate personal protective equipment to avoid exposure to the agent. Casualties' clothing is removed and surface decontamination using soap and water to remove the agent that has not yet bound to tissues is performed without scrubbing so that systemic uptake of the sulfur mustard can be avoided. Skin creases in the groin, buttocks, and axilla should be particularly cleansed because condensed vapor in these areas causes unusually deep wounds, and eyes must be irrigated [27]. Severe cases of inhalation may require intubation and ventilator support. Steroids do not help alter the tissue injury. Wound care is the same as with scald burns, which includes debridement and treatment with topical antimicrobial agents. Systemic preventive antibiotics are inappropriate.

Lewisite is another arsenical chemical that was developed as a potential vesicant for military application [28], although it has not yet been used. It is a more potent vesicant than sulfur mustard and is also a liquid at room temperature and dispersed as a vapor. It does not have immunosuppressive effects. Management of lewisite exposure follows the same guidelines as sulfur mustard exposure.

Other agents

Riot control agents and other incapacitating agents have been developed by the military to temporarily incapacitate individuals without causing permanent injury. These are called *tear gas* but in reality are aerosolized solids. Other incapacitating agents that have been evaluated include cannabinoids, indoles (eg, lysergic acid diethylamide [LSD]), and various anticholinergics. These agents are only identified for completeness, because temporary incapacitation without major injury or death does not give theses agents much approval for terrorist activity.

Summary

Chemical agents have been developed as military weapons during the past century. Some have now been used for civilian terrorist threats. Dispersal of vapors or gases seems to be the strategy most likely to be used for chemical weapons. Incidents occurring in auditoriums or arenas where wind and climate conditions would not affect delivery of the vaporized agent are the most likely scenario. Because chemicals, biologics, or radioactive contamination may be added to conventional explosive devices, those who care for traumatic injury must be sensitive to the possibility of exposure, even though it may not be readily apparent, when managing injured patients. Cyanide salts remain a potential threat for contamination of food, water, and even medications. A working knowledge and understanding of the potential chemical agents is now a requirement for surgeons and emergency health personnel.

References

[1] Beck M, Monroe S. The Tylenol scare: the death of seven people who took the drug triggers a nationwide alert-and a hunt for a madman. Newsweek 1982;100:32–6.
[2] Okumura T, Suzuki K, Fukuda A, et al. The Tokyo subway sarin attack: disaster management, part 1: community emergency response. Acad Emerg Med 1998;5:613–7.
[3] Okumura T, Suzuki K, Fukuda A, et al. The Tokyo subway sarin attack: disaster management, part 2: hospital response. Acad Emerg Med 1998;5:618–24.
[4] Okumura T, Suzuki K, Fukuda A, et al. The Tokyo subway sarin attack: disaster management, part 3: national and international responses. Acad Emerg Med 1998;5:625–8.
[5] Baskin SI, Brewer TG. Cyanide poisoning. In: Zajtchuk R, Bellamy RF, editors. Textbook of military medicine: medical aspects of chemical and biological warfare. Washington (DC): US Department of the Army; 1997. p. 271–86.
[6] Hall AH, Rumack BH. Clinical toxicity of cyanide. Ann Emerg Med 1986;15:1067–74.
[7] Chen KK, Rose CL. Nitrite and thiosulfate therapy in cyanide poisoning. JAMA 1952;149: 113–9.
[8] Marrs TC. Antidotal treatment of acute cyanide poisoning. Adverse Drug React Acute Poisoning Rev 1988;7:179–206.
[9] Evans CL. Cobalt compounds as antidotes for hydrocyanic acid. Br J Pharmacol 1964;23: 455–75.
[10] Sauer SW, Keim ME. Hydroxocobalamin: improved public health readiness for cyanide disasters. Ann Emerg Med 2001;37:635–41.

[11] Baud FJ, Borron SW, Megarbane B, et al. Value of lactic acidosis in the assessment of the severity of acute cyanide poisoning. Crit Care Med 2002;30:2044–50.

[12] Sidell FR. Nerve agents. In: Zajtchuk R, Bellamy RF, editors. Textbook of military medicine: medical aspects of chemical and biological warfare. Washington (DC): US Department of the Army; 1997. p. 129–79.

[13] Volans AP. Sarin: guidelines on the management of victims of a nerve gas attack. J Accid Emerg Med 1996;13:431–2.

[14] Lee EC. Clinical manifestations of sarin nerve gas exposure. JAMA 2003;290:659–62.

[15] Taylor P. Anticholinesterase agents. In: Hardman JG, Limbird LE, Gilman AG, editors. Goodman and Gilman's the pharmacological basis of therapeutics. 9th edition. New York: McGraw-Hill; 1996. p. 161–70.

[16] Yokoyama K, Yamada A, Mimura N. Clinical profiles of patients with sarin poisoning after the Tokyo subway attack. Am J Med 1996;100:586.

[17] Karczmar AG. Acute and long lasting central actions of organophosphorus agents. Fundam Appl Toxicol 1984;4:S1–17.

[18] Diller WF. Pathogenesis of phosgene poisoning. Toxicol Ind Health 1985;1:7–15.

[19] Borak J, Diller WF. Phosgene exposure: mechanisms of injury and treatment strategies. J Occup Environ Med 2001;43:110–9.

[20] Evison D, Hinsley D. Chemical weapons. BMJ 2002;324:332–5.

[21] Diller WF, Zante R. A literature review: therapy for phosgene poisoning. Toxicol Ind Health 1985;1:117–28.

[22] Sidell FR, Urbanetti JS, Smith WJ, et al. Vesicants. In: Zajtchuk R, Bellamy RF, editors. Textbook of military medicine: medical aspects of chemical and biological warfare. Washington (DC): US Department of the Army; 1997. p. 197–228.

[23] Karnofsky DA, Graef I, Smith HW. Studies on the mechanism of action of the nitrogen and sulfur mustards in vivo. Am J Pathol 1948;24:275–91.

[24] Mol MAE, van de Ruit AMBC, Kluivers AW. NAD^+ levels and glucose uptake of cultured human epithelial cells exposed to sulfur mustard. Toxicol Appl Pharmacol 1989;98:159–65.

[25] Papirmeister B, Gross CL, Petrali JP, et al. Pathology produced by sulfur mustard in human skin grafts on athymic nude mice. I. gross and light microscopic changes. J Toxicol Cutan Ocular Toxicol 1984;3:371–91.

[26] Gentilhomme E, Neveux Y, Hua A, et al. Action of bis(betachloroethyl) sulphide(BCES) on human epidermis reconstituted in culture: morphological alterations and biochemical depletion of glutathione. Toxicol In Vitro 1992;6:139–47.

[27] Safarinejad MR, Moosavi SA, Montazeri B. Ocular injuries caused by mustard gas: diagnosis, treatment, and medical defense. Mil Med 2001;166:67–70.

[28] Goldman M, Dacre JC. Lewisite: its chemistry, toxicology, and biological effects. Rev Environ Contam Toxicol 1989;110:75–115.

ELSEVIER
SAUNDERS

SURGICAL
CLINICS OF
NORTH AMERICA

Surg Clin N Am 86 (2006) 649–663

Biological Weapons: An Introduction for Surgeons

Lt Col W. Brian Perry, MD[a,b,*]

[a]*Department of Surgery, Wilford Hall Medical Center,
859 MSGS/MCSG, 2200 Bergquist Drive, Suite 1, Lackland AFB, TX 78236, USA*
[b]*University of Texas Health Science Center, 7703 Floyd Curl Drive,
San Antonio, TX 78229, USA*

Although the actual threat of a widespread bioterrorism event is relatively low, the successful deployment of any of these agents is likely to wreak havoc on local and regional medical systems. Those truly affected will be largely outnumbered by the "worried well." This article introduces the history of biological weapons, the methods used to recognize and begin to ameliorate the effects of an attack, and some specifics of the various agents available, with emphasis on the possible roles for surgeons. There are several excellent recent reviews that eloquently cover more of the details of these potential weapons. The US Army Medical Research Institute of Infectious Diseases (USAMRIID) at Ft. Detrick, Maryland, has published handbooks on the medical management of biological weapon casualties [1]. These handbooks have perforated tear-out cards on the major agents for rapid reference. The *Journal of the American Medical Association* recently published a series of consensus statements on the medical and public health management of the major biological weapons [2–7]. In *Critical Care Medicine*, Karwa and colleagues [8] offered a detailed summary that includes a thoughtful discussion of hospital preparations for a bioterrorist attack.

History

The use of biologic agents dates to the ancient Assyrians who poisoned their enemies' wells with rye ergot (a vasoconstrictor and precursor for

---

This work represents the views of the author and does not represent an official doctrine of the United States Air Force or the Department of Defense.

* Corresponding author. Department of Surgery, Wilford Hall Medical Center, 859 MSGS/MCSG, 2200 Bergquist Drive, Suite 1, Lackland AFB, TX 78236.

E-mail address: william.perry@lackland.af.mil

0039-6109/06/$ - see front matter. Published by Elsevier Inc.
doi:10.1016/j.suc.2006.02.009

lysergic acid diethylamide), and to Solon who used hellebore (a purgative) in the siege of Krissa. During the fourteenth century, an outbreak of plague in the Tartar army laying siege to Kaffa in the Crimea was turned to the attackers' advantage when they hurled infected corpses over the city walls. The ensuing epidemic forced the defenders to surrender and may have started the Black Death that later engulfed Europe. Smallpox, intentionally spread through gifts of contaminated clothing or blankets, was used by Pizzaro and by the English against Native Americans in Pre-Revolutionary North America [1].

In 1937, Japan opened a laboratory complex code-named Unit 731 in Manchuria dedicated to the development of biological weapons. Postwar inquiries revealed that a number of organisms were investigated for their potential as weapons, including anthrax and plague. Up to 3000 victims, primarily prisoners of war, died in the facility, many due to aerosolized anthrax. An epidemic of plague in China and Manchuria in 1940 has been attributed to the airborne dispersal of plague-infested fleas by Japanese warplanes. By the time the laboratory was destroyed in 1945, more than 400 kg of anthrax had been stockpiled for use in fragmentation bombs [9].

The United States began research on the offensive use of biological weapons in 1943 in response to a perceived German, not Japanese, threat. All research was stopped by President Nixon's executive order in 1969. The weapons stockpiles, which included anthrax, botulinum toxin, *Francisella tularensis, Coxiella burnetii, Brucella suis,* and staphylococcal enterotoxin type B (SEB) were destroyed by May 1972. Also in 1972, the Convention on the Prohibition of the Development, Production, and Stockpiling of Bacteriological (Biological) and Toxin Weapons and on Their Destruction was signed by many countries including the United States, the Soviet Union, and Iraq. The medical defensive research program at USAMRIID began in 1953 and continues today [1].

Despite the Conventions, there were several incidents with biological weapons agents in the late 1970s and early 1980s. The "yellow rain" attacks in Laos, Kampuchea, and Afghanistan were possibly aerial dispersals of T-2 mycotoxins. There is considerable controversy over these, but the geographic and temporal pattern of affected people and animals fits a biological weapon use profile (similarly affected individuals in close proximity in time and location). In 1978, the Bulgarian dissident Georgi Markov was assassinated in London with ricin toxin delivered from a device disguised in an umbrella. The agent was later traced through the Bulgarian government to the former Soviet Union [1].

In April 1979, there was an accidental release of aerosolized anthrax from Soviet Military Compound 19 in Sverdlovsk (now Yekaterniburg). Residents in a classic cloud-plume distribution downwind from the microbiology facility developed fever and respiratory failure, and many died. The Soviet Ministry of Health initially blamed contaminated meat, but in 1992, Russian President Boris Yeltsin acknowledged that the event was due to the unintentional release of anthrax spores from the facility. A detailed analysis of the incident by Meselson and colleagues [10] identified 77 patients, with 66 fatalities.

United Nations inspectors found in 1991 that Iraq had conducted research into several biological warfare (BW) agents including anthrax and botulinum toxin. Further information gathered in 1995 confirmed this biowarfare work. Testing in delivery systems was followed by the deployment of numerous bombs and missiles with anthrax, botulinum toxin, and aflatoxin by the Iraqi military in January 1991 [11].

One of the latest uses of BW agents occurred in the United States in September 2001, with the delivery of anthrax-laden letters in Washington, DC, and New York. Most of the cases have been traced to letters heavily contaminated with anthrax spores that were sent through the United States mail. All strains recovered from mail and from clinical specimens reportedly have the same molecular fingerprint, indicating their dissemination from a single source. Seven of these mail-related cases occurred among the intended recipients of the letters or others in their work environment; 11 were among postal workers. In addition, there were 4 other cases (2 cutaneous and 2 inhalational, both fatal) in elderly women, in which the victims appear unrelated to the intended recipients or the postal system [12].

Current risk

Although state-sponsored offensive biological weapons are unlikely to be deployed, terrorist attacks using these agents remain a possibility. The effectiveness of any attack is related to the virulence of the agent and the dispersal mechanism. The World Health Organization in a 1970 publication estimated that 50 kg of aerosolized anthrax spores dispersed by a line source such as a crop duster under ideal meteorologic conditions would kill nearly half the population of a city of 500,000; a similar dispersal of *F tularensis* would kill one third. The medical care system of the affected region would be quickly overwhelmed.

The most effective agents are those that can be dispersed as aerosols of particles between 1 and 5 μm in size, which allows for penetration to the distal bronchioles if inhaled [13]. Commercial pesticide sprayers can be modified to produce particles of this size. Airborne transmission is the most likely; huge quantities are required to affect food or water supplies. Cutaneous absorption of most agents is also unlikely because most are inactivated by soap and water or a mild hypochlorite solution. Even the relatively smaller quantities needed for widespread airborne use would be difficult for non–state-sponsored groups to obtain. Historical accounts of the BW weapons programs in the United States and the former Soviet Union have shown that it takes a huge investment in personnel and equipment to weaponize these agents.

The Centers for Disease Control and Prevention (CDC) categorizes BW agents into three groups (A, B, and C) based on several criteria, including virulence, environmental stability, ease of production and delivery, person-to-person transmission, potential for public panic, and probable effects on the public health system. Group A agents such as smallpox and anthrax are easily disseminated or are highly transmissible person-to-person. Group B agents like the biologic toxins are more difficult to weaponize and have lower mortality rates, making them a lower priority for detection and amelioration; however, they could cause major public health disruptions if successfully deployed. Group C agents are currently limited by availability and production difficulties but may be important in the future.

Event detection and surveillance

The deployment of BW agents by terrorists will almost certainly be covert, with discovery of the event coming only after the target population is affected. Several features could distinguish a BW attack from a naturally occurring disease outbreak. A rapid rise and fall of cases in the epidemic curve over a short time (hours to days) or the steady rise of cases suggests an attack. A large number of patients who have the same symptoms from the same geographic area and a large number of rapidly fatal cases may also signal the deployment of a BW agent. A relative protective effect of those who are indoors or a large number of similarly affected animals may also be seen. Finally, the appearance of an uncommon disease with BW potential, such as anthrax or smallpox, would almost certainly be from a malicious dispersal.

Detection of a BW agent release relies on surveillance of symptoms in the population at risk, regional laboratory data, or direct detection of the agent in the environment. Syndromic surveillance collects data over large segments of the population, collating unusual illnesses, hospital and emergency room use rates, patient complaints, medication purchases, unusual deaths, and animal incidents in the hopes of recognizing an attack early in its course. The CDC recently conducted a national demonstration project using aggregate data from multiple health plans covering 20 million covered lives. If a suspicious cluster of symptoms or diagnoses was identified from these overlapping segments, then more detailed information on individual events could be extracted. There are significant logistic hurdles and a built-in level of uncertainty with any syndromic surveillance system, making such an undertaking complementary to other forms of detection [14].

The CDC in conjunction with the Association of Public Health Laboratories established the Laboratory Response Network in 1999 to provide a system for handling potential BW agents. Level A laboratories are found in hospitals and clinics and will likely be the first to encounter specimens from an attack. They need to be able to distinguish BW pathogens from the vast numbers of nonweaponized organisms they see on a daily basis.

Level B and C facilities, found at county and state public health laboratories, provide confirmatory testing and initial susceptibility analysis. Level D laboratories are national resources for further agent characterization and, potentially, source identification. The Laboratory Response Network also works to develop protocols for specimen handling and reporting to national security agencies.

Environmental surveillance attempts to detect BW agents after release but before they affect the target population. Correct agent identification is balanced against speed; culture and sensitivity analysis of material collected in the field are the most accurate but can be very slow. Remote or standoff detection systems attempt to determine whether an aerosol cloud contains BW agents. The US Army has developed long-range and short-range systems using infrared laser and ultraviolet reflectance to offer warnings of potential BW agent clouds out to 30 km, giving enough time for those in the cloud's path to don personal protective equipment. Pollen clouds or other airborne organic material is difficult to distinguish from BW agents, making these systems complementary to other methods of detection. The Biological Integrated Detection System is a vehicle-mounted sensor apparatus that concentrates particles of the appropriate size for BW agents and attempts to identify them using antibody and genetic testing. On the civilian side, the Biowatch program employs 500 air filters deployed in 31 cities that are analyzed every 12 hours for the presence of BW agents. Although impractical to deploy in sufficient numbers to cover the entire country, such systems can be used in high-threat situations or in response to a specific threat.

The final piece of the detection and surveillance problem is prerelease intelligence. Numerous national and international agencies are dedicated to assessing potential adversaries for capability and intent [1,8].

Specific agents

Anthrax

Anthrax is one of the most serious of the bacterial forms of biological weapons potentially available to terrorists. The organism *Bacillus anthracis* is an encapsulated bacterium commonly found as a zoonotic disease in cattle and sheep. The spores are very hardy and can survive many years in the environment; however, the vegetative form is incapable of surviving outside the host. Clinically, there are three forms of anthrax: cutaneous, gastrointestinal, and inhalational. Cutaneous anthrax occurs when the spores are seeded into breaks in skin; this commonly occurs in farm workers in endemic areas. The rate of this naturally occurring process is very low. This form of disease is rarely fatal and easily treated with antibiotics. The gastrointestinal form of the disease occurs when contaminated meat products are ingested. The most serious form of anthrax from the point of biological weapons is inhalational anthrax. This form occurs after aerosolized, inhaled spores are transported by regional lymphatics to the mediastinal lymph nodes. The spores germinate to the vegetative bacilli over 2 to 5 days, but germination can be delayed as much as 60 days. The antiphagocytic capsule and three toxic components cause edema hemorrhage and necrosis and produce anthracic lymphangitis and hemorrhagic mediastinitis. After these manifestations occur, the process is rapidly fatal, even with excellent supportive care and antibiotics.

To weaponize anthrax, spores must be dispersed in an aerosol form so that they will reach the distal airways. Following a large aerosol dispersal, a large number of patients will present with nonspecific symptoms including fever chills, weakness, headache, vomiting, abdominal pain, dyspnea, cough, and chest pain. There may be a period of short recovery, and then a sudden resurgence of fever, shortness of breath, and shock. Deterioration is rapid and may be accompanied by hemorrhagic mediastinitis and hemotogenous spread to the bowel, causing necrotizing enteritis. Ventricular arrhythmias and fatal pericardial effusions have also been seen. Diagnosis, especially early on, is difficult because it may often be confused with a seasonal viral syndrome. Confirmatory testing is necessary, as is a clinical index suspicion. Empiric treatment of presumptive inhalational anthrax includes streptomycin or doxycycline, combined with one or two other antibiotics with activity, such as imipenem or clarithromycin. Ciprofloxacin is the drug of choice for postexposure prophylaxis and should be continued for up to 60 days. Inhalational anthrax is not spread from patient to patient, so standard precautions are adequate; decontamination of potential victims of an aerosol spread, however, must be accomplished before entry to the health care system.

There are several aspects of inhalational anthrax or gastrointestinal anthrax that may require the services of a general surgeon. Pleural effusions are common and there have been reported cases of fatal pericardial effusions, so thoracic drainage for diagnostic or therapeutic purposes may be required. Although gastrointestinal anthrax is not considered to be an important entity in a biological weapons arena, the hemotogenous spread of the bacillus to the gastrointestinal tract may lead to abdominal pain and regionalized enteritis that may progress to necrosis and require a full exploratory laparotomy. Patients who have cutaneous anthrax may need aggressive local wound care or reconstruction of the damaged tissues with skin grafts or localized flaps [1,2,8].

Plague

The causative agent of plague, *Yersinia pestis*, is a gram-negative coccobacillus that displays a typical safety pin appearance. Historically, plague has been the cause of massive pandemics throughout history. The first began in AD 541 in Egypt and swept through Europe with an estimated population loss of 50% to 60%. The second plague pandemic was the Black Death in Europe, which began in 1346 and lasted approximately 130 years. Nearly one third of the population of Europe succumbed during this time. Attempts of weaponization of plague have primarily included dispersal of infected fleas and aerosolization of the plague bacteria [3].

Clinically, plague takes several forms. The most common is bubonic plague, the form passed from infected fleas to humans. Before human outbreak, there is often a large number of rodent deaths, which causes the fleas to leave their primary host and attack humans. Several thousand of the plague organisms can be transmitted to the human victim by bites of the infected flea. The organisms are then phagocytized and travel in subcutaneous lymphatics to the regional lymph nodes where buboes form. These buboes are 1 to 10 cm in diameter and extremely painful, often limiting the motion of the limb. Following bubo formation, septicemia occurs through hemotogenous dissemination of the organism throughout the host, leading to vascular collapse. Of the patients who have plague from flea transmission, a small percentage progresses to a septicemic form without bubo formation. Bubonic plague may be followed by secondary pneumonic plague as the lungs become infected with blood-borne organisms. This form of plague is the only one that displays person-to-person transmission through the respiratory droplet route [8].

Primary pneumonic plague occurs after inhalation of the organism directly through aerosol forms in a BW attack or from droplets from patients who have primary or secondary pneumonic plague. Clinically, primary pneumonic plague is a rapidly progressing form of bronchopneumonia with high fevers and chills and variable gastrointestinal symptoms. These symptoms may appear clinically similar to inhalational anthrax; however, the presence of hemoptysis and typical organisms in the sputum differentiate this from an episode of anthrax. Diagnosis is made by the identification of the organism in sputum or lymph node aspiration; Gram stain may show the typical safety pin appearance of the coccobacillus. Cultures usually take 2 to 6 days; antibody detection is a late finding.

Prompt use of antibiotics has reduced the case fatality rate of plague from nearly 100% to between 5% and 14% in late-treated pneumonic plague. Streptomycin has traditionally been the antibiotic of choice, but its widespread availably in a mass exposure situation is uncertain. Doxycycline or gentamicin may also be used with good results. Postexposure treatment of affected individuals includes doxycycline as the first choice; ciprofloxacin may be used as a second choice and would likely be more readily available for mass distribution in a mass exposure event. Respiratory isolation is critical when a patient is suspected to have pneumonic plague because patient-to-patient transmission is very common. Health care workers need protection from exposure through ruptured buboes or surgical procedures that aerosolize organisms. Environmental decontamination is not necessary with plague because there is no spore form of the organism. A World Health Organization study concluded that a dispersal of aerosolized plague would last only approximately 1 hour; after this point, environmental degradation of the organism, mostly through exposure to sunlight, would render the organisms nonviable. A commercial vaccine for plague was available, but due to a large number of side effects and the lack of protection provided for the inhalational or primary pneumonic plague, it was discontinued in 1999. A substitute has not recently been produced. Surgical involvement in a plague outbreak would be unusual because an aerosol dispersal of the organism is the most likely form of BW attack. Should an outbreak of bubonic attack occur, surgeons may be consulted initially for incision and drainage of buboes, especially if the plague was not suspected early on. In general, however, surgical drainage of buboes is not indicated [1,3,8].

Tularemia

Tularemia is a zoonotic disease caused by the small aerobic, gram-negative coccobacillus *F tularensis*. This organism is highly resistant, surviving for long periods in soil, water, and animal carcasses. Humans are affected by direct contact with mucus membranes, broken skin, ingestion, or inhalation of as few as 10 to 50 organisms; person-to-person transmission has not been documented. Weaponization of *F tularensis* would occur primarily as an aerosolized dispersal of the agent. Following an aerosol release, most patients would present with a nonspecific febrile illness. The manifestations of tularemia occur where the organisms enter the body. Following entry to the body, the bacteria are ingested by macrophages and transported to regional lymph nodes where they multiply. Typical incubation is 3 to 5 days, after which the patient develops a sore throat, abdominal pain, and arthralgias. Eighty-five percent of naturally occurring cases are the ulcer glandular form in which tender ulcers measuring 0.5 to 3 cm are found at the inoculation site. Regional adenopathy is common, and these nodes may suppurate. Occasionally, the glandular form without overlaying skin involvement is seen. Oculoglandular and pharyngeal forms are similar, based on the site of the inoculation. Typhoidal tularemia occurs in 15% of the cases found naturally and would be the predominant form seen in an aerosolized attack. This primary pneumonic process occurs when the inhaled organisms are phagocytized by polymorphonuclear leukocytes and become granulomas. Patients may also develop hemorrhagic inflammation of the airways. Diarrhea and abdominal pain can occur in these patients, and high fever, chills, and aches are common. Diagnosis is somewhat difficult because patients will have laboratory findings consistent with a significant systemic illness. The organisms are notoriously difficult to grow in culture. Antibody detection is useful for prior exposure but is not timely and would not be of great benefit early on in an exposure. Streptomycin is the drug of choice for treating tularemia; gentamicin is an acceptable alternative. In a mass exposure situation, oral doxycycline, chloramphenicol, or ciprofloxacin can be used effectively. Recovery occurs in 5 to 7 days with appropriate antibiotic therapy, and permanent immunity is conferred. There is a vaccine; however, it is limited to microbiology workers or to those at extreme risk of exposure. Again, human-to-human transmission does not occur. Mortality may approach 35% in untreated forms, but with prompt institution of antibiotics, case fatally rates of less than 5% would be expected. The biggest difficulty in this process would be identifying it from an underlying naturally occurring upper respiratory illness or distinguishing tularemia from plague or inhalational anthrax in an attack situation. Surgical manifestations of this disease are uncommon; fluctuant lymph nodes may need treatment. The presence of abdominal pain in the face of a pneumonic process, especially in the large number of patients seen at the same time, may result in surgical consultation. There is little need, however, for laparotomy in the management of this disease. Environmental decontamination is not necessary [1,4,8].

Smallpox

Smallpox is caused by Orthopoxvirus variola and is highly contagious, spreading rapidly from person to person through inhalation of respiratory droplet nuclei that contact mucus membranes; it can also be spread by way of fomites. Since its eradication in 1980, smallpox vaccination has ceased throughout the world except in special populations. Because of its high person-to-person infectivity, its viability outside the human host, and high case fatality rate, the intentional release of the smallpox virus would lead to colossal damage.

Clinically, deposition of the virus particles on the pharyngeal mucosa leads to migration to regional lymph nodes. Viremia occurs 3 to 4 days following infection. With further dissemination, a secondary viremia occurs on the 8th to 12th day and is marked by fever and systemic symptoms. Virus localizes in the pharyngeal mucosa and in the small blood vessels in the dermis, leading to the first cutaneous manifestations. It is not until this point that a patient is infectious to others. Classic smallpox, when clinically manifest, is characterized by 2- to 3-mm reddish macules beginning on the face, hands, and forearms. These macules progress to papules and vesicles and spread centrally to cover the whole body. All of the lesions in smallpox erupt at the same stage, which distinguishes it from chickenpox in which the vesicles occur in crops and can be of differing clinical ages in the same region of the body. Further in the course, the lesions begin to crust and separate. Patients remain infectious until all scabs have completely separated; secondary bacterial infection is uncommon. Death in the classic form of smallpox is most common during the second week and is proportional to the amount of confluence of the skin lesions. There is no specific antiviral therapy, and supportive measures compromise the primary treatment.

Two other forms of smallpox are extremely lethal. The hemorrhagic type, which has a predilection for pregnant women, is characterized by a shorter prodromal phase and marked prostration. It is manifested by defuse hemorrhagic lesions involving mucus membranes and the skin. Pulmonary edema and hemoptysis are common, with a 100% fatality rate within a week. The other unusual form is the malignant type or flat type. At the outset, toxicity is profound; however, the skin lesions remain flat, soft, and velvety to the touch and never progress to the pustular stage. The case fatality rate of this form is 95% [5].

Any confirmed case of smallpox would be considered an international health emergency. Strict quarantine with respiratory isolation should be applied for at least 17 days for all suspected contacts. Because of the long incubation period, spread could be very wide before it is recognized as smallpox. Smallpox vaccination is indicated in the postexposure period up to 3 to 4 days and confers good protection. The United States military has begun to revaccinate personnel who are deploying; however, the vaccination is not without risk. Postexposure vaccination and appropriate public health control measures would be rapidly necessary within a large-scale outbreak. Surgical measures of smallpox cases would be problematic, especially in hemorrhagic and confluent cases in which large areas of skin is sloughing and may need the care of specialized centers such as burn units [1,5,8].

Viral hemorrhagic fever

The viral hemorrhagic fevers (VHF) are a group of human illnesses that are caused by a diverse family of RNA viruses. These viruses include Filoviridae (Ebola and Marburg viruses); Arenaviridae (Lassa virus and Argentine and Bolivian hemorrhagic fever viruses); Bunyaviridae (hantaviruses and Congo-Crimean fever); and Flaviviridae (yellow fever virus and the dengue viruses). As a group, these viruses are transmitted to humans though various animals and arthropod vectors, although for many, the exact natural repository is unclear. They are included in the discussion of bioterrorism weapons because several have been weaponized in the past and have shown good infectivity in an aerosolized form. Person-to-person transmission is more variable, with many showing clear transmission through blood, body, and tissue fluid contact.

VHF viruses target the endothelium, casing problems in the microcirculation and altering vascular permeability. Patients commonly present with fever, myalgias, flushing, and a variable amount of bleeding, which is usually not life-threatening alone but is a marker of disease severity. The course of each virus is similar, with progression to vascular collapse, varying degrees of neurologic, pulmonary, and hepatic involvement, and eventual multisystem organ failure. Case fatality rates are also variable but may approach 80% in Ebola virus outbreaks.

Definitive identification depends on isolation in cell culture or by immunohistochemical techniques. Presumptive diagnosis is suggested by thrombocytopenia and coagulation disorders in the setting of an acute viral illness. ELISA or polymerase chain reaction has also been successfully used.

Treatment is largely supportive. Aspirin, antiplatelet drugs, and steroids are contraindicated. Invasive monitoring, mechanical ventilation, and hemodialysis are sometimes necessary, with dopamine being the inotrope of choice in most cases. Ribavirin is a nonimmunosuppressive nucleoside analog that has shown some efficacy in treating VHF. The only commercially available vaccine is targeted to yellow fever, which is considered to have very little potential as a BW agent. Isolation is crucial, especially before definitive identification. Autoclaving or incineration of linens and other contaminated materials is necessary. Decontamination requires bleach or detergent. Surgical involvement is likely limited but may become necessary for exsanguinating internal bleeding, which is rare [1,7,8].

Botulinum toxin

Botulinum toxin is the single most poisonous substance known to man. As little as 0.1 μg administered intravenously or intramuscularly is fatal in a normal-sized person. It also has the unique distinction as the only potential BW agent that is Food and Drug Administration–approved: botulinum toxin type A is currently used for a variety of disorders featuring abnormal muscle contraction, from cervical torticollis to anal fissures. *Clostridium botulinum* is a spore-forming anaerobic bacillus commonly found in the soil worldwide. Four genetically distinct strains each produce one or more of seven potent neurotoxins, types A to G. Preformed toxin may be ingested or inhaled or the toxin may be produced by the bacteria in the gastrointestinal tract or in devitalized wounds. After it is absorbed, the toxin is carried to neuromuscular junctions where it is endocytosed. After it is inside the nerve cell, cleaved light-chain fragments prevent the fusion of vesicles containing acetylcholine with the cell membrane, thus inhibiting their release. This lack of release of the acetylcholine vesicles causes flaccid paralysis of the affected muscle and is irreversible. Recovery depends on regeneration of new motor axon twigs.

BW use of botulinum toxin would likely take the form of aerosolized dispersion of 0.1- to 0.3-μm particles, ideal for deposition in the distal airways. Following Gulf War I, Iraq admitted to having produced over 19,000 L of botulinum toxin and to equipping 13 missiles with a range of up to 600 km with the toxin. The Aum Shinrikyo cult in Japan attempted to use aerosolized toxin at least three times in the early 1990s; none of the attempts were successful. Food or water-borne contamination is thought to be less likely because the quantity needed and distribution difficulties make this route less attractive.

Following an incubation period of 12 to 72 hours, patients begin to present with an acute, afebrile descending flaccid paralysis. Cranial nerves are often affected first, causing dysphonia, dysphagia, and dysarthria, followed by hypercapnic respiratory failure. Diagnosis is made clinically initially and can be confirmed with mouse neutralization bioassay. Intubation and mechanical ventilation are usually required (for an average of 97 days in one series), thus making a large-scale attack particularly devastating to the medical infrastructure. Antibiotics may be necessary for ventilator-acquired pneumonia, but aminoglycosides and clindamycin should be avoided because they may exacerbate neuromuscular blockade. Early administration of antitoxin limits the severity of the disease but does not affect established paralysis. Postexposure prophylaxis in the absence of symptoms is not warranted. A vaccine is available in limited quantities and is currently used in laboratory and military personnel who have an exposure risk. Decontamination would be minimal because the toxin is impermeable to intact skin and is rapidly degraded in ambient environmental conditions. The toxin cannot be passed from patient to patient or to other health care workers. In a BW event, botulinum toxin release may mimic nerve agents or naturally occurring illnesses such as Guillain-Barré syndrome, stroke, or intoxication.

Surgical involvement in a botulinum toxin attack would be primarily for durable airway access for prolonged ventilation (tracheotomy) and feeding access (gastrostomy). Botulism from infected wounds would require prompt and adequate debridement [1,7,8].

Other potential agents

A number of other toxins and diseases may pose a BW threat but are limited by their lack of infectivity or toxicity or by difficulties in manufacture or delivery. A substance that is very unstable and hard to aerosolize is a poor choice, regardless of how toxic it is. Three additional toxins—SEB, ricin, and the T-2 mycotoxins—are less lethal but have been weaponized or used before.

SEB is a one of a number of heat-stable pyrogenic exotoxins produced by *Staphylococcus aureus*. It has caused countless cases of food poisoning, but its utility as a BW agent is based on its ease of production and stability in an aerosol. Although the median lethal dose is large, its incapacitating effects are seen at doses 100-fold smaller. A variety of toxic effects occur following inhalation, primarily mediated by binding to the major histocompatibility complex, which begins a cascade of cytokine release. After an incubation period of 3 to 12 hours, victims develop high fevers, cough, chills, headache, and gastrointestinal distress from additional swallowed toxin. Specific diagnosis would be difficult initially because SEB intoxication shares many clinical features with a host of other processes; ELISA detection from nasal swabbing is possible within the first 24 hours. Supportive care is the only current therapy, and there are no vaccines or postexposure prophylactic measures currently available.

Ricin is a potent protein toxin derived from castor beans. Production of large quantities of castor beans, which are grown worldwide, is relatively easy. On the cellular level, ricin inhibits protein synthesis; clinical manifestations are determined by route of entry. Deposition in the airways causes a necrotizing tracheobronchitis and pneumonia, leading to acute respiratory distress syndrome. Ingestion causes visceral hemorrhage, perforation, and organ necrosis. Intramuscular injection, as was seen in the case of the Bulgarian dissident Georgi Markov, causes local pain and necrosis, followed by systemic involvement leading to vascular collapse and end-organ failure that is similar to septic shock. Diagnosis may be made with ELISA detection. No specific antidote is known, and a vaccine is under development.

Trichothecene mycotoxins are a group of more than 150 compounds produced by filamentous fungi that are extremely stable to attempted heat or ultraviolet inactivation. They are dermally active and highly toxic to rapidly dividing cells through inhibition of protein and nucleic acid synthesis. After skin or eye contact, these toxins cause pain, redness, blistering, necrosis, and sloughing. Inhalation causes similar effects on the airways, with chest pain and hemoptysis. Ingestion leads to nausea, vomiting, and profuse watery or bloody diarrhea. Severe exposure is followed by prostration, collapse, and death. Alimentary toxic aleukia is a protracted lethal illness caused by chronic ingestion and characterized by abdominal complaints followed by myalgias, bone marrow suppression, and sepsis. This illness progresses to a third stage, with painful skin and mucosal ulcers with skin and visceral hemorrhage. Diagnosis is made clinically and should be considered following an attack of "yellow rain" or an attack that includes green, red, or white smoke. Blood, urine, fecal, or environmental sampling using gas-liquid chromatography/mass spectrometry confirms the presence of toxin. Superactive charcoal can absorb swallowed toxin, but there is no other specific therapy or vaccine [1,8].

Hospital preparedness

Preparation for a potential BW attack is based on sound disaster planning currently in place in most hospitals and communities. Several features of an incident of this nature, however, warrant further scrutiny. The public response, if such a BW agent release were to occur, would truly be phenomenal, with the potential for a huge number of worried well or non–agent-affected "casualties" in addition to those actually exposed seeking access to the health care system. In distinction to a physical disaster such as an earthquake or explosion, there may be little or no external evidence of the event before victims begin to show up at hospitals where the nature of the calamity may first be appreciated. The patient population is likely to be homogeneous, rapidly overwhelming local resources. In addition, the threat of person-to-person transmission of some agents adds a level of complexity not seen in a conventional mass-casualty scenario.

Regional and national cooperation will be essential in the effective handling of a BW event. The National Disaster Medical System has been established to provide a cooperative effort for responding to large-scale disasters, bringing together the Department of Health and Human Services, the Department of Defense, the Federal Emergency Management Agency, the Department of Veterans' Affairs, and state and local governments. Approximately 150 teams within the National Disaster Medical System can respond, in addition to a network for evacuation to more than 100,000 pre-committed beds throughout the country. This system was put to use following Hurricane Katrina, with mixed results.

A BW event, especially one with a bacterial agent, will quickly empty all the local and regional pharmacies of specific medications. The Strategic National Stockpile, managed jointly by the Department of Homeland Defense, the Department of Health and Human Services, and the CDC, aids local communities faced with such a disaster by providing push-packages within 12 hours. These caches, strategically located in secure warehouses, contain commonly needed pharmaceuticals, antidotes, and other supplies to replenish those used in the initial response. After 24 to 48 hours, more specific items can by delivered [1,8].

Summary

It is hoped that none of us will ever have to treat victims of a BW attack. Recognition of such an attack will require considering its possibility when the epidemiology of an illness outbreak is unusual. The effects of many of the agents can be at least partially ameliorated with prompt treatment or postexposure prophylaxis. Surgeons need to be active participants in hospital, local, and regional disaster planning.

References

[1] US Army Medical Research Institute of Infectious Diseases. Medical management of biological casualties handbook. Fort Detrick (MD): USAMRIID; 1996.
[2] Inglesby T, Henderson D, Bartlett J, et al. Anthrax as a biological weapon: medical and public health management. JAMA 1999;281(18):1735–45.
[3] Inglesby T, Dennis D, Henderson D, et al. Plague as a biological weapon: medical and public health management. JAMA 2000;283(17):2281–9.
[4] Dennis D, Inglesby T, Henderson D, et al. Tularemia as a biological weapon: medical and public health management. JAMA 2001;285(21):2763–73.
[5] Henderson D, Inglesby T, Bartlett J, et al. Smallpox as a biological weapon: medical and public health management. JAMA 1999;281(22):2127–37.
[6] Borio L, Inglesby T, Peters C, et al. Hemorrhagic fever viruses as a biological weapon: medical and public health management. JAMA 2002;287(18):2391–405.
[7] Arnon S, Schecter R, Inglesby T, et al. Botulinum toxin as a biological weapon: medical and public health management. JAMA 2001;285(8):1059–70.
[8] Karwa M, Currie B, Kvetan V. Bioterrorism: preparing for the impossible or the improbable. Crit Care Med 2005;33(Suppl 1):S75–95.

[9] Gomer R, Powell J, Rolling B. Japan's biological weapons: 1930–1945—a hidden chapter in history. Bull At Sci 1981;17(6):3434–42.

[10] Meselson M, Guillemin J, Hugh-Jones M, et al. The Sverdlovsk anthrax outbreak of 1979. Science 1994;266(5188):1202–8.

[11] United Nations Security Council. Tenth report of the Executive Chairman of the Special Commissions established by the Secretary-General pursuant to paragraph 9(b)(1) of Security Council Resolution 687 (1991), and paragraph 3 of resolution 699(1991) on the Activities of the Special Commission. New York: United Nations Security Council; 1995. Publication #S/1995/1038.

[12] Webb F, Blaser M. Mailborne transmission of anthrax: modeling and implications. Proc Natl Acad Sci U S A 2002;99(10):7027–32.

[13] Morrow P, Yu C. Models of aerosol behavior in airways. In: Moren F, editor. Aerosols in medicine: principals, diagnosis, and therapy. New York: Elsevier Science; 1985. p. 149–91.

[14] Platt R, Bocchino C, Caldwell B. Syndromic surveillance using minimum transfer of identifiable data: the example of the national bioterrorism surveillance demonstration program. J Urban Health Bull N Y Acad Med 2003;80:i25–31.

SURGICAL
CLINICS OF
NORTH AMERICA

Surg Clin N Am 86 (2006) 665–673

Civilian Application of Military Resources

LTC Seth Izenberg, MD

*Trauma Services, Emanuel Hospital, 2801 North Gantenbein Street,
MOB 130, Portland, OR 97227, USA*

The chapter for disaster response in the book *Resources for Optimal Care of the Injured Patient: 1999* notes, "demands intrinsic to disaster situations often exceed the resources, capabilities, and orderly procedures of any single hospital" [1]. In every hospital, there is a finite limit to the number of operating rooms, surgeons, anesthesiologists, nurses, beds, and other resources. The need for further assistance is paramount; the resources of immediate aid are limited. This article discusses the availability of military resources and the prescribed interaction with civilian authority. A list of commonly used acronyms is given in the Appendix.

System of information flow and requests

During a mass-causality or disaster event, each hospital is expected to activate its incident command system. An example of such a system is the Hospital Emergency Incident Command System (HEICS) [2]. The flow chart of HEICS defines the role of medical liaison for the hospital [2]. This individual is indispensable for obtaining information about the event, expected casualties, and expected disease or trauma types so hospital resources can be coordinated to meet the demand. This individual also has the job of communicating the hospital's requirements and capabilities up the chain of command (it clearly does no good to have 100 injured people arrive where there is no capability to care for them). In the HEICS there must be constant communication between the various departments as the event unfolds. Only through constant feedback and reassessment can the individual hospital maintain its function.

The views expressed in this article are those of the author and do not reflect the official policy of the United States Army, Department of Defense or the United States Government.

E-mail address: Lastizzy41@comcast.net

Inherent in the Incident Command System is an operations section that has the responsibility of continuing health care support. Local Metropolitan Medical Response Systems perform that function, tying together the hospital resources of a defined region and then reporting back to the overall Incident Commander [3]. It is possible that within a state the Office of Emergency Management will be able to request from the state's governor the activation of National Guard resources (as discussed later) without declaration of an Incident of National Significance (also discussed later). In some states (eg, Washington) the Office of Emergency Management (or equivalent) is contained with the state military department.

The National Response Plan (NRP) [4] is the result of the coordination of a presidentially directed effort to organize the federal response to domestic incident management. It is an all-hazards and all-discipline approach to unified decision making based on the National Incident Management System (NIMS) [5]. The main goal is improved coordination among the responding agencies, whether governmental or nongovernmental. This plan defines the use of federal assets for incident management. As discussed in the plan, the NIMS applies to designated Incidents of National Significance, high-impact events that require a coordinated and effective response by an appropriate combination of federal, state, local, tribal, private-sector, and nongovernmental entities to save lives, minimize damage, and provide the basis for long-term community recovery and mitigation activities [6].

Homeland Security Presidential Directive 5 sets four criteria for declaring an event an Incident of National Significance, and the NRP definition of Incidents of National Significance relates to these four criteria:

1. A federal department or agency acting under its own authority has requested the assistance of the Secretary of Homeland Security.
2. The resources of state and local authorities are overwhelmed, and the appropriate state and local authorities have requested federal assistance. Examples include major disasters or emergencies as defined under the Stafford Act [7] and catastrophic incidents.
3. More than one federal department or agency has become substantially involved in responding to an incident. Examples include credible threats, indications, or warnings of imminent terrorist attack or acts of terrorism directed domestically against the people, property, environment, or political or legal institutions of the United States or its territories or possessions and threats or incidents related to high-profile, large-scale events that present high-probability targets such as National Special Security Events and other special events as determined by the Secretary of Homeland Security, in coordination with other federal departments and agencies.
4. The Secretary of Homeland Security has been directed to assume responsibility for managing a domestic incident by the President [6].

These incidents make national military assets available to civilian authorities. Self-maintenance is part of the initial plan. Lessons learned from events such as Hurricane Katrina will be applied, and the plan will be updated on a regular basis. This plan guides the military in the support of domestic civilian authorities. Events outside the scope of the plan must be assessed on another basis. All catastrophic events are Incidents of National Significance [6].

The NRP contains the expanded version of the NIMS and designates the role of the various agencies involved. In addition, the NRP contains multiple annexes to define the Emergency Support Functions (ESFs) needed to carry out a multilayer and coordinated response. These annexes include everything from transportation (ESF #1; logistics obviously play a major role in incident recovery and mitigation) to oil and hazardous material response (ESF #10). Fifteen ESFs are defined. The section of most interest to surgeons is ESF #8, public health and medical services. The avowed purpose of ESF #8 includes "the mechanism for coordinated Federal assistance to supplement State, local, and tribal resources in response to public health and medical care needs for potential or actual Incidents of National Significance or during a developing potential health and medical situation" [6]. The support includes medical care personnel, medical equipment, and supplies [6]. Supporting agencies, which include the Department of Defense (DOD), are responsible for "conducting operations, when requested by the Department of Homeland Security (DHS) or the designated ESF primary agency, using their own authorities, subject-matter experts, capabilities, or resources; ... furnishing available personnel, equipment, or other resource support as requested by DHS or the ESF primary agency" [6].

Also, "When requested, and upon approval of the Secretary of Defense, the Department of Defense (DOD) provides Defense Support of Civil Authorities (DSCA) during domestic incidents" [6]. This mechanism allows DOD assets to be requested and made available to the Incident Commander and his ESF #8 coordinator, the Assistant Secretary for Public Health Emergency Preparedness (ASPHEP).

The Health and Human Services (HHS) Secretary Operations Center facilitates coordination of the overall ESF #8 response. "Persons representing an ESF #8 organization are expected to have extensive knowledge of the resources and capabilities of their respective organizations and have access to the appropriate authority for committing such resources during the activation" [6].

The reporting lines back to the ASPHEP include personnel at the National Response Coordination Center, the Interagency Incident Management Group, the Regional Response Coordination Center/Joint Field Office, the National Emergency Response Team, and the Emergency Response Team. The ASPHEP also may maintain a liaison to the Joint Information Center to allow outflow of information from HHS about the incident.

Fig. 1 shows the complexity of the organization of response. At all levels there is an interaction back and forth between the agencies and their representatives on the ground and the response centers. This multilevel interaction is necessary because the local Incident Commander must be able to request assets from the state and higher operation centers, and the higher operation centers must notify the local authorities of resources committed. Finally, the local authorities must prepare to receive the assistance.

Military medical organizations

To understand the deployment of medical assets as requested by the Defense Support of Civilian Authorities Liaison, the regional civilian liaison officer must be familiar with the current organization of the Medical Department. This organization varies with service, so that the assets of each are not interchangeable. This article discusses the Army organization as an example, but assets from the Navy or the Air Force may be first to respond. The decision will be based on available resources and the discretion of the Secretary of Defense and must, of necessity, consider other commitments of the DOD.

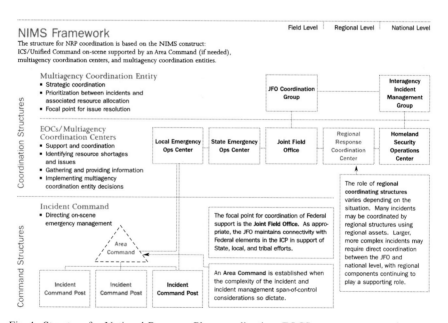

Fig. 1. Structure for National Response Plan coordination. EOCS, emergency operations center; JFO, joint field office; NIMS, National Incident Management System; NRP, National Response Plan.

Organization of care

The organization is based on the different needs of the different services. The Air Force has defined its capabilities on small units needed for providing medical services at forward air bases and therefore has small modules ready to go. The Navy, on the other hand, traditionally has been involved with large invasions and therefore has obtained assets for handling large number of casualties. The Army's capabilities lie between those of the two other services.

Organizations

Doctrinally, the Air Force Medical Service will provide a tiered and tailored medical capability that is driven by mission, threat scenario, airlift availability, and population at risk. The initial package may be a squadron medical element progressing to the Air Force Theater Hospital [8]. The Expeditionary Medical Support (EMEDS) package starts very simply but can be augmented by personnel or equipment based on the assessment. The base package is designed to gather casualties and to provide only emergent surgery. The EMEDS + 10 package is designed to have 10 inpatient beds and to provide up to 7 days of care. The EMEDS + 25 package is designed to have significantly more capability, with 25 inpatient beds (cumulative, because the EMEDS + 10 package is embedded into the EMEDS + 25 package), also for 7 days of care. All EMEDS packages contain anesthesia and general and orthopedic surgery capability.

Currently, there are plans to have equipment sets immediately available in all 10 Federal Emergency Management Agency regions. Regional supplies allow much shortened response times. Personnel will have to be allocated from other sites, and available reserve and National Guard components may be mixed. At the current operational tempo, it may be necessary to move personnel for longer distances, because some units may be committed to other incidents or conflicts.

The DOD also may be tasked with coordination of movement of patients in conjunction with the Department of Transportation [6]. Currently the Air Force operates a worldwide patient-movement control center for evacuation of sick and wounded DOD personnel. This system may be used for civilian disasters if deemed appropriate by the Secretary of Defense. Evacuation of the injured and sick is one of many priorities that must be juggled by the Incident Commander and the Secretary of Defense.

Army medical resources are provided by both the National Guard and the Army (Reserve and Active components). In most states, the Army National Guard contains Medical Companies that are part of Support Battalions. These companies do not contain the necessary equipment or personnel to perform surgery or provide inpatient therapy but may be used in support roles for housing, food, sanitation, and even triage roles. The medical personnel attached to these units have been trained as combat medics and physicians to provide such services. The National Guard can function under either Title 10 or Title 32. Title 10 is the US Code, which defines the role of the Active Army and the Reserve. Title 32 defines the role of the National Guard. Once troops have been placed on orders; the orders define the command authority. Under Title 32 such actions are at the command of the governor of the state. Troops may be mobilized as state active duty in one state to assist another state, as defined by the Emergency Management Assistance Compact [9]. This compact allows the governors of the several states to assist each other with state-level military resources even without the intervention of the Secretary of Defense. Hawaii is not currently a participant (but may be a member by time of this publication). This compact also allows the governors to act without a federal declaration of an Incident of National Significance.

To understand the system and units available, one must understand the organization of Army Medicine. Army Medicine must provide continuous and effective care for injured and sick solders from the site of injury (active battle) all the way through rehabilitation services. The breakdown is shown in Fig. 2. Active Army and Reserve components contain medical units that may have special roles in time of disaster. The Army Medical Department contains echelon two and three units that may be deployed.

Echelon two units correspond to the Air Force EMEDS and can perform gathering and emergent operations but provide no significant bed or holding space. These teams are called Forward Surgical Teams (FSTs). The current force mix includes FSTs assigned to brigades as organic medical assets. FSTs are designed to be deployed, fully mobile, and staffed for a maximum of 30 operations in 72 hours [10]. Beyond that level of employment the FST must be resupplied, allowed to sterilize equipment, repair any broken equipment, and repack for another mission. The normal complement of FST physicians is three general surgeons and one orthopedic surgeon. There are two nurse anesthetists and nurses for resuscitation, operating room, and recovery. The unit is not designed for holding patients; patients are intended to be evacuated to the next-higher level of care.

Echelon three units provide hospital care. The Combat Support Hospital (CSH) as defined by the Army contains 296 patient beds in two separate packages [11]. The CSH has the capability of performing 120 operating room table-hours in a 24-hour period when configured as the Hospital Unit Base and Hospital Unit Surgical in one combined setting. The surgical staffing includes two general surgeons and two orthopedic surgeons, with provisions for attached oral maxillofacial, neurosurgical, thoracic, urologic, ophthalmologic, and obstetric/gynecologic surgeons as dictated by mission. Additional physician resources include internists, emergency physicians, primary care physicians, and psychiatrists. Ideally the CSH is located at a site where resupply and evacuation are straightforward; in contrast to the FST, the CSH is not designed to be self sufficient in transportation, rations, and

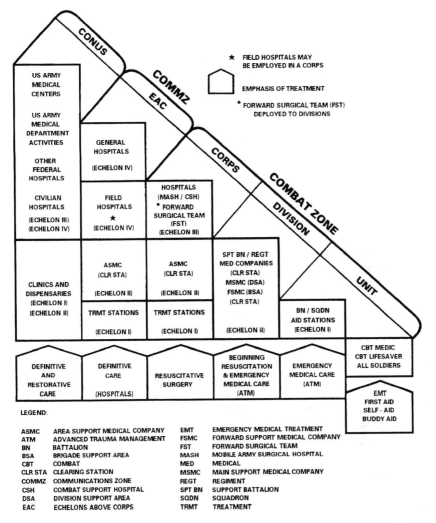

Fig. 2. Echelons of combat health support. ASMC, area support medical company; ATM, advanced trauma management; BN, battalion; BSA, brigade support area; CBT, combat; CLR STA, clearing station; COMMZ, communications zone; CSH, combat support hospital; DSA, division support area; EAC, echelons above corps; EMT, emergency medical treatment; FSMC, forward support medical company; FST, forward surgical team; MASH, mobile army support hospital; MED, medical; MSMC, main support medical company; REGT, regiment; SPT BN, support battalion; SQDN, squadron; TRMT, treatment.

site preparation. The estimated time needed to prepare for deployment is 72 hours or less [11]. Realistically, once the unit is deployed, it may take up to 5 days to be ready to undertake full-scale operations. The size of the package for deployment is considerable: 604 officers and enlisted personnel and 1,794,726 pounds of personnel, basic assigned equipment, and additional allowed deployable equipment (personal weapons and check-in baggage). This package requires the equivalent of 38 railcars (80 feet) or 11 C5A aircraft [11]. Transportation to a site within the United States for domestic use would require no less.

Class VIII (medical) supplies must be resupplied often and may need to be propositioned on an area-wide basis.

Because of the large footprint and needs of the CSH, and because the threat analysis has changed since the 1990s, a medical reengineering initiative has been taking place [11]. The current plan is to provide a unit that can be deployed within 24 to 96 hours of activation. This unit will be smaller and more mobile, consisting of a 44-bed early-entry hospital unit. The larger, more familiar CSH is made up of combinations of units and teams currently being assembled. Mobility will be the key feature of the 44-bed early entry unit. Moving 11 C5A aircraft during a disaster is not easy. These early-entry units are being fielded currently and will become more available within the next few years.

Additionally, the NRP allows propositioning of assets before the event [12] so that initial response resources may be more easily available. It is clear that this authority for the DHS will include medical assets as needed.

Finally, the Navy maintains two hospital ships (normally one on either coast), which may be directed to be available in time of emergency. These ships require sailing time and would not be available to the entire country but may be useful in coastal cities. The *USNS Mercy* and the *USNS Comfort* maintain 1000 beds each that could be activated if needed. Each ship contains modern medical suites and equipment for both basic and advanced life support as well as the ability to provide evacuation platforms for helicopter arrival and departure. The Secretary of Defense would activate this resource.

Military assistance will occur in other areas as well. In all 15 ESF, the DOD is a supporting agency. National Guard and active duty servicemen were deeply involved in search and rescue, security, logistics, and reengineering in the aftermath of Hurricane Katrina. The DOD is singularly well configured to take ground and hold it in wartime, with all the potential natural and manmade catastrophes that can occur. Activation for support (not replacement) of civil authorities is a natural extension. In conclusion, the DOD will support local authorities with assets within the framework of the NRP and in support of local civilian authorities. The assets used may vary, the service of origin may vary, the component may vary, but the commitment to serve the people of the United States will remain constant.

Appendix

Acronym list

ASPHEP Assistant Secretary (of Health and Human Services) for Public Health Emergency Preparedness

CSH Combat Support Hospital
DHS Department of Homeland Security
DOD Department of Defense
DSCA Defense Support of Civilian Authorities
EMEDS Expeditionary Medical Support
ESF Emergency Support Function
FEMA Federal Emergency Management Agency
FST Forward Support Team
HHS Health and Human Services
HIECS Hospital Emergency Incident Command System
ICS Incident Command System
INS Incident of National Significance
MMRS Metropolitan Medical Response System
NIMS National Incident Management System
NRP National Response Plan
OEM Office of Emergency Management
SOC Secretary's Operations Center
USNS United States Naval Ship

References

[1] Resources for optimal care of the injured patient: 1999. American College of Surgeons; 1998. p. 87.
[2] Emergency medical services authority (California). Available at: http://www.emsa.ca.gov/Dms2/HEICS98a.pdf. Accessed February 14, 2006.
[3] Metropolitan medical response system. Available at: http://www.mmrs.fema.gov/default.aspx. Accessed February 14, 2006.
[4] National response plan. Available at: http://www1.va.gov/emshg/docs/national_response_plan/start.htm. Accessed February 14, 2006.
[5] Federal emergency management agency. Available at: http://www.fema.gov/nims. Accessed February 14, 2006.
[6] Department of homeland security. Available at: http://www.dhs.gov/interweb/assetlibrary/NRP_FullText.pdf p. 4. Accessed February 14, 2006.
[7] Federal emergency management agency. Available at: Stafford Act. http://www.fema.gov/library/stafact.shtm. Accessed February 14, 2006.
[8] Brooks City (Air Force Base). Available at: http://www.brooks.af.mil/web/html/EMEDS/. Accessed February 14, 2006.
[9] Council of State governments. Available at: http://ssl.csg.org/terrorism/98ssl21.pdf. Accessed February 14, 2006.
[10] Medical reengineering initiative. Available at: http://www.findarticles.com/p/articles/mi_m0IAV/is_2_92/ai_114783372. Accessed February 14, 2006.
[11] Field manual, no. 8–10–14, section 1–2c; section 4–3 a 6; appendix B. Washington (DC): Department of the Army; 1994.
[12] Available at: http://mrimedforce.amedd.army.mil/links.htm. Accessed February 14, 2006.

SURGICAL
CLINICS OF
NORTH AMERICA

Surg Clin N Am 86 (2006) 675–688

Introduction to Military Medicine: A Brief Overview

COL Stephen P. Hetz, MD

Department of Surgery, William Beaumont Army Medical Center, 5005 N Piedras St, El Paso, TX 79920-5001, USA

Military medicine encompasses the entire spectrum of health care—from prenatal to end-of-life care. World-class, cutting-edge research, equipment, facilities, and education are all part of the military health care system of the United States of America. What makes United States military medicine unique, however, is the ability to project and sustain this care to soldiers, sailors, airmen, and marines in virtually any location on the planet and in the most chaotic, difficult, and hostile circumstances imaginable, specifically during combat operations. This ability has become possible because the structure of the military medical forces has evolved with every military operation since the Revolutionary War. This article provides an overview of the current organization and structure of the United States military medical forces. The levels of care (also known as "echelons" or "roles" of care, denoted 1–5 or I–V) are presented, with a specific focus on how this structure works to provide the military forces with the best combat medical care in the history of the world. The "glue" that binds the five levels of care together—medical evacuation, including the introduction of the Critical Care Air Transport Teams (CCATT)—is briefly discussed. The logistics system/structure that sustains military medical systems in remote locations is summarized. Finally, the overall command and control of in-theater combat medical assets, the initiative to establish a Joint Military Trauma System, and the ongoing efforts to collect real-time casualty data with the goal of enhancing combat care through improved training and early equipment fielding are described.

Brief historical perspective

Military medical care has evolved with the warfare it was designed to support. As the weapons of war became more destructive and lethal, medical

---

E-mail address: stephen.hetz@amedd.army.mil

0039-6109/06/$ - see front matter © 2006 Elsevier Inc. All rights reserved.
doi:10.1016/j.suc.2006.02.011
surgical.theclinics.com

care necessarily adapted and became more effective in treating the wounded. Likewise, as medicine advanced, wounded soldiers (who previously were beyond the capabilities of the care available) became salvageable. Near the beginning of the twentieth century, the concept of military triage was developed because, for the first time, improved evacuation systems resulted in more severely wounded soldiers reaching medical care than ever before and the rudimentary military medical systems of the time had never had to contend with the overwhelming volume of casualties being presented. Subsequently, military medical systems and structure had to adapt to the magnitude and volume of wounded produced by modern warfare. Before the introduction of general anesthesia, surgical salvage of severe intraperitoneal, intracranial, and intrathoracic wounds was a rarity, with most surgical care directed toward the extremities [1]. Because amputation was the major surgical intervention, rarely was there a need for significant sorting of casualties to make sure those who had a chance to survive would. With the introduction of general anesthesia into the mainstream of medicine, along with the improved initial treatment and evacuation of salvageable casualties from the battlefield to forward hospitals, the concept of triage of the wounded was an essential step in efficiently managing combat casualties. With more wounded surviving their initial injuries, military medical systems had to be developed to safely transport patients from the site of wounding back to a point of relative safety for stabilization and ultimate transport to a definitive-care facility. This system of combat casualty care has been refined to its current state over the greater than two-century history of the United States Armed Forces.

Basic military structure

Briefly, to understand the military combat medical structure, it is necessary to have a rudimentary understanding of conventional military combat organization. Although specific for an infantry combat unit, other US Army and Marine Corps maneuver combat units are similarly organized. Currently, although undergoing significant transformation, infantry soldiers are grouped in squads (led by a noncommissioned officer) of 10 men, with four squads in a platoon (led by a lieutenant). An infantry company, commanded by a captain, consists of four such platoons, with additional soldiers in leadership and staff positions. Five companies of similar composition constitute an infantry battalion (commanded by a lieutenant colonel), and three to five battalions make up a brigade. Other units of platoon, company, or battalion size are attached to this brigade to form a brigade combat team (commanded by a colonel), giving this team the necessary equipment, additional specialized weapons systems, logistics support, and soldiers to conduct independent combat operations. A typical brigade combat team has approximately 4000 to 5000 soldiers. Several brigade combat teams can be grouped under a division (commanded by a two-star general), and several divisions can be grouped under a corps headquarters (commanded by a three-star general). The combat medical structure necessarily parallels this organization. Specifically, combat medics (level 1), found in an infantry company, are often assigned down to the squad and platoon level as necessary to support combat patrols and missions. The Battalion Aid Station (BAS, level 1), found at the battalion level, is the collection point for casualties from the different companies and the first level at which physicians or physician assistants are found. At the brigade level, the medical company (referred to as Charlie Med, level 2), with radiography, laboratory, and casualty holding capability, often augmented by a Forward Surgical Team (FST, level 2+) in the maneuver phase of the combat operation, is the first surgical capability found on the battlefield. Combat Support Hospitals (CSHs) are generally found in support of a division's several brigade combat teams (level 3). Specially augmented CSHs (level 4) are found at and above the corps and are generally far removed from actual combat operations. Finally, level 5 care is found in continental United States–based military medical centers.

Overview

In the ensuing paragraphs, a brief overview of battlefield medical care is presented. Although this overview is most typical of the capabilities found in the US Army Combat Health Care System, the setup is typical of the ground forces of all three services (Army, Navy [which includes the Marine Corps], and Air Force). Each level is elaborated on more fully in the remainder of this article, although the levels most closely associated with the combat zone (levels 1, 2, and 3) are presented in greater detail. Combat medical care occurs in a continuum, starting at the location of the combat wound and extending back to stateside medical centers. "Levels of medical care describe the five levels of treatment within the military health care system. Each level has the same capabilities as the level before it, but adds a new treatment capability that distinguishes it from the previous level" [2]. Care is usually initiated by the wounded soldier's compatriots, a combat lifesaver, or the combat medic (military occupational specialty designation 91W) assigned to that particular combat unit. This care is commonly referred to as level 1 care. Level 1 care continues at the BAS, a casualty collection point where physicians or physician assistants are first found and are capable of delivering Advanced Trauma Life Support care. Level 2 care begins at the brigade level where the Charlie Med, with basic radiography, laboratory, and holding capability, first appears. In recent decades, the FST has been inserted as level 2+ care, which introduces resuscitative surgical care to the battlefield and augments the Charlie Med. The CSH is the first surgical hospital capability and is designated as level 3 care. CSHs can add different modules to enhance surgical and other medical modality care and can constitute level 4 care. Level 4 capability can also be found outside of the immediate vicinity of the combat theater. Landstuhl Army Regional Medical Center in Germany functions as a level 4 hospital in support of the current combat theater. Finally, level 5 care includes stateside Army Medical Centers (AMC) like Walter Reed AMC, Brooke AMC, Madigan AMC, William Beaumont AMC, and Dwight David Eisenhower AMC. Particularly at Walter Reed AMC and Brooke AMC, definitive care and rehabilitation of war wounded have become a significant focus of those respective facilities.

Levels of care

Level 1

The concept of fellow soldiers or assigned combat medics providing lifesaving care at the forward location of wounding is a concept that was not always doctrinally accepted by the US Army Medical Department. Following the Civil War, the combat medic became a more constant presence on the battlefields of the United States. The combat medic has historically been expected to render immediate first aid, including stopping bleeding, splinting fractures, dressing wounds, and administering pain medication. The use of intravenous fluids was introduced during World War II, with the use of plasma. During the Korean and Vietnam Wars, medics were also able to give crystalloid fluids. Antibiotic powder was introduced during World War II and has occasionally been part of the armamentarium of combat medics. Medical training for the common soldier has also been a staple of army training since the First World War, with significant emphasis in the past 2 decades. The emphasis of this training has been similar to that of combat medics: control of hemorrhage, wound dressing, and fracture splinting. Although there have been several attempts over the history of the Army Medical Department to collect information with respect to wounding and the common causes of death on the battlefield, the picture of precisely what kills soldiers on the modern battlefield did not emerge until COL (Retired) Ron Bellamy [3] published his landmark article in 1984. Although the database used by COL Bellamy was specifically designed to evaluate the effects of certain weapons on the human body, he used the data to give a clearer picture of why soldiers die. Although many of the reasons for death on the battlefield were not surprising, a startling discovery was the percentage of potentially preventable deaths from extremity hemorrhage, from apparently unsuspected tension pneumothorax, and from airway obstruction. These revelations, along with further observations of possibly preventable deaths that occurred during combat operations since the Vietnam War, began a transformation in the Army Medical Department educational system for combat medics. In addition, combat lifesavers, a group of nonmedical soldiers who receive additional training in initial combat wounding care, were trained in more advanced first aid techniques. A shift toward placing a greater capability for dealing with hemorrhage, pneumothorax, and airway problems in the hands of combat medics began. With the advent of the current Global War on Terrorism, including Operation Enduring Freedom (OEF) in Afghanistan and Operation Iraqi Freedom (OIF) in Iraq, combat medics have been given more advanced tools, with a focus on hemorrhage control [4]. For example, in the past, the use of an extremity tourniquet was frequently taught to be the procedure of last resort after direct pressure and other methods to control bleeding were exhausted. This teaching has been modified significantly, with tourniquet control of bleeding extremity wounds often being used as the initial hemorrhage control method. Hemorrhage control of wounds not amenable to tourniquet application has also undergone intense research over the past decade [5]. Medics are now supplied with "active" dressings designed to control bleeding in these previously often-fatal wounds. Training for combat medics in the control of a compromised airway and treatment for tension pneumothorax, along with the necessary equipment for both, is ongoing. Given the historically high rate ($\sim 20\%$) of soldiers who are killed in action, this focus on the combat medic seems to have had an impact on the killed-in-action rates in the current war, with the current rate almost 25% lower (approximately 15% overall). Augmenting the level 1 care provided by combat medics is the closely located BAS, the first medical treatment facility found in the combat military health care system. The BAS acts as a casualty collection point and is staffed with primary care physicians, emergency medicine physicians, or physician assistants. This continuation of level 1 care brings Advanced Trauma Life Support capabilities close to the battle and provides further stabilization and resuscitation to allow further transport through the medical system.

Level 2

After a wounded soldier has been initially treated and stabilized by the combat medic and the BAS (level 1) to the extent possible, the wounded soldier's next stop depends on the tactical situation and the available assets for transport to the next level of care. Air and ground ambulances provide this transport capability. In general, when the patient is deemed stable enough to tolerate transport and it is likely that surgery is necessary, the patient is transported to the nearest level 3 facility (CSH), bypassing level 2. When the patient is too unstable to travel the distance to a CSH or does not require further resuscitation or surgery, the patient is transported to the nearest level 2 facility. This facility will typically be a brigade-level Charlie Med, with similar professional capabilities (primary care or emergency medicine physicians) as the BAS but with additional equipment including basic radiography, laboratory, and holding capability. In a highly mobile battlefield, the distances involved and the potential delay in obtaining lifesaving surgical care at the CSH spawned the development of FSTs. FSTs are attached to the Charlie Med at the brigade level and are typically attached to the combat maneuver brigades involved in the rapidly moving battle. This highly mobile level 2 capability is a 20-man team consisting of 4 surgeons and the necessary support soldiers and equipment to perform lifesaving surgery on wounded who would not survive transport to the next level of care (level 3, CSH). Up to 50 units of packed red blood cells are carried with the unit. Various "soft" shelters including special rapidly erectable tents are used for the triage/resuscitation, operating, and recovery areas (Fig. 1). The FST is 100% mobile and capable of setting up quickly (Fig. 2). In addition, they are also capable of breaking down quickly and following closely behind the battle. Not all casualties presented to the FST who require surgery undergo surgery at that location. Only those wounded soldiers deemed too unstable to survive transport to level 3 facility undergo intervention at the FST. Even those patients who are operated on at the FST rarely undergo extensive operations. Damage-control procedures for the control of bleeding, minimizing contamination, and restoring blood flow to compromised extremities are rapidly performed. FSTs fielded at the onset of Operation Iraqi Freedom were provided with specially equipped vehicles capable of providing chemically sealed self-inflating shelters, allowing operations in a contaminated (chemical, biological, or nuclear warfare) environment. After the patient is resuscitated and stable enough to survive transport, she is then rapidly evacuated to the next level of care.

Level 3

The first level of full surgical and hospital capability occurs at level 3, the CSH. In the past, various levels of theater hospitals were available. As recently as Desert Storm (1991), the Mobile Surgical Hospital, the CSH, the Evacuation Hospital, the Field Hospital, and the General Hospital—each different in configuration and capability—were found at different levels

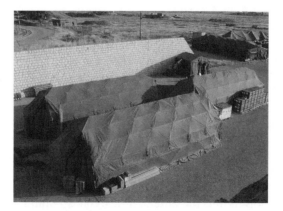

Fig. 1. FST setup in three rapidly deployable tents.

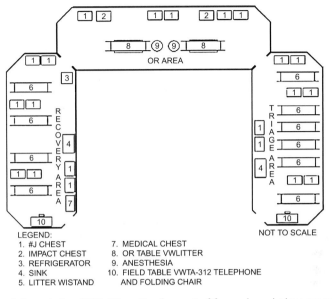

Fig. 2. Sample layout of an FST. (*From* Employment of forward surgical teams: tactics, techniques and procedures. FM 4–02.25. Washington, DC: Headquarters, Department of the Army; 2003.)

within the combat theater. Although the last active Mobile Surgical Hospital (the 212th Mobile Surgical Hospital) was effectively deployed during the initial maneuver phase of OIF, the US Army has moved to a single, modular hospital—the current Medical Re-engineering Initiative (MRI) CSH. The basic configuration is a 248-bed facility consisting of composite endoskeleton modular tentage (temper tents) with climate control, lighting, and water and power systems. Initial triage, resuscitation, and patient holding capacity including ICUs, intermediate care wards (ICWs), and minimal care wards are contained in various-sized "sections" of these temper tents. Eight-section temper tents provide a standard-sized 12-patient ICU or a 20-patient ICW. These tents interconnect with uniquely designed International Organization for Standards shelters, which are expandable metal "boxes" in which completely contained operating theaters, radiography (including CT), laboratory (including blood banking), and pharmacy operations are performed. This entire system is known as DEPMEDS (**dep**loyable **med**ical systems). This transportable and entirely self-contained and self-sufficient hospital has a modular design that allows the appropriate number of beds to support the medical mission assigned. Modules of the MRI CSH allow a 44-bed, an 84-bed, a 164-bed, and a full 248-bed configuration as needed. Fig. 3 is a photograph of an 84-bed CSH currently being used in Iraq. The full 248-bed hospital has six operating room tables capable of providing 96 hours of operating capability daily. The professional capability of the basic

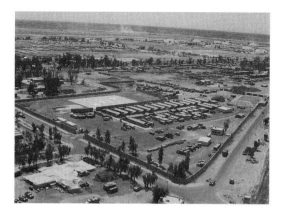

Fig. 3. Photograph of an 84-bed CSH in Iraq.

CSH includes general, thoracic, orthopedic, and oral and maxillofacial surgeons; anesthesia providers (anesthesiologists and nurse anesthetists); internists; emergency medicine physicians; other primary care physicians; a radiologist; and a psychiatrist. This professional capability can be augmented as necessary (see the level 4 section that follows). Approximately 500 soldiers are assigned to an MRI CSH and provide the necessary medical and support activities required to carry out the broad spectrum of level 3 medical care.

Level 4

This same MRI CSH, in the 248-bed configuration, also provides the next level of care in the military health care system. Typically located in the communications zone, far from the area of active combat operations, the 248-bed hospital is augmented by various modules that easily integrate into the existing structure. Most commonly, a head and neck augmentation team is added, which provides neurosurgical, eye, ear, nose, and throat surgery capabilities. Renal dialysis and infectious disease modules are also available, as is the special-care module that includes pediatric, family practice, preventive medicine, obstetrics/gynecology, and community nursing services. A pathology module is also available to provide anatomic pathology services and enhanced laboratory and microbiology capabilities as needed. Finally, a minimal-care module provides additional holding capacity, rehabilitation services, nutritional care support, and emergency nursing augmentation along with administrative support that might be needed by this larger CSH. When the tactical situation does not permit establishing a level 4 facility in the region of combat operations, level 4 care may require fixed-wing transport to a location and fixed facility far removed from the combat zone. Currently, Landstuhl Army Regional Medical Center in Germany functions as a level 4 facility for both OIF and OEF.

Level 5

The highest level of care available for combat wounded is in the United States, which is the final destination for soldiers who cannot be returned to duty. Typically, these casualties include those who undergo major abdominal, thoracic, vascular, brain, head and neck (including eye), and extremity operations and treatment for major burns. They may require prolonged intensive care or rehabilitation at the military's Centers of Excellence for Extremity wound care. This care may extend to the Veterans Administration Health Care System for soldiers unable to continue on active duty. The ultimate goal is to reintegrate these individuals into society with the highest level of function possible.

Medical evacuation

The five levels of care function as a continuum due to the capability of the medical evacuation system to deliver casualties from a lower level to a higher level of care without a decrement in the casualty's condition. Ground evacuation is available on the battlefield, and these vehicles assist in evacuating casualties from the site of wounding back to the first medical treatment facility available. Casualties are stabilized and evacuated to the next level of care as soon as possible. Often, helicopter evacuation is available to take seriously wounded soldiers from the site of wounding directly to level 2 care (Charlie Med or FST if the patients would not survive transport to the CSH) or level 3 care (CSH). Patients evacuated in this manner by ground and by air are kept stable by the accompanying combat medics; however, treatment (other than emergent airway, breathing, or hemorrhage control) en route is extremely difficult on the aforementioned evacuation platforms. This form of evacuation is labeled casualty evacuation (CASEVAC). After patients arrive at level 3, they undergo the appropriate surgery to resuscitate and stabilize them for transport to level 4, which in the current theater is Landstuhl Army Regional Medical Center in Germany. The evacuation times by fixed-wing transport aircraft (US Air Force) can be up to 10 to 12 hours. This form of evacuation is labeled medical evacuation (MEDEVAC). Before the Global War on Terrorism, limited en route care during MEDEVAC was available. Severely wounded patients who could be stabilized [6] but not rendered absolutely stable could not be transported unless accompanied by a physician capable of providing surgical critical care (typically a general surgeon from the sending hospital). Lessons learned from the previous conflicts (particularly from Somolia) contributed to the transformation of the MEDEVAC system, with the development and introduction of the CCATT (phonetically referred to as "see cat team") [7]. The CCATT is a three-person team that includes a physician (usually one with critical care skills—typically a general surgeon, an anesthesiologist, or a pulmonary-critical care physician), a respiratory therapist, and a critical care nurse. Critically ill, stabilized patients are routinely transported from Iraq to Germany with excellent results and safety. It is not unusual for a critically ill patient who has a temporary abdominal closure and who is on a ventilator to undergo transport in the hands of a CCATT. At the level 4 fixed facility, patients are further cared for until well enough to undergo MEDEVAC back to the United States for ultimate recovery and rehabilitation.

Medical logistics

Although medical assets (from combat medics to CSHs) are required to carry enough medical supplies to perform their missions during the initial phase of combat operations, this effort cannot be sustained without almost immediate resupply. During the maneuver phase of combat, resupply can prove extremely challenging because of the rapid movement and vast distances covered on the modern-day battlefield. Medical equipment, supplies, and blood are handled entirely separately from the rest of the logistic needs of the US Army (ammunition, fuel, food, water, repair parts, and so forth), with entire units devoted to medical logistics resupply. Medical supply specialists are found at each level of care (1–5) to ensure that each level's unique requirements are filled in a timely manner. Points of delivery and distribution are established, and entire information systems including satellite uplinks are dedicated to this mission. Ultimately, success of the medical mission depends on timely and appropriate medical resupply.

Command and control

Although having appropriate medical assets (with the ability to deliver the five levels of medical care), a logistics stream, and evacuation capabilities is essential to deliver world-class combat casualty care, it is not sufficient. Coordinating this effort in the most chaotic environment imaginable is essential to mission success. The Medical Brigade (MB) is the unit responsible for orchestrating this effort. The MB is the headquarters with the staff and communications assets necessary to coordinate the main-theater medical plan, including the deployable hospitals, evacuation assets, and medical logistics resupply system. The MB commander generally works directly for the theater commander as his senior medical officer and typically advises the theater commander on theater hospitalization and medical care. In conjunction with the combat maneuver brigades (who own all of the level 1 and much of the level 2 assets), it falls to the MB to ensure that level 3 assets are properly deployed to support the war fight and help coordinate FST placement in the theater. In addition, the MB is responsible for medical regulation throughout the theater of operations. Medical regulation involves identifying patients requiring evacuation, coordinating this evacuation using appropriate assets (ground transportation, helicopter, or fixed-wing aircraft), and ensuring that patients are appropriately distributed to facilities with the appropriate capacity and type of medical care required by those patients. Before the Global War on Terrorism, most coordination by the MB was done without direct input from physicians trained in trauma systems. Recently, an initiative has been instituted to place a senior clinician (specifically a general/trauma surgeon) on the MB commander's staff to specifically develop and organize a theater trauma system. The first phase of this initiative focused on data acquisition. It has always been extremely difficult to obtain prospective data on combat casualties, so to accomplish this, a data sheet was developed that would capture the essential data points of combat wounded (Fig. 4). Using

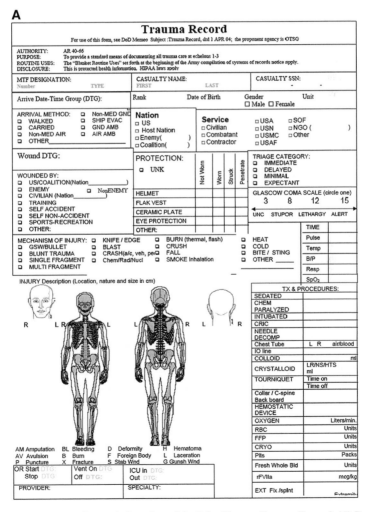

Fig. 4. (*A*) Front page of an early iteration of the Joint Theater Trauma Record. (*B*) Back page of an early iteration of the Joint Theater Trauma Record.

B

Trauma Record DISCHARGE SUMMARY

MEDICATIONS:	LABS:	XRAYS:	PMH: Allergies:

REGION	DIAGNOSIS, PROCEDURES and COMPLICATONS
Face	
Head & Neck (incl C-spine)	
Chest (incl T-spine)	
Abdomen (incl L-spine)	
Pelvis	
UPPER /LOWER Extremities	
Skin	

DISPOSTION DTG:	□ EVAC to _____ □ RTD □ DECEASED (see below)	Evacuation Priority □ ROUTINE □ PRIORITY □ URGENT

Damage Control Procedures? Y / N   Hypothermic (< 34°C)? Y / N   Coagulopathy?   Y / N

Cause of Death at _DTG_____.

ANATOMIC:
□Airway □Head □ Neck □ Chest □Abdomen □Pelvis □ Extremity (Upper/Lower)
□Other

PHYSIOLOGIC:
□ Breathing □CNS □Hemorrhage □Total Body Disruption □Sepsis □Multi-organ failure

COMMENTS:	SURGEON: (printedName)

MEDCOM Test Form 1381, JAN 2004

Fig. 4 *(continued)*

what is known as the Joint Theater Trauma Record (JTTR), initial data was retrospectively abstracted from the busiest CSHs in the theater by reviewing patient records. Then, similar to stateside trauma centers, each CSH was staffed with a trauma nurse coordinator whose principle job was to insure that the JTTR was being properly filled out, in addition to collecting the information from the JTTR and forwarding it to the trauma surgeon at the MB for collation and analysis. Virtually all casualties in the current conflict have been abstracted from records or prospectively recorded, giving a real-time picture of wounding types and rates and some insight into causes of mortality. Ongoing evaluation of autopsy data of war dead has given additional insight into the principle causes of death in this conflict, with the main focus on analyzing potentially preventable deaths. Using the JTTR and the autopsy information, medical training for deploying medical soldiers can and has been tailored to reflect current conditions.

Disaster relief

The actual practice of medicine on the battlefield, especially as it pertains to trauma care, is similar to the care available in trauma systems around the United States. What is unique, however, is the fact that this care can be projected and sustained in the most austere and remote locations on the earth and can be conducted under extremely chaotic and hazardous conditions. The combat military health care system has been developed over its 2 centuries of responding to the nation's wars in foreign and domestic settings. As previously described, this care is tiered so that casualties receive care almost immediately after wounding and are rapidly returned to duty or continued along the continuum of care until they reach the level appropriate to their medical need. By necessity, the military health care system has developed the appropriate structure and command/control to be rapidly deployable, mobile, modular, flexible, and sustainable in almost any environment. These qualities also allow the military medical system to respond to noncombat disasters. Many national and international disasters in the past, natural and manmade, have required a rapid medical response. There is no organization comparable to and as capable as the United States military in responding to and providing the medical care necessary in such scenarios. As has been extensively described in the previous text, the military medical structure can be configured, mobilized, and deployed forward with the appropriate medical, evacuation, and logistics assets along with the necessary command and control elements to rapidly respond to virtually any medical need. As recently as the disaster resulting from hurricane Katrina, the military, when alerted, had medical assets on the ground and functioning within 48 hours. No other local, state, or federal agency had the capability of responding in a similar manner. Over the past decade, military medical systems have had the opportunity to train such deployments and have been deployed on many occasions for combat and noncombat medical operations. Most medical soldiers used in the Katrina response had recently returned from Operation Enduring Freedom/Operation Iraqi Freedom or were awaiting departure for the current combat theater.

Summary

Combat medical care has evolved since the Revolutionary war to its current state in the midst of the Global War on Terrorism. The five levels of care have been designed to ensure that our combat wounded receive immediate and lifesaving treatment virtually at the moment of wounding and that this care continues with safe and timely evacuation until final recovery and rehabilitation is completed. The ability to place and sustain this system of care in any location and environment and to coordinate the many elements necessary for effective health care delivery is the precise mission that military medicine is uniquely designed to accomplish. Given this capability and the current tempo of disasters (manmade and natural), it is likely that our military medical forces will have many opportunities in the future to project this care at home and around the globe.

References

[1] Kuz JE. The ABJS presidential lecture, June 2004: our orthopaedic heritage: the American Civil War. Clin Orthop 2004;429:306–15.
[2] Health service support in corps and echelons above corps. FM 4-02.12. Washington, DC: Headquarters, Department of the Army; 2003.
[3] Bellamy RF. The causes of death in conventional land warfare: implications for combat casualty research. Mil Med 1984;149:55–62.
[4] Basu S. First aid skills revised for soldiers. US Med 2005;41(5).
[5] Holcomb J, MacPhee M, Hetz SP, et al. Efficacy of a dry fibrin sealant dressing for hemorrhage control after ballistic injury. Archives of Surgery 1998;133:32–5.
[6] Burris DG, Hetz SP, Holcomb JB, et al. Emergency war surgery. In: Third United States Revision. Washington, DC: Borden Institute; 2004. p. 4.7.
[7] Chishom P. Critical care in the sky. Mil Med Technol 2006;10(1).

ELSEVIER
SAUNDERS

SURGICAL
CLINICS OF
NORTH AMERICA

Surg Clin N Am 86 (2006) 689–709

United States Military Surgical Response to Modern Large-Scale Conflicts: The Ongoing Evolution of a Trauma System

MAJ Alec C. Beekley, MD

*Madigan Army Medical Center, 9040 Fitzsimmons Avenue, Fort Lewis,
Tacoma, WA 98431, USA*

In the past 15 years, the United States military has been involved in conflicts that have varied in size from small peacekeeping and stabilization missions, such as Operation Restore Hope in Somalia, to large-scale conflicts such as Operation Desert Shield/Desert Storm and Operation Iraqi Freedom. Several operations have fallen somewhere in the middle in terms of scale, such as Operations Uphold and Restore Democracy in Haiti, peacekeeping and stabilization operations in Balkans, and Operation Enduring Freedom. In Operations Uphold and Restore Democracy, the geographic area and amount of combat involved was small, but the number of troops involved was large (22,000 multinational troops, of which approximately 20,000 were from the United States) [1]. Operation Enduring Freedom was large in terms of geographic areas involved and political and military goals set, but small in terms of number of United States military forces committed. The global and domestic political impacts of these missions have varied (eg, Operation Restore Hope in Somalia, Operation Enduring Freedom in Afghanistan), and this and the success of the missions are not always commensurate with the number of troops involved.

Hence, differentiating a large-scale conflict from one of a smaller scale is sometimes difficult. This article analyzes the United States military's trauma

---

The views expressed in this paper are those of the author and do not reflect the official policy or position of the Department of the Army, the Department of Defense, or the United States Government.

E-mail address: alec.beekley@amedd.army.mil

surgical.theclinics.com

surgical posture and response to large-scale conflicts. For the purpose of this analysis, *modern large-scale conflicts* is defined as

1. Conflicts that occurred after 1990
2. Conflicts involving more than 50,000 United States or coalition combatants
3. Conflicts involving invasion of foreign soil during United States military combat operations

Using these definitions, the large-scale conflicts that meet these criteria are Operations Desert Shield/Desert Storm and Operation Iraqi Freedom. This article provides a brief description of the evolution of trauma surgical care since Desert Storm and the ongoing evolution of the trauma system in Operation Iraqi Freedom.

Operations Desert Shield and Desert Storm

Operations Desert Shield and Desert Storm were the first massive deployment of United States Military personnel since the Vietnam era, with more than 200,000 personnel deployed for Desert Shield and more than 500,000 for Desert Storm. At the start of Desert Storm, 44 hospitals were set up in Saudi Arabia and other supporting Gulf states to support the coalition's military efforts (COL William E. Eggebroten, MD, MC, USA, personal communication, 2005). The hospital support consisted of four types of facilities: the combat support hospital (CSH), field hospital, evacuation hospital, and general hospital. Frequently, the hospitals were large (a Desert Storm-era CSH had 296 beds), and one criticism of these units was that they were too cumbersome to meet the mobility needs of the modern combat maneuver elements and too heavy to airlift in concert with combat units [2]. Hence, they were frequently left in the far rear of the advancing ground forces, lengthening evacuation times and distances. Because of size and mobility issues, Field, evacuation, and general hospitals were decommissioned after Desert Storm and a single, modular concept, the medical re-engineering initiative (MRI) CSH was instituted. This MRI CSH was designed to provide improved mobility and flexibility and is well described elsewhere in this issue.

Before Desert Storm, mobile Army surgical hospitals (MASHs) provided forward surgery. As King and Jatoi [4] point out in their thorough review of the evolution of the MASH, auxiliary surgery groups (ASGs), consisting of small detachments of surgeons, anesthesiologists, surgical nurses, and technicians from a larger evacuation hospital, were created during World War II to provide resuscitative surgical support a few miles from the front lines. These installations showed improved outcomes and enabled the salvage of previously unsalvageable, severely wounded casualties. These units gradually evolved into the concept of the MASH unit used during the Korean and Vietnam Wars and are the grandfathers of the modern forward surgical teams (FSTs) and forward resuscitative surgical systems (FRSSs).

During Desert Storm, the MASH, made famous in the 1970s television program of the same name, was a 60-bed hospital that required 24 hours to establish full trauma support services. This unit also required ships or multiple aircraft to deploy into theater, and substantial ground transportation assets to be truly mobile. To move a 60-bed MASH required "organic transport to haul 63 containers configured in fifty 40-foot truckloads" [9]. Another drawback of trauma surgical care during Operation Desert Storm was the inability of the MASH to keep up with the accelerated pace of modern mechanized and armor combat operations [2,3]. The "quick fix" response during the Gulf War itself was to break up the MASH into smaller units to improve mobility and keep pace with the maneuver units. Hence, the MASH was divided into the FST, an approximately 20-person, two-operating table unit designed to advance just behind the maneuver elements and be prepared to perform resuscitative surgery within 2 hours; the forward surgical element (FSE), a larger forward surgical unit (110 persons, four operating tables) designed for more robust and sustained trauma surgical support; the MASH(-), a 36-bed hospital with 3 to 4 operating tables that was intended to be a more rapid and streamlined version of the full MASH; and the main body of the MASH, a 60-bed, 6-operating table, full-service medical and surgical unit [4].

The 5th MASH is one example of the creation and use of MASH subunits. The 5th MASH FSE was the first such unit to deploy into Iraq during Desert Storm, and sustained operations for 48 hours. This FSE then rejoined the 5th MASH(-), advanced further with the ground troops, and remained in Iraq for 7 days. Finally, an FST from the 5th MASH deployed and moved deeper into Iraq and remained operational for 1 week [4]. The success of these units and segments of units validated the concept of these smaller, highly mobile teams and served as the templates for the modern FST. The 212th MASH, deployed to Iraq at the beginning of Operation Iraqi Freedom, is the only unit that remains active. As recently as October 2005, it deployed to Pakistan to provide humanitarian assistance (earthquake relief) (MAJ Tommy Brown, MD, MC, USA, personal communication, 2005).

The history of the World War II-era ASGs and the MASH shows that the concept of far-forward resuscitative surgery is not new to the military. What is new during warfare over the past 15 years is the pace and distance combat maneuver elements travel to engage the enemy. Use of and response to *asymmetric warfare*, defined as "the leveraging of inferior tactical or operational strength against a nation's vulnerabilities to achieve disproportionate effect with the aim of undermining a nation's will to achieve the asymmetric actor's strategic objectives" [5], requires increasingly mobile and flexible trauma surgical support to a degree not historically seen.

The anticipated large numbers of casualties (25,000–65,000) from Operations Desert Shield and Desert Storm did not materialize. An estimated 382 total coalition military deaths occurred. The Department of Defense reported that United States forces had 148 battle-related and 145 non–battle-related deaths and 467 wounded in action [6]. The United Kingdom had 47 deaths, the supporting Arab states had about 40 killed, and the French had 2 killed in action. Total coalition wounded was estimated as fewer than 1000 [7–9]. Most reviews found that the combat casualty care provided was adequate. However, a more thorough review by United States congressional analysts found substantial deficiencies in training, evacuation, communications, and mobility of medical units, which might have caused suboptimal combat casualty care if casualty rates met the predicted levels [10].

Analysis of the limited number of wounded personnel from Desert Storm provided vital information regarding body armor and casualty care. First, compared with prior wars, Desert Storm had smaller percentages of casualties with severe wounds to the head and chest and a concomitant increase in casualties with severe wounds to the extremities. This predominance of extremity injuries was documented by the US Army's Casualty Data Assessment Team (CDAT) and in Carey's [11] review of US Army's Seventh Corps' wounded personnel [11]. This shift in wound location was attributed to improvements in helmets and body armor and to the predominance of wounds from fragmentation munitions (95%) compared with gunshot wounds (5%). Carey's analysis of wounded personnel showed an even higher percentage of extremity injuries than the CDAT, and an unexpected finding that the predominant cause of death for patients treated at Seventh Corps Hospitals was exsanguinating extremity wounds.

These identified problems with prehospital and inhospital compressible hemorrhage control were consistent with Bellamy's [12,13] landmark findings from his analysis of killed-in-action personnel from Vietnam, and the experiences reported by Mabry and colleagues [14] and Holcomb [15] 2 years later involving casualties from the Battle of the Black Sea in Mogadishu, Somalia. The focus on compressible extremity hemorrhage as the main cause of preventable deaths in wounded soldiers continued to drive Army research for the decade leading up to Operations Enduring and Iraqi Freedom.

Operation Iraqi Freedom

Operation Iraqi Freedom can be divided into two phases.

First phase—maneuver warfare

The first phase was the primary invasion and maneuver phase, which lasted from March 19, 2003, to May 1, 2003, when President George W. Bush announced the completion of main combat operations. This phase featured the initial air bombardment of key Iraqi military formations, installations, communications, and command centers, combined with a rapid ground phase that placed armor, infantry, and marine units around Baghdad. The expected intense, urban, house-to-house infantry fighting for the capital did not materialize, primarily because of the "thunder runs" up

Highway 8 in mid-April 2003 by the 2nd Brigade (Spartan Brigade) of the 3rd Infantry (Mechanized). These runs first went to Baghdad International Airport (which had already been captured by American forces), then into the heart of Baghdad 3 days later to seize and hold Saddam Hussein's seat of power. This bold and unprecedented use of combined arms centered on an armor formation, effectively toppling Hussein's regime [16].

Role of level II surgical units in the first phase

Army FSTs and Marine FRSSs provided initial trauma surgical support for the rapidly advancing ground forces. The composition and organization of these forward surgical units is well described in the published literature [3,17–19] and in this issue. In their article on the experience of the 555th FST, Patel and colleagues [18] provide one of the best descriptions of a US Army FST's employment during this early maneuver phase (assigned to the Spartan Brigade). In a 23-day period, the authors evaluated 154 casualties and performed 25 major operations. Although most of these operations consisted of extremity wound irrigation and debridements, applications of external fixators, or debridement amputations, several damage-control abdominal operations and several vascular repairs were performed. Patel documented that during approximately the first 10 days of the conflict, the nearest higher echelon of surgical support was located at the Kuwaiti border, which was more than a 1-hour flight by helicopter [18].

Bohman and colleagues [20] presented the experience of six Marine FRSSs in the first phase of Operation Iraqi Freedom. These FRSSs teams were designated as *forward* or *jump* teams, depending on their role. The forward FRSSs operated 5 to 15 km from the battlefield and served much in the same manner as the Army FSTs, whereas the jump FRSSs were subunits of a larger Marine surgical company that would establish preliminary surgical support 2 to 3 days before the surgical company arrived. These jump FRSS teams were usually located farther from the combat (∼20 km), and therefore evacuation times to these units were longer and the acuity of patients lower. The number and distribution of injuries encountered at these units were comparable to those documented by Patel and colleagues [18]. Casualties treated at these units were evacuated to a Marine Alpha Surgical Company, which, like the Army Combat Support Hospitals, was located in Kuwait for the maneuver phase of the war [19]. Bohman and colleagues concluded that the presence of the FRSS teams decreased evacuation times of seriously wounded casualties, and the combination of the FRSSs with a Shock Trauma Platoon (STP), which was essentially a mobile emergency medicine team, enhanced the FRSS's capability [20]. The Marine FRSS/STP teams and Army FSTs likely provided the best chance for life and limb salvage for many of the patients treated in this early phase of the war.

Far-forward deployments of surgical assets during the first (maneuver) phase were designed to positively influence the morbidity and mortality of casualties wounded in action. These deployments had some risk for combat loss of these assets, and the forward surgical units were occasionally required to engage in activities outside the traditional roles of past surgical units. For example, two Army FSTs (the 250th and the 274th) are designated airborne units, capable of jumping with maneuver elements into combat zones. The 250th FST performed an airborne jump with combat units of the 173rd Infantry, the first airborne insertion of an FST since World War II [21]. In one of the most dramatic cases, members of the 555th FST took seven prisoners of war and cleared a mosque of numerous enemy weapon systems [18]. A reserve FST, the 915th, was required to move seven times in 4 months (most of the moves occurring in the first month), taking down their equipment and quickly setting it up again after the move in preparation for casualties (MAJ Daniel Hamre, MD, MC, USAR, personal communication, 2003).

Many of these units experienced direct fire from small arms and rocket-propelled grenades, and indirect fire from mortars and rockets. On July 3, 2003, an incoming mortar round struck the camouflage netting of the 915th FST, a reserve unit from the Pacific Northwest, injuring 14 of the 20 soldiers in the unit, including the commander [24]. On March 20, 2004, two members of the 782nd FST, LTC Mark Taylor, a general surgeon, and Specialist Matthew J. Sandri, a medic and scrub technician, were killed during a rocket attack near Al Fallujah, Iraq [26,27]. These dead and wounded medical personnel emphasize the need to develop or use hardened facilities whenever possible when forward surgical units are placed in stable locations. For example, the 912th FST was able to use a deserted office building in their location near Al Mussayib. This reinforced concrete building protected team members during an attack in which eight mortar rounds landed directly on their position in June 2004. These experiences illustrate the danger to the theaters in the Global War on Terror and the need for FSTs to have adequate training in basic soldier skills and small unit tactics.

By the time the main maneuver phase was completed, 17 forward surgical units from active duty and reserve components were deployed into the theater. These units were typically under operational control (OPCON) of the combat maneuver commanders (at the brigade level), and kept pace with the line units and their direct supporting units. This arrangement allowed brigade combat team commanders to have far-forward trauma surgical support under their direct control during the violent and rapidly fluid maneuver phase. The continuation of this OPCON during the second, more static, and more prolonged phase of operations contributed to early redundancy and underuse of trauma surgical assets [22], which was gradually corrected as the theater matured and a joint theater trauma system was instituted.

Second phase—security and stabilization operations

The second phase of Operation Iraqi Freedom, which began after May 1, 2003, featured stability and support operations (SASOs) and counterinsurgency operations. In this phase, combat maneuver units established forward operating bases in individual areas of responsibility (AORs) to conduct these SASOs. The current insurgency developed and grew during this phase. In late 2003 and 2004, Operation Iraqi Freedom featured this growing and evolving insurgency, with United States military forces periodically returning to offensive combat operations, such as the Marine assault on Al Fallujah in April 2004, the joint military assault on An Najaf in August 2004, and the second Marine assault on Al Fallujah in November 2004, to name a few of the larger operations.

Role of level III surgical units in the second phase

During this second phase of operations, CSHs were established in or near the cities of Mosul, Tikrit, Balad, Baghdad, and Tallil. In the fall of 2004, an Air Force Expeditionary Medical Group took over the level III mission in Balad because this was the main fixed-wing airfield for evacuation of casualties out of theater. These level III hospitals varied in size and capability to fit the support missions and expected casualties in the various AORs in Iraq and were based on the modular concept discussed previously. Some of these units (eg, 28th and 31st CSHs) used a deserted building as a hardened, fixed facility; for example, the deserted Ibn Sina Hospital in the "Green Zone" in central Baghdad was used by coalition forces as a combat support hospital (Fig. 1). The use of this facility provided improved security for CSH personnel from rocket and mortar attacks. In addition, the restoration of this facility will allow eventual turnover of a fully functional hospital to the Iraqi people. The 86th CSH, currently at the Ibn Sina Hospital, began a program to help train Iraqi medical students, residents, and fellows in trauma and emergency medical care (LTC Kelly Blair, MD, MC, USA, personal communication, 2005). The arrangement of hospitals provided robust trauma surgical support within a 1-hour helicopter flight for most of the theater. For areas of operation beyond a 1-hour helicopter flight to a CSH,

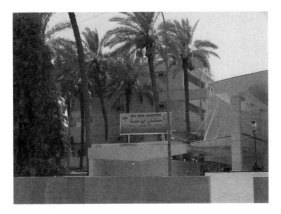

Fig. 1. The deserted Ibn Sina Hospital in the "Green Zone" in central Baghdad was converted into a Combat Support Hospital by coalition forces.

forward trauma surgical support remained in the form of an FST, an FRSS, or a combination of these elements.

Established air superiority, which coalition forces experienced from the onset of combat operations, is critical to the success of a combat theater trauma system. Air superiority has allowed rapid evacuation of casualties in theater from point of injury to surgical care (Fig. 2) and out of theater to level IV hospitals (the primary one being Landstuhl Regional Medical Center). This practice of rapidly moving casualties, even critically ill ones, out of theater has allowed the creation of more mobile surgical units and combat support hospitals with smaller "footprints" (ie, fewer personnel and physical structures and less equipment). Establishment of Air Force Critical Care Transport Teams, discussed elsewhere in this issue, has allowed critically ill casualties to have near state-of-the-art intensive care management during air transport on fixed-wing aircraft. Evacuation times from theater to level V hospitals in the continental United States decreased from an average of 8 days at the beginning of Operation Iraqi Freedom to an average of 4 days by early 2005. In extreme cases, this evacuation time has been as short as 36 hours [23].

Once CSHs were established, many casualties were flown directly to these hospitals from the battalion aid stations or even points of injury. Numbers of casualties treated at the level III hospitals far exceeded the numbers treated at FSEs (level II). For example, the 31st CSH, which divided its personnel and operations between facilities in Balad and Baghdad for part of its year deployment, treated more than 3400 trauma patients. Numbers of casualties reported by other CSHs are expected to be comparable. The shift of the casualty care burden from level II to level III facilities was an expected and desired result of instituting strategically-placed robust hospitals within a 1-hour flight of most areas in Iraq.

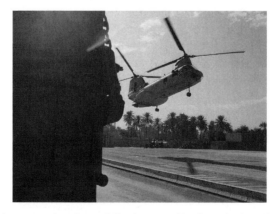

Fig. 2. Rotary wing evacuation shown delivering casualties from the front lines or FSTs to the 31st CSH at the Ibn Sina Hospital, Baghdad.

Role of level II surgical units in the second phase

Level II surgical assets (eg, FSTs) remained in Iraq under the control of maneuver brigade commanders, and these teams were usually positioned in their commanding brigades' tactical areas of operation [22]. These locations were often coincidentally well within the 1-hour flight radius of the combat support hospitals. For example, the 912th FST spent most of its 15 months in Iraq at Baghdad International Airport, a location that was approximately 5 minutes by helicopter and 15 minutes by ground to the 28th and later the 31st CSH, located in the Green Zone in downtown Baghdad. For the remainder of their time in Iraq, the 912th FST moved to the vicinity of Al Mussayib, which was still only about a 15-minute helicopter flight from the 31st CSH. Similarly, the 8th FST spent their nearly 12 months in Iraq in the vicinity of Babylon and Al Diwaniyah, approximately 30 to 35 minutes from the 31st CSH in Baghdad. In addition, they were only 10 miles from a Marine FRSS (MAJ James A. Sebesta, MD, MC, USA, personal communication, 2005). The 915th FST spent a short period of their deployment within 5 miles of the 250th FST and later moved onto the same base (Balad) as the 1st FST and the 21st CSH [24]. The 240th FST spent some of their deployment in Baqubah, approximately 30 miles northeast of Baghdad [25] (again, easily within a 1-hour helicopter flight of the 28th/31st CSH in Baghdad). As documented by Rush and colleagues [22], the 250th FST was co-located at Kirkuk Military Airfield with a 60-bed Air Force Expeditionary Medical Support (EMEDS) hospital.

The proximity of many of these forward surgical units to a more robust hospital resulted in frequent overflight of the forward units with consequent underuse of these assets. Reported months in theater and the operative caseloads of five forward surgical teams are listed in Table 1. Some of these data are derived from press reports or interviews and may not be entirely accurate. Many of these trauma operations occurred in clusters at specific times corresponding with active combat on the ground (eg, the Marine assault on Al Fallujah in April 2004). Large numbers of nontrauma operations were

Table 1
Numbers of surgical operations for select forward surgical teams

Unit	Months in theater	Total operations	Trauma operations
912th FST	15	355	103
2nd ACR FST	8	235	164[a]
250th FST [22]	11	59[b]	43
8th FST[c]	12	42	31
915th FST [28]	5	10	10
782nd FST [45]	3	16	16

Abbreviations: ACR FST, armored cavalry regiment forward surgical team; FST, forward surgical team.

[a] LTC Richard Ellison, MD, MC USA, personal communication, 2005.

[b] Does not include 105 operations performed in conjunction with Iraqi surgeons as part of a civil affairs/humanitarian assistance effort [22].

[c] MAJ James A. Sebesta, MD, MC USA, personal communication, 2005.

performed, many on Iraqi civilians, particularly in the 912th and 250th FSTs. The 250th FST's totals do not include 105 operations that were performed with local surgeons at two local public hospitals as part of a civil affairs and humanitarian assistance effort [22]. These initiatives helped build bridges to the local Iraqi communities while maintaining the surgical teams' skills. Overall, however, the number of trauma operations performed during the periods shown illustrate these teams' minor trauma surgical role for much of the time in theater during the second phase of operations.

The problems with FST locations involved not only the physical distances and evacuation times from the larger hospitals but also the small numbers of ongoing combat operations and casualties in some of the areas. The case numbers reflect this issue. FSTs positioned in more peaceful areas, such as the Kurdish-controlled north (250th FST) and the Shi'ite-controlled south (8th FST), had smaller trauma case loads than FSEs in the Sunni-dominated regions where insurgent activity was highest (912th FST and the Marine Surgical Shock Trauma Platoon [SSTP]).

The Marines' experience in Al Anbar province highlighted the advantage of a robust, task-oriented surgical unit being close to the action. The Marines combined two FRSS teams with an STP to create a Marine SSTP, a robust surgical element that resembles a MASH more than an FST. This element, positioned between Al Fallujah and Al Ramadi, had four surgeons (three general and one orthopaedic) and twice the support personnel of a single FRSS. Although positioned slightly more than 30 minutes by helicopter from the 31st Army CSH in Baghdad, this unit was task-oriented to support Marine combat operations in Al Fallujah and Al Ramadi. Casualty evacuation from the points of wounding occurred by ground and air and occasionally took 30 minutes or more because of tactical considerations or delays at level I facilities. The SSTP provided initial evaluation and treatment for more than 500 casualties over 6-months [46]. The Navy and Marine surgeons concluded in postdeployment analysis that several casualties treated at the SSTP probably would not have survived the additional 30-minute evacuation to the CSH. Whether the delays at level I facilities (some deemed avoidable and some unavoidable) would have allowed these casualties to survive the flight to the CSH is debatable. The Navy and Marine surgeons nevertheless concluded the sources of these level I delays must be identified and corrected (LCDR Lowell W. Chambers, MD, MC, USN, personal communication, 2005).

The perceived underuse of forward surgical units for trauma surgery has several implications. First, patient outcomes at small, lower-volume units may be poorer than higher-volume forward surgical units or CSHs. Unfortunately, rigorous scientific study of these correlations in a combat theater has limitations. Obstacles unique to the battlefield environment make accurate data collection difficult. These obstacles include incomplete or inaccurate data on mechanism of wounding, time to first treatment, evacuation times from point of wounding to initial surgical care, treatments administered, number of casualties treated at any time, and long-term outcomes in patients evacuated out of theater. Nevertheless, studies examining patient outcomes of these forward surgical units are ongoing, and some early results suggest that patient outcomes may be comparable to those for a similar patient population at a state-side level I trauma center, at least for augmented, four-surgeon teams (LCDR Lowell W. Chambers, MD, MC USN, personal communication, 2005). The same outcomes have not been shown to extend to smaller (two-surgeon) teams, and no data correlating patient volume to outcomes are available.

Several modern studies in civilian medical literature have suggested a positive correlation between hospital and physician volume and improved patient outcomes [28]. Admittedly, this correlation has not been as clear when specifically analyzing trauma patient outcomes, and the limitations in the ability to clearly study this correlation have been described [29–32]. However, fairly consistent positive correlations have been shown between the implementation of urban and state trauma systems and the reduction of injury-related mortality [33,34].

Most United States military surgeons with whom the author discussed combat trauma surgical experiences described a learning curve in developing the skills required to care for multiple casualties with severe penetrating wounds who arrive simultaneously. The surgeons believed this learning curve existed (to some degree) regardless of level of training. In fact, regarding the treatment of combat casualties, fellowship-trained trauma surgeons reported the same learning curve as non–fellowship trained general surgeons (COL Kenneth Azarow, MD, MC, USA, personal communication, 2005). This anecdotal evidence suggests a relationship between combat casualty volumes and providers' self-perceived proficiency in caring for these casualties. Although common sense would suggest that units and surgeons that treat higher volumes of combat casualties would have improved patient outcomes compared to lower volume units, the available data and literature is not yet conclusive. The relationship between hospital volume, surgeon experience, and trauma patient outcomes continues to be studied in military and civilian settings.

Current warfare in Iraq features an insurgency that uses improvised explosive devices, ambushes, and hit-and-run tactics as primary means of attack. This type of warfare creates casualties in discrete events, and therefore victims tend to arrive in groups rather than individually. As a result, surgical elements will have stretches of inactivity punctuated by multiple casualties arriving simultaneously. Regardless of the quality and training of the personnel, this scenario suggests that skills may degrade during slow periods, resulting in less streamlined performance of the team with each intense event.

These problems are often amplified by other factors, such as rotation of surgeons every 3 months on reserve FSTs, lack of continuous trauma exposure for active duty Army community hospital surgeons (and many Army tertiary medical center surgeons) during their nondeployed periods, and the occasional reduction of FSTs to only two general surgeons or having the FST perform *split operations*. A split operation divides an already small ($\sim$20-person) unit into even smaller units, providing only one to two surgeons and one operating table per FST segment. In this author's experience, the arrival of three to four seriously wounded casualties constitutes a mass casualty for a one- to two-surgeon FST. Current US Marine experience has shown that these smaller, one- to two-surgeon FSEs do not perform as well as four-surgeon units (LCDR Lowell W. Chambers, MD, MC, USN, personal communication, 2005).

Another problem with the FST redundancy is the "Field of Dreams" phenomenon, "if you build it, they will come" [35], even when evacuation to the closest unit is not necessarily best for a casualty. Early in the second phase of operations, the medics on the ground or in the evacuation helicopters often decided the location of a casualty's evacuation. Based on this author's experience, these personnel had varying degrees of guidance and training with which to make these decisions, and many medics tended to direct the casualty to the nearest surgical element. This decision caused some patients to be evacuated from the point of injury by helicopter and taken to an FST instead of directly to a CSH (which was frequently only another 5–20 minutes away). In a civilian scenario, this decision is comparable to evacuating a patient injured in a car accident to a small community hospital 15 minutes away rather than a level I trauma center 30 minutes away. Although skilled surgeons may be on call at the community hospital, these smaller hospitals are not equipped with the hospital system of level I trauma centers that enables improved patient outcomes. This system includes multiple, in-house, highly-trained subspecialty providers; robust blood bank support; and full ICU capabilities, all of which many community hospitals (and FSTs) have only in limited quantities.

The number of patients treated at level II facilities also amplified the problems with care on medical evacuation (MEDEVAC) transports between level II and level III facilities. These problems were particularly evident in patients who were critically injured and underwent post–damage control surgery (DCS). Anecdotal reports describe patients who were stabilized, normothermic, and post-DCS leaving level II facilities and being in extremis on arrival at level III facilities. Identified problems during transport have included loss of airway, tension pneumothorax, loss of critical intravenous lines, lack of adequate oxygen supply, and casualty heat loss. Frequently, the highest level of provider on helicopters carrying patients from FSTs or FRSSs to CSHs were combat medics who had varying degrees of skills and experience with which to recognize these problems. FSTs were often reluctant to release one or two certified registered nurse anesthetists (CRNAs), nurses, or surgeons to escort a patient on the helicopter, particularly when military operations were ongoing, for fear of compromising the team's ability to care for more trauma patients.

A study examining the effect of interfacility transfer on patient outcomes in an urban trauma system found that although mortality and length of stay were not necessarily affected, resource use was significantly higher for patients who required transfer between facilities. The investigators attributed this increase in resource requirements to the nature of the injuries or to "delays in reaching definitive care" [36]. They also note that "in...environments where transport times are relatively short, there is little doubt that there is a survival benefit associated with the bypass of nearer...centers in deference to the care provided at regional designated Level I centers" [36]. These conclusions are applicable to Iraq, particularly considering that small FSEs were located less than a 30-minute helicopter flight from a CSH.

The belief that the most proximate surgical element is the best place to take a casualty largely stems from continued reliance on the "golden hour" concept. However, few objective scientific data support this concept [37]. Martinowitz and colleagues [38], in their review and endorsement of pushing advanced hemorrhage control techniques (such as recombinant Factor VIIa) onto the battlefield, suggest that rather than a "golden hour," many combat casualties have only a "platinum 5 minutes." Bellamy's [12] data from the Vietnam War and Gofrit's [39] data from the Lebanon War suggest that after an initial group of injured individuals dies within 5 to 15 minutes of being wounded, many of the remaining trauma patients will have well more than an hour before they bleed to death. Other research suggests that the "golden hour" can likely be extended, at least in patients who have experienced blunt trauma [40]. Hence, current research has focused on extending the time before a casualty reaches physiologic exhaustion through using better tourniquets, hemostatic dressings, judicious use of volume expanders, and permissive hypotension. However, evacuation strategies should always be designed to deliver casualties to the most robust trauma surgical care as quickly as possible.

Evolution of a trauma system

Fortunately, many steps have been taken to solve the problems. For example, the Army Medical Command continues to update Tactical Combat Casualty Care courses, which are administered to all combat medics within 6 months of their next deployment to the combat zones. These courses include didactic sessions, practical exercises with simulation mannequins, and, in some institutions, practical exercises with live animals in laboratory and simulated tactical environments. These courses focus on the prehospital treatment of preventable causes of death on the battlefield, such as exsanguination from compressible hemorrhage, tension pneumothorax, and airway problems. Other education initiatives (which existed before Operation Iraqi Freedom) include the Army Trauma Training Center at the Ryder Trauma Center in Miami, Fla, and the Navy Trauma Training Center at Los Angeles County Trauma Center in California. FSEs rotate through these centers before deployment for the purposes of unit team building and gaining real-world experience for treating civilian trauma patients. These training initiatives have not been shown to decrease the learning curve that is required to care for combat casualties, but they do provide an opportunity for individuals to hone technical and cognitive skills and function better as a team.

Additionally, by mid-2004 the number of FSTs was reduced to four to six teams in the theater, and the placement of these teams integrated into a joint theater trauma system. The goal is to place the teams in locations that are a 60-minute-or-more flight from the nearest CSH, or to place task-oriented units (for finite periods of time) close to anticipated combat, such as during major offensives (eg, the second Marine assault on Al Fallujah). This joint theater trauma system initiative has integrated trauma surgical elements and personnel from the Navy, Marines, Air Force, and Army into a sensible and cohesive system. Personnel from less-active forward surgical units rotate through busier CSHs to learn and maintain the skills needed for effective combat trauma surgical care. Guidance on positioning of surgical assets and evacuation strategies to streamline the flow of casualties have been provided to MEDEVAC assets. Since November 2004, military trauma physicians and nurses have been deployed with dedicated roles for creating standardized guidelines for trauma care; training and updating surgical units and medics on these guidelines and latest techniques; identifying unit and system problems at all levels of care; and collecting and analyzing combat casualty data.

The collection and analysis of combat casualty data has been critical. Historically, most trauma publications from wars have included level III or IV data. One of the main goals of the theater trauma system is to expand the Joint Theater Trauma Registry (JTTR), a database of all trauma patients from Operations Enduring and Iraqi Freedom that is patterned after civilian trauma registries. Analysis of the data from the JTTR produces level II data. Using the data collected, several problems with combat casualty care have been identified and measures to improve these problems instituted. Examples of these issues and solutions are provided in Box 1.

Box 1 lists just a few examples of problems identified by providers at various echelons of care and the steps taken within a system to solve those problems. More than 30 systemic issues have been identified since implementation of the theater trauma system [42]. Deeper analysis of some of these problems is provided elsewhere in this issue and in other forums. The institution of a theater-wide trauma system and dedicated personnel to collect and evaluate combat casualty data allow for a systematic review of the impact of such initiatives. Ongoing research is being conducted on patient outcomes based on factors such as initial level of surgical treatment and use of (1) recombinant Factor VIIa, (2) fresh whole blood (MAJ Jeremy Perkins, MD, MC, USA, and LTC Philip Spinella, MD, MC, USA, personal communication, 2005), (3) prehospital tourniquets, (4) an intensivist-directed ICU model (LTC

Box 1. Combat casualty care issues and solutions

Issue

Early in Operation Iraqi Freedom, not every soldier had his own tourniquet in some units.

Solution

By August 2005, more than 275,000 Combat Application Tourniquets (CAT-1) had been sent to Iraq (COL John B. Holcomb, MD, MC, USA, personal communication, 2005).

Issue

Hypothermia, particularly in patients treated surgically initially at level II facilities (FSEs), is a recurring problem. Patients develop hypothermia en route to the level III facilities despite outside temperatures of more than 100°F.

Solutions

Small portable fluid warmers are being approved for use on helicopters. Critically ill patients are frequently placed in vinyl body bags to conserve heat. Education initiatives for surgeons at level II and III facilities are being undertaken to emphasize recognition of hypothermia and to install guidelines for the prevention of heat loss. Some CSHs have ordered devices for Continuous Arterio-Venous Rewarming (CAVR). The impact of CAVR on decreasing rewarming times and blood product requirements has been shown [41].

Issue

Transmission of data among echelons of care was frequently incomplete. Paper charts were blown out of helicopter doors by the rotor wash or data were lost during patient transfer.

Solutions

Surgeons frequently wrote operative findings and treatments directly on the patient's dressings (Fig. 3). Thousands of USB thumb drives (flash memory cards) were sent to theater, with the idea that an electronic copy of a standardized Theater Trauma Registry sheet could be placed in the thumb drive and attached directly to the patient. E-mail chains were initiated among surgeons in theater to discuss ongoing problems with combat casualty care and disseminate lessons learned. Surgeons were encouraged to communicate about patients transferred and to provide feedback on the care. Finally, a weekly teleconference between the CSH in Baghdad, Walter Reed Army Medical Center, and Brooke Army Medical Center now occurs, allowing feedback between continental United States and theater surgeons.

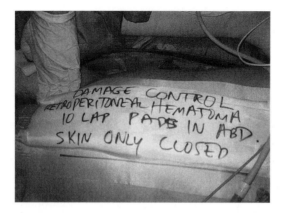

Fig. 3. Typical operative report written on dressing of casualty operated on at a forward area who arrived at the CSH after a damage control procedure.

Kurt M. Grathwohl, MD, MC, USA, personal communication, 2005), (5) the thromboelastogram (TEG) to guide trauma resuscitation (LTC Donald L. Jenkins, MD, MC, USAF, personal communication, 2005), and (6) ultrasound-guided placement of intra-aortic and intracaval occlusion balloons to treat abdominal vascular injuries (LTC Kelly Blair, MD, MC, USA, personal communication, 2005). Many different injuries, injury patterns, and related outcomes are also being evaluated.

The number of United States military fatalities as of December 13, 2005, was 2150. The number of United States military wounded in action reported by the Department of Defense as of December 13, 2005, was 16,061 (8567 returned to duty), for a total of 18,211 United States military casualties [43]. This number does not include other coalition member casualties or the Iraqis, who by all estimates have suffered the most casualties. Review of the JTTR has identified that 1886 (12.4%) of those wounded in action underwent an initial surgical procedure at an FSE. The accuracy of this number may be limited by incomplete data in the JTTR, but current data indicate that most casualties are being evacuated directly to level III surgical facilities (CSHs). Although the data are not complete enough to see the entire picture, the percentage of patients being treated at level II facilities (FSEs) is expected to be higher in the maneuver phase and lower in the second, more static phase. This expected finding is consistent with the development of a theater-wide trauma system that integrates trauma surgical support from all branches of military service.

Future considerations

Future theaters of operations have the potential to be substantially different from the current theater in Iraq. Unchallenged air superiority must not be taken for granted when planning future combat casualty care missions. The current luxury of secure air space like that which exists today in Iraq and Afghanistan may not be present in future theaters. In these situations, military leaders must be prepared to plan for more robust in-theater patient holding and treating capabilities unitl secure evacuation patterns can be established. Stateless terrorist organizations have increased the potential for nuclear, radiologic, biologic, and chemical attacks, and medical and surgical units and personnel must continue to train for this possibility. An unforeseen conflict in another country has the potential to strain the United States military's already committed combat and combat support units. Because of the potential for terrorist attacks home and abroad, military surgeons must be prepared to respond to civilian emergencies and integrate with organizations such as the Federal Emergency Management Agency (FEMA) and other relief organizations [44,45].

Lessons learned

Approximately 130 active-duty surgeons and comparable numbers of CRNAs, anesthesiologists, and critical care nurses are in the US Army. These personnel, with their counterparts in the Navy, Air Force, Marines, and Reserves, continue to support operations in two geographically large theaters (Afghanistan and Iraq) and numerous smaller peace-keeping, humanitarian assistance, and Special Operations engagements. Hurricanes Katrina and Rita in the late summer/early fall of 2005 and an earthquake in Pakistan in October 2005 caused other deployments of military medical and surgical assets. The personnel and unit requirements identified in this article emphasize the need for optimal deployment of these limited assets. Attempts should be made to avoid the underuse of forward surgical units, such as what occurred in the first half of 2004. To prevent repeating this issue in future conflicts, surgeons should make a greater effort to educate combat unit commanders on how surgical assets are best used. Once level III surgical assets are established such that most evacuation times are less than 1 hour, FST volume should be routinely analyzed. Low-volume units should be redeployed home, used to augment level III facilities, or consolidated into task-oriented teams, as in the marine experience. These redeployments require combat unit commanders to yield operational control of these surgical assets to a theater trauma coordinator once primary maneuver phase ends.

The Joint Theater Trauma Coordinator must have the seniority and experience with trauma systems to establish how each unit, regardless of branch of service, fits into the whole joint theater trauma system. These individuals and their staff should have the authority to shift medical and surgical assets, particularly forward surgical units, to locations where they will be maximally used. The redistribution of surgical assets requires consistent communication between combat commanders and trauma coordinators about upcoming operations, so that forward surgical support can be placed where it is needed in anticipation of a spike in casualties. Thorough knowledge of average evacuation times from various AORs is crucial in making these decisions.

This knowledge can best be gained through improvements in prehospital data acquisition and transfer. Novel use of hand-held computers and hands-free or voice-activated recording devices, and improved use of USB drives (flash memory cards) to transmit prehospital data may be the key. After-action reviews between prehospital personnel and theater trauma personnel may provide important insights into problems medics have faced, and allow for more rapid changes in policy and training.

MEDEVAC helicopters require improved critical care, primarily for severely injured patients who have undergone surgery and are being transported between level II and level III facilities. Possible solutions to this requirement include creation of a MEDEVAC critical care transport team, augmentation of forward surgical units with additional personnel for this mission, or enhanced training for the medics already on these helicopters. Dedicated helicopter teams could be created whose primary mission is the transport of critically ill patients. Reducing the number of deployed forward surgical units will allow these limited assets to be focused where they are needed most.

Casualty data collection must begin with the onset of combat. Personnel who are trained in and dedicated to casualty data collection and who report to a central authority (eg, Theater Trauma Coordinator) must be deployed with surgical units. Casualty databases will therefore be centrally compiled rather than remain only with the unit or collecting individual. Continued analysis of the data will allow the ongoing institution of more rapid, evidence-based changes. This policy is already largely in effect.

Summary

The adaptation of a theater-wide trauma system and integration of trauma surgical units from all branches of military service, combined with the initiative of the Joint Theater Trauma Registry, have allowed the rapid collection and analysis of combat casualty data. The collection of combat casualty data during a large-scale conflict is not new to the military; it was performed by United States surgeons in almost every conflict since World War I. However, the way the global communications network has allowed this data to be transmitted and analyzed, and has enabled the lessons and conclusions from that analysis to be disseminated to the medics, nurses, and surgeons in the combat zone or preparing to deploy, is revolutionary. Analysis of the data during collection has helped identify problems that in turn spawn new basic science and research initiatives. More importantly, updated guidelines for casualty treatment (eg, resuscitation of patients with hemostatic products), use of new or better devices and products (eg, tourniquets and hemostatic dressings), and adjustment of unit placement and personnel are being driven by data and evidence supporting these changes. Hence, military surgeons are evolving and adjusting to the current war, in real-time, as the conflict unfolds. The number of casualties and the severity of their injuries have provided a wealth of trauma experience for those medics, nurses, and physicians responsible for combat casualty care. The innovations and research initiatives of these individuals will catapult the military to the forefront of trauma research for the next decade.

References

[1] Globalsecurity. org. Operation uphold democracy. Available at: http://www.globalsecurity. org/military/ops/uphold_democracy.html. Accessed October 16, 2005.

[2] US General Accounting Office. Wartime Medical Care: DOD is addressing capability shortfalls, but challenges remain. Report to the Chairman, Subcommittee on Military Personnel, Committee on National Security, House of Representatives. Washington, DC: US General Accounting Office; 1996. Publication GAO/NSAID-96-224.

[3] Pratt JW, Rush RM. The military surgeon and the war on terrorism: a Zollinger legacy. Am J Surg 2003;186:292-5.

[4] King B, Jatoi I. The Mobile Army Surgical Hospital (MASH): a military and surgical legacy. J Natl Med Assoc 2005;97(5):648-56.

[5] McKenzie KF Jr. Quote from address to USMC National Defense University. Available at: http://www.iwar.org.uk/military/resources/aspc/text/aa/def.htm. Accessed October 31, 2005.

[6] US Department of Defense. The Operation Desert Shield/Desert Storm Timeline. Available at: http://www.defenselink.mil/news/Aug2000/n08082000_20008088.html. Accessed October 20, 2005.

[7] Veterans Museum and Memorial Center. Operations Desert Shield and Desert Storm, 1990–1991. Available at: http://www.veteranmuseum.org/desertstorm.html. Accessed October 20, 2005.

[8] Gulf War. Available at: http://en.wikipedia.org/wiki/Operation_Desert_Storm. Accessed October 20, 2005.

[9] Persian Gulf War. Available at: http://democracyrising.us/content/view/50/74/. Accessed October 19, 2005.

[10] Smith AM. Joint medical support: are we asleep at the switch? Joint Force Quarterly 1995;102-9.

[11] Carey ME. Analysis of wounds incurred by U.S. Army Seventh Corps personnel treated in Corps hospitals during Operation Desert Storm, February 20 to March 10, 1991. J Trauma 1996;40(3 Suppl):S165-9.

[12] Bellamy RF. The causes of death in conventional land warfare: implications for combat casualty care research. Mil Med 1984;149:55-62.

[13] Champion HR, Bellamy RF, Roberts CP, et al. A profile of combat injury. J Trauma 2003; 54:S13-9.

[14] Mabry RL, Holcomb JB, Baker AM, et al. United States Army Rangers in Somalia: an analysis of combat casualties on an urban battlefield. J Trauma 2000;49:515-29.

[15] Holcomb JB. Fluid resuscitation in modern combat casualty care: lessons learned from Somalia. J Trauma 2003;54:S46-51.

[16] Zucchino D. Thunder run. New York: Atlantic Monthly Press; 2004.

[17] Beekley AC, Watts DM. Combat trauma experience with the United States Army 102nd Forward Surgical Team in Afghanistan. Am J Surg 2004;187(5):652-4.

[18] Patel TH, Wenner KA, Price SA, et al. US Army Forward Surgical Team's experience in Operation Iraqi Freedom. J Trauma 2004;57:201-7.

[19] Marshall TJ Jr. Combat casualty care: the Alpha Surgical Company experience during Operation Iraqi Freedom. Mil Med 2005;170:469–72.

[20] Bohman HR, Stevens RA, Baker BC, et al. The US Navy's forward resuscitative surgery system during Operation Iraqi Freedom. Mil Med 2005;170(4):297–301.

[21] Stinger HK. College plays pivotal role in Operation Iraqi Freedom. Bull Am Coll Surg 2004; 89(3):8–15.

[22] Rush RM, Stockmaster NR, Stinger HK, et al. Supporting the Global War on Terror: a tale of two campaigns featuring the 250th Forward Surgical Team (Airborne). Am J Surg 2005; 189(5):564–70.

[23] Gawande A. Casualties of war—military care for the wounded from Iraq and Afghanistan. N Engl J Med 2004;351(24):2471–5.

[24] Boivin J. No safe haven: Army surgical team injured in mortar attack. Nursing Spectrum Career Management Magazine [serial online] September 2003. Available at: http://community. nursingspectrum.com/MagazineArticles/article.cfm?AID=10388. Accessed October 21, 2005.

[25] American Academy of Orthopaedic Surgeons Bulletin. In the heart of the Sunni Triangle. Interview with Greer E. Noonburg, MD, Lieutenant Colonel, US Army Medical Corps. Available at: http://www.aaos.org/wordhtml/bulletin/feb04/feature2.htm. Accessed October 21, 2005.

[26] United States Department of Defense New Release. Available at: http://www.defenselink. mil/releases/2004/nr20040322-1108.html. Accessed October 26, 2005.

[27] Adobe GoLive5. Injured Army man receives Purple Heart. Interview with Sergeant Jeremey Wellman, US Army, 915th Forward Surgical Team. Available at: http://www.thereflector. com/PAGES/STORIES/Old%20Stories/2004/02-17-04.html. Accessed October 24, 2005.

[28] Gandjour A, Bannenberg A, Lauterbach KW. Threshold volumes associated with higher survival in health care: a systematic review. Med Care 2003;41:1129–41.

[29] Cooper A, Hannan EL, Bessey PQ, et al. An examination of the volume-mortality relationship for New York State trauma centers. J Trauma 2000;48(1):16–24.

[30] Marcin JP, Romano PS. Impact of between-hospital volume and within-hospital volume on mortality and readmission rates for trauma patients in California. Crit Care Med 2004;32(7): 1477–83.

[31] Tepas JJ, Patel JC, DiScala C, et al. Relationship of trauma patient volume to outcome experience: can a relationship be defined? J Trauma 1998;44(5):827–31.

[32] Richardson JD, Schmieg R, Boaz P, et al. Impact of trauma attending surgeon case volume on outcome: is more better? J Trauma 1998;44(2):266–72.

[33] Nathens AB, Jurkovich GJ, Rivara FP, et al. Effectiveness of state trauma systems in reducing injury-related mortality: a national evaluation. J Trauma 2000;48(1):25–31.

[34] Mann NC, Mullins RJ, MacKenzie EJ, et al. Systematic review of published evidence regarding trauma system effectiveness. J Trauma 1999;47(3):S25–33.

[35] Robinson PA. Field of Dreams [motion picture] . Universal Studios, 100 Universal City Plaza, North Hollywood, CA, 91608. 1989.

[36] Nathens AB, Maier RV, Brundage SI, et al. The effect of interfacility transfer on outcome in an urban trauma system. J Trauma 2003;55:444–9.

[37] Lerner EB, Moscati RM. The Golden Hour: scientific fact or medical "urban legend"? Acad Emerg Med 2001;8:758–60.

[38] Martinowitz U, Zaarur M, Yaron BL, et al. Treating traumatic bleeding in a combat setting: possible role of recombinant activated Factor VII. Mil Med 2004;169(12 Suppl):16–8.

[39] Gofrit ON, Leibouci D, Shapira SC. The Trimodal death distribution of trauma victims: military experience from the Lebanon War. Mil Med 1997;162:24–6.

[40] Osterwalder JJ. Can the "golden hour of shock" safely be extended in blunt polytrauma patients? Prospective cohort study at a level I hospital in eastern Switzerland. Prehospital Disaster Med 2002;17(2):75–80.

[41] Gentilello LM, Cobean R, Offner P, et al. Continuous arterio-venous rewarming: rapid reversal of hypothermia in critically ill patients. J Trauma 1992;32:316–27.
[42] Jenkins D, Eastridge B, Schiller H, et al. Trauma system development in a theater of war: experiences from Operation Iraqi Freedom [abstract]. J Trauma 2005;59(2):529.
[43] Operation Iraqi Freedom (OIF) U.S. Casualty Status. Available at: http://www.defenselink.mil/news/casualty.pdf. Accessed December 15, 2005.
[44] Peck M. "Golden Hour" Surgical Units Prove Worth. Military Medical Technology, Online Edition. Available at: http://www.military-medical-technology.com/print_article.cfm?DocID=176. Accessed October 29, 2005.
[45] Eiseman B, Chandler JG. Sheriff's surgeon's alert: a trauma surgeon's responsibility. J Trauma 2003;54:156–60.
[46] Chambers LW, Gillingham BL, Green DJ, et al. Experience of the US Marine Corps Surgical Shock Trauma Platoon with 304 operative combat casualties during a 6 month period of Operation Iraqi Freedom [abstract]. J Trauma 2005;59(2):529.

SURGICAL
CLINICS OF
NORTH AMERICA

Surg Clin N Am 86 (2006) 711–726

Special Lessons Learned from Iraq

MAJ James Sebesta, MD[a,b,*]

[a]Uniformed Services University of the Health Sciences, Bethesda, MD, USA
[b]Department of Surgery, Madigan Army Medical Center,
Bldg 9040 Fitzsimmons Drive, Tacoma, WA 98431, USA

Since the beginning of recorded history, wars have forced military medical systems to revamp practices proven in prior conflicts. The war on terrorism is no different. The large number of casualties produced as a result of Operation Iraqi Freedom (OIF) and Operation Enduring Freedom (OEF) has stimulated the military medical community to retrain and rethink traditional battlefield trauma management. Because of changing weapons systems and numbers of personnel engaged, everyone from the combat medic to surgeons at combat support hospitals (CSH) to stateside fixed medical centers are exposed to types of injuries and casualty numbers that are uncommon in nondeployed daily practices. Surgeons located at small community hospitals, who rarely see trauma, may find themselves in the middle of a mass-casualty situation with multiple critical patients. Damage-control techniques or various subspecialty procedures such as vascular repairs that have not been practiced since the surgeon was a resident may first appear as daunting tasks. After working in a motor pool for most of their careers, medics may find themselves as the first line of treatment for patients who have complex injuries including mutilating amputations As a result, military medical departments provide refresher courses to medics before deployment. A greater effort is made to ensure that medical teams such as Forward Surgical Teams train in civilian trauma centers before deploying. This training allows them to hone trauma skills and management algorithms. In an effort to improve outcomes, the function and use of all medical units is evaluated and redefined continually in the combat theater. Data collection is now a priority and is performed for each casualty. The data are placed in the Theater Trauma Registry (TTR) to study injury patterns, treatment practices, and outcomes. Data from the TTR can be used by research teams,

---

* Correspondence. Department of Surgery, Madigan Army Medical Center, Tacoma, WA 98431, USA.
E-mail address: james.sebesta@amedd.army.mil

0039-6109/06/$ - see front matter © 2006 Elsevier Inc. All rights reserved.
doi:10.1016/j.suc.2006.03.002
surgical.theclinics.com

such as the 31st CSH research group, to establish practice guidelines and change policy for types and numbers of personnel. Communication between combat zones and the higher-echelon rear-area treatment facilities in Germany and the United States has improved dramatically, allowing trends to be identified rapidly, addressed, and corrected at the forward area and along the medical evacuation route The following discussion outlines some of the lessons learned in OIF and OEF.

The 31st CSH deployed in support of OIF from January 2003 to January 2004. The hospital was divided between two sites, Balad and Baghdad. Located within the International Zone, the Baghdad portion of the 31st CSH operated out of the Ibna Sina hospital and was staffed with approximately 300 active-duty and reserve soldiers. This hospital was a three-story building that provided a fixed hardened structure perfect for continued operations in the combat theater. The hospital was connected to a five-story dormitory-like building used to house the staff. A separate area of the hospital that once served as Saddam Hussein family's private hospital was converted into a 10-bed emergency department and triage area. The hospital was renovated and provided approximately 60 inpatient ward beds for coalition troops, Iraqi nationals, and insurgents. Three operating suites provided five operating tables. A 20-bed ICU, CT and MRI scanners, and a basic radiology suite were available. During the yearlong deployment, approximately 3600 trauma patients and 700 medical patients were treated. Sixty percent of trauma patients were American (Fig. 1). The average patient age was 28 years (range, 9 months to 77 years). There were more than 100 pediatric patients and 29 patients over the age of 60 years (Fig. 2). Penetrating injuries from blasts or gunshot wounds were the most common mechanism of injury (Table 1). The CSH treated patients who were evacuated directly from the site of injury and also acted as higher level of care for forward surgical units. The CSH performed definitive treatment and coordinated evacuation out of theater. United States and Coalition troops treated at the CSH were evacuated to higher echelons of care in Germany and stateside locations when stable. Iraqi patients stayed until they were near ready for discharge and were transferred to an Iraqi facility to arrange follow-up care. In addition to the care of patients injured as a result of the ongoing

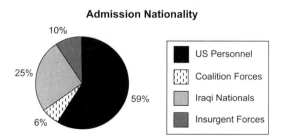

Fig. 1. Admission to 31st Combat Support Hospital by nationality.

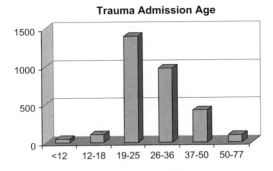

Fig. 2. Trauma admissions to 31st Combat Support Hospital by age (in years).

conflict, the 31st CSH provided medical treatment for new or existing medical conditions in Coalition troops, embassy personnel, contract company employees, Iraqi detainees, and some Iraqi nationals. There was also a focused humanitarian mission for children who had medical conditions that could not be cared for in the Iraqi medical system.

Prehospital care

A review of the causes of death at the CSH showed findings similar to those of prior conflicts. Non-survivable injuries were present in 49% of the deaths. The remaining 51% had potentially survivable injuries; the most common mechanisms were penetrating injuries from small arms fire and fragmentary devices. The most common cause of death was hemorrhage, which accounted for 76%. In this group, 68% had torso injuries, 13% had axillary/groin or neck injuries, and 19% had extremity injuries;

Table 1
Causes of injury

Primary mechanism	No, if injuries (%)
IED/blast	1246 (36.7)
Gunshot wound	997 (29.4)
Indirect fire	443 (13.0)
Motor vehicle crash	329 (9.7)
Fall	126 (3.7)
Crush	76 (2.2)
Stab wounds	47 (1.4)
Burns	42 (1.3)
Assault	35 (1.1)
Aircraft crash	12 (<1)
Electrical injuries	8 (<1)
Other	7 (<1)
Unknown	26 (<1)

Abbreviation: IED, improvised explosive device.

68% had noncompressible hemorrhage, whereas 32% had hemorrhage that could be compressed or controlled with a tourniquet (Cuaddrado D, et al. Cause of death analysis from Operation Iraqi Freedom. Abstract submitted for presentation). The knowledge of the distribution of the injuries and especially that soldiers die from hemorrhage that could be stopped with simple pressure applied to the wound pointed out the need to improve battlefield treatment techniques, especially in the area of hemorrhage control.

This information has changed the training of medics and other medical staff at the first level of care. Combat medics are sent to courses such as the Tactical Combat Casualty Care course conducted at Ft. Lewis, Washington. This course includes short didactic sessions, case-based scenarios, team-building exercises, medical simulation, and live tissue training combined into a hybrid, weeklong review of treatment and triage principals specific to battlefield trauma. This course provides needed refreshment of training and skills that may not be used in the medic's day-to-day function while stationed in the United States. Courses now are being added to unit training schedules as a skill that is as important as firing a weapon. Commanders understand that these skills must be practiced and the knowledge refreshed in a periodic fashion.

In most cases combat medics do not have the skills or equipment to perform intubations in the field, and they are not afforded the luxury of being able to participate in anesthesia rotations as are doctors, physician's assistants, and paramedics. Only a small portion of salvageable patients die from airway injuries, and the loss of airway in the field carries a poor prognosis. Airway issues were found to be the cause of death in 10% of the patients who reached the CSH, although it is not clear how many patients who had airway issues died and were never transferred to the CSH (Cuaddrado D, et al. Cause of death analysis from Operation Iraqi Freedom. Abstract submitted for presentation). Medics have a very short time to address airway issues before death, and doing so may be impossible if the tactical environment prevents rapid extraction and treatment. The largest group of potentially salvageable patients is those who have compressible hemorrhage. After the shooting stops, medics are to use the mnemonic MARCH (Box 1) to direct treatment priorities [1].

Box 1. MARCH mnemonic for directing treatment priorities

M Massive hemorrhage
A Airway
R Respiration
C Circulation
H Head injury/hypothermia

There is now an emphasis on treating life-threatening compressible hemorrhage first. Treatment includes the use of direct pressure, pressure dressings, tourniquets, and hemostatic dressings, including HemCon, QUIKCLOT, and dry fibrin sealant. The MARCH mnemonic also is used in mass-casualty situations to prioritize the treatment of patients. Tourniquets are taught as a first-line treatment to control bleeding, which then allows the time to identify other injuries in that patient and to triage other patients in the area. After the hemorrhage is controlled, airway issues are addressed. Medics are given instructions on the use of a Combitube, although it was more common for a patient to arrive at the 31st CSH after a cricothyroidotomy than with a Combitube in place. Medics are instructed in performing cricothyroidotomy and practice this skill using simulators and live-tissue models. This training is followed by the identification and treatment of tension pneumothorax and sucking chest wounds. Medics learn to perform needle decompression of tension pneumothorax, the use of an occlusive dressing or Asherman chest seal valves for sucking chest wounds, and chest tube insertion. Circulation is evaluated, and the idea of permissive hypotension is now emphasized. In patients who have a radial pulse and normal mentation, intravenous fluids are not given. Intravenous access is obtained but not used unless the radial pulse is lost or mental status changes are present. Intravenous fluids are then given but in small, controlled volumes, and the patient's response is monitored closely. This protocol is a change from prior resuscitation practices in which all patients received fluids that may lead to continued losses because of higher blood pressure, dilution of the remaining red cells and coagulation proteins, and increased hypothermia. The final treatment involves preventing additional injuries and loss of body temperature.

Tourniquets

Tourniquet use was restricted primarily to military prehospital prevention of exsanguination from extremity wounds. Opinions about tourniquets range from it being an "instrument of the devil that sometimes saves a life" [2] to the current teaching of the military. Some believe that the tourniquet should be prohibited except to allow extraction of the patients and placement of a long compression dressing out of fear that additional ischemic injury occurs to the tourniqueted extremity and reperfusion injuries to the limb and other vital organs occur upon removing the device. Some of these concerns are based on experience with improvised tourniquets that were applied improperly [3]. Tourniquets are almost never used in civilian trauma systems. Dorlac and colleagues [4] reviewed deaths from isolated extremity injuries in a civilian trauma system and found that there was a small number of patients who potentially could benefit from early hemorrhage control of extremity injuries. Approximately 10% of all combat deaths are caused by extremity injuries that are potentially preventable with proper tourniquet use. Lakstein and colleagues [5] reported a 4-year review of tourniquet use in the prehospital setting by the Israeli defense forces. Of 550 soldiers treated in the prehospital setting, 91 had tourniquets applied. Of these tourniquets, 78% were effective in controlling hemorrhage, but 47% of the applied tourniquets were not medically indicated. Five patients experienced neurologic complications in seven limbs, ranging from paralysis to paresthesias and weakness, that were thought to be related to the tourniquet use. The authors concluded that use of a tourniquet in the prehospital setting is technically easy, cheap, and effective for the control of extremity hemorrhage.

Tourniquets are an essential therapy based on recent experience in Iraq. The 31st CSH saw 67 patients with documented tourniquets between January 2003 and January 2004 [6]. The average tourniquet time was 70 minutes. For the patients for whom tourniquet effectiveness was documented, 83% of the tourniquets were effective. Tourniquets at the thigh level were much more likely to be ineffective than those applied to the lower leg or arm. The tourniquet was not indicated in 20.9% of cases, and only one tourniquet was improperly placed. There were no known complications associated with tourniquet use. A review of patients who died at the CSH with extremity injuries without tourniquets found that four of seven patients were potentially salvageable if a tourniquet had been used. The data point that is missing in the 31st CSH tourniquet database is the number of patients who had extremity injuries and who died from compressible extremity exsanguination before evacuation to a treatment facility. This information would provide the denominator to show a difference in the tourniquet versus no-tourniquet outcome. It is hoped that reducing the number of deaths caused by extremity hemorrhage now that every soldier has a tourniquet as part of the first aid pack will show the true effectiveness of tourniquets.

The use of a tourniquet at the CSH was universal. Patients arrived hypotensive with multiple fragmentation wounds distributed throughout their bodies. It was common for these patients to start bleeding from multiple extremity injuries as the resuscitation ensued. If the patient arrived with a tourniquet, it was rapidly converted to a pneumatic tourniquet for better control. A tourniquet was placed on any patient who had multiple-level fragmentation wounds and hypotension. The evaluation of the head, chest, and abdomen then was performed without concern of further blood loss from an extremity injury. The extremity evaluation and removal of tourniquets occurred after the completion of this evaluation. In patients who had life-threatening abdominal or thoracic injuries, the tourniquets remained in place until the completion of the damage-control procedure for these injuries.

Tourniquets should be used in all patients who have extremity hemorrhage or penetrating injuries to facilitate rapid control that allows extrication or triage and treatment of other patients. When the patient reaches a medical treatment facility, the need for the tourniquet can be reassessed, and it can be left in place or replaced with a pressure dressing.

Triage at the combat support hospital

Rapid effective triage of multiple patients is a skill that is vital to the success of a CSH. In his article reviewing his experience as the Chief of Surgery at the 67th evacuation hospital in Vietnam, Sebesta [7] writes that the skill of triage cannot be taught. The basic principals of triage can be taught in residency programs, but the implementation of those principals and the ability to identify injury patterns is a skill that is developed and polished in the combat environment. To triage a patient effectively, a simple and rapid evaluation without the use of additional instrumentation is required. McManus and colleagues [8] showed that the character of a trauma patient's radial pulse is prognostic. Patients who had a strong radial pulse had a mortality of 3% compared with 29% if the pulse was weak. Holcomb and colleagues [9] reported that the character of the radial pulse, combined with the motor and verbal components of the Glasgow Coma Scale, is effective at predicting the need for prehospital life-saving interventions in patients who do not have head injuries. Checking a radial pulse and making a quick assessment of the motor and verbal components of the Glascow Coma Scale by asking patients to raise two fingers and state their names provided a rapid triage tool that differentiated urgent from delayed patients. This assessment could be made in a few seconds as the patient was rolled through the door. Patients who had weak radial pulses or who were unable to comply with the directions were taken into more urgent treatment areas for closer assessment and triage.

Triage for the CSH involved stratifying patient needs at multiple levels. The triage officer had the ominous task of directing patient evaluations and use of hospital assets in the chaos of a mass-casualty event. In the emergency department, triage of the patients was done first to determine their place in the line for evaluation. Within the emergency department, patients were again triaged for the use of the CT scanner, ultrasound, and emergency department–level treatments including the use of emergency-release blood products. As patients reached the operating theater, the use of blood products again was triaged because of the limited capacity to thaw products or draw and prepare whole blood. The use of hospital beds and the need for evacuation of stable, treated patients to the next echelon of care was assessed continually. All of this coordination required accurate, timely communication and retriage at all levels to optimize the care of the injured.

Evaluation of the patient who has multiple fragmentation injuries

The introduction of the improvised explosive device has created injury patterns not seen before. These weapons create casualties with multiple, in some cases hundreds, of fragmentation injuries from head to toe (Fig. 3). In addition, blast injuries, burns, and inhalation injuries commonly are seen in the same patient. The evaluation of these patients who have literally

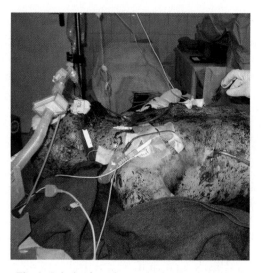

Fig. 3. Injuries from improvised explosive device.

hundreds of penetrating injuries is complex, and frequently there are several patients from the same event. The depth of penetration depends on the size of the weapon, the type of material that was fragmented, and the patient's distance from the explosion. The sensitivity and specificity of physical examinations, focused abdominal sonography for trauma (FAST), and the CT scan for identifying fascial penetration and the need for laparotomy were reviewed retrospectively at the 31st CSH. The first lesson learned was that physical examination and estimation of penetration based on the entrance wound was not effective, with a sensitivity of 28% and specificity of 94%. Patients would present with a tiny, scratchlike injury to the head, and CT evaluation would reveal intracranial fragments. Abdominal examinations and palpation often were misleading because of the diffuse nature of the injuries and because small fragments may create localized perforations that are not evident clinically for hours. The use of FAST examination was found to be useful only in the quick evaluation of the abdomen in the unstable patient who had multilevel injuries. A positive FAST scan confirmed that the probable source of instability was in the abdomen, and the patient was taken directly to the operating theater. With a sensitivity of 12% and a specificity of 100%, FAST was not effective at identifying fascial penetrating injuries in stable patients. The most effective tool for the rapid assessment of multiple fragmentation injuries was the CT scanner, which demonstrated a sensitivity of 96% and a specificity of 85%. It provided rapid, accurate assessment of the depth of penetration of fragments and the need for operative exploration of the head, chest, and abdomen. The use of the CT scanner prevented the unnecessary exploratory laparotomy that would waste precious operating theater time and hospital assets. The

CT scanner also was extremely effective in determining which patients required a neck exploration for penetrating neck injuries.

Damage-control surgery

Pringle [10] championed the technique of damage-control surgery for the treatment of hepatic hemorrhage for trauma in 1908. These techniques had been used through World War II but fell out of favor because of poor outcomes. The techniques were reintroduced in 1981 by Feliciano and colleagues [11] and were described in detail by Stone and colleagues [12] in 1983. Since then, the use of damage-control surgery has gained widespread support in the treatment of trauma patients. Eiseman and colleagues [13] expressed concerns about the use of damage-control techniques in a combat environment, especially in highly mobile forward surgical units. They believed that these techniques were resource intensive and limited unit mobility. Recent experiences in OIF and OEF have mirrored the results found in the urban trauma centers and re-emphasized the importance of damage-control surgery in combat. In the current combat theater, most medical assets are in fixed positions, and evacuation channels are well established. Even in the absence of these factors, damage-control surgery allows rapid stabilization and transfer to higher echelons of care for definitive treatment. The constellation of injuries, evacuation times, and limited resources in the face of multiple casualties made damage-control techniques essential to avoid physiologic burnout in severely injured patients. Data from the 31st CSH showed that 18% of casualties were hypothermic (temperature $< 36°C$) at presentation and that these patients had lower pHs and hematocrits, higher base deficits, required more blood products, and had a higher mortality. Temperatures below 34°C were associated with nearly 100% mortality, a finding consistent with the data reported by Jurkovich [14].

From January 2003 to January 2004, the 31st CSH performed 333 primary laparotomies for penetrating trauma. Damage-control techniques were performed on 92 (27.6%) of the initial laparotomies. The overall survival rate was 72.8%. For the most part, the use of damage control was the default operative plan, and the surgical team had to decide during the case to change to a definitive-treatment procedure. In the forward surgical facilities, damage control allowed stabilization of the patient for transportation. The patient could then be transferred to a CSH with more robust resources for the evaluation and definitive treatment. In the author's experience, patients transferred from forward surgical units after properly applied damage-control techniques had outcomes similar to those of patients who had their primary procedure performed at the CSH, 66.6% versus 72.8%.

The decision to perform damage-control surgery was based primarily on the status of the patient. The initial point considered was the type and severity of injuries. In patients who had injury complexes such as penetrating head and abdominal injuries or major extremity vascular and complex abdominal injuries, damage-control procedures allowed rapid assessment and temporization of the abdominal wounds, making possible treatment or damage control of the other injuries. Temperature, pH, and base deficit then were used to help direct the operative plan. The deadly triad of hypothermia, acidosis, and coagulopathy was avoided at all costs. The final factor was the current backlog of surgical cases, the severity of their wounds, and the current number of inbound casualties. During extremely busy times, damage-control procedures were performed in a relatively stable patient to limit operative times to allow the operative management of a more severely injured patient who had arrived after the case had started. The planned second-look and definitive repairs could occur within 1 to 2 hours or be delayed for as long as 36 hours. The patient was returned to the operating theater as soon as the patient's physiologic status improved and time was available.

The basic damage-control procedure was based on the principals of controlling bleeding, limiting contamination, and preventing additional injuries or worsening of the physiologic status. The initial step was incision, packing, and allowing anesthesia to "catch up" with the resuscitation. Proper packing of the abdomen temporarily controlled most injuries and allowed time for resuscitation and for the operative team to prepare for the procedure by obtaining staplers, packs, and other equipment. After the patient was resuscitated, the abdomen was explored. Depending on the injuries, vascular injuries were treated first, as they were identified. Injuries to minor veins were treated with ligation. Major venous structures including the inferior vena cava and portal vein can be ligated, but the goal was repair or shunting. Most venous injuries can be treated initially by packing or by shunting. Bowel injuries were controlled by using a stapler or umbilical tape to prevent further contamination. Mesenteric defects required the isolation and control of the individual vessels and then a running suture to over-sew the free edge of the mesentery. Duodenum and pancreatic injuries were drained. Spleen and kidney injuries that were complex or had arterial bleeding usually required rapid removal. Liver injuries generally could be controlled with packing. Rarely, hepatic injuries had to be explored to control bleeding from a hepatic artery branch. Ureter injuries could be treated with ligation or simple drainage. Bladder injuries were over-sewn and drained. If a rectal injury was present, the distal sigmoid colon was divided with a stapler, and drains were placed, including a presacral drain. After these injuries were treated, the abdomen was irrigated with warm fluids to remove gross contamination and repacked. A radiograph cassette cover was fenestrated and then placed between the bowel and the fascia. A Kerlix (The Kendall Company, Mansfield, Massachusetts) roll was unrolled in the defect, and two 10-mm Jackson-Pratt (JP) drains were placed in the layers of the Kerlix. The skin on the abdomen was dried, and Mastisol (Ferndale Laboratories, Ferndale, Michigan) was placed in a wide swath around the wound. An

Ioban (3M, St. Paul, Minnesota) was then placed to create a seal, and the drain tubes were enclosed in a mesentery of the Ioban. The drains were placed quickly on suction. This dressing configuration allowed continued swelling of the abdominal contents without forming an abdominal compartment syndrome. The fenestrations and the JP's allowed fluid loss and ongoing hemorrhage to be monitored. This dressing was inexpensive, durable, and allowed patient movement and other treatments without losing its integrity. It also prevented injury to the surrounding skin or fascia that can occur with other closures.

The importance of damage-control techniques was demonstrated again in the complex set of injuries created by a high-velocity, trans-pelvis penetrating injury. Casualties who had this injury were some of the most challenging to treat. These patients had a complex injury including pelvic fracture and major vascular, ureter, bladder, and colorectal injuries. Often the exit wound would contain aerosolized stool in the extensive soft tissue injury. These patients generally presented with hypothermia and acidosis and were hypotensive. Any attempt at anything other than damage control resulted in sliding down the slippery slope of huge blood losses and physiologic burnout. Major pelvic veins can be controlled with packing. Internal iliac arteries were ligated, and common and external iliac arteries were stented or were repaired very rapidly with an abdominal aortic cross-clamp and femoral vessel clamps in place. Vessel loops were left in place at the closing to facilitate future dissections and rapid control if arterial bleeding restarted. The distal sigmoid colon was stapled, and a distal washout was performed because of the degree of destruction of the rectum and associated structures. Ureters were ligated, and bladder injuries were over-sewn. Most of the bleeding from the pelvic fractures was controlled with packing and rarely required internal iliac artery ligation on the side of the fracture. The packing of the pelvis required forceful packing of sponges into the pelvis. Additional packs were placed in the lower abdomen, and the skin of the lower abdomen was closed to help with the tamponade affect. Standard damage-control closure was performed in the upper abdomen.

The second-look procedure was performed as soon as the patient was resuscitated and rewarmed. In several cases, the patient was so unstable that the resuscitation and rewarming occurred in the OR. After several hours, a second-look damage-control procedure was performed before taking the patient to the ICU. In general, second-look procedures occurred between 12 and 24 hours after damage control. The average number of procedures was 3.4 for each patient, and 77% of patients who survived had definitive treatment of their injuries and closure of the abdomen. Average time to closure was 3.3 days [15].

Damage-control techniques often were used outside the abdomen. Vascular injuries of the extremities often were treated with shunting in forward surgical units. Tourniquets are a variation of vascular damage control that allows the patient to be stabilized and transported for definitive treatment. Thoracic damage control included tractotomy and packing of the thoracic cavity for diffuse soft tissue injuries.

Knowledge of damage-control surgery techniques in the management of complex trauma patients is essential for the surgeon in the combat environment. The use of damage-control techniques can avoid the lethal triad and allows rapid treatment of larger numbers of casualties in mass-casualty situations. The author's experience shows outcomes similar to that of urban trauma centers in both the forward surgical units and at the CSH.

Transfusion services

One of the most precious resources at the CSH was blood products. Within the combat theater, adequate stores of blood products, including packed red blood cells, cryoprecipitate, and frozen fresh plasma (FFP) were available. During times of high-intensity combat, stores of blood products at the CSH could be limited. Part of the issue with availability of blood products at the CSH was the limited staff and equipment to prepare blood products for transfusion. Thawing of FFP and cryoprecipitate was particularly difficult. During the 31st CSH deployment, platelets rarely were available. Blood product use commonly was triaged to the most severely injured until the blood bank could process enough units for all patients. A review of all the patients who received blood products during the first 24 hours at the CSH revealed that the average number of units administered per patient was 5.5, less than half the units required for patients undergoing damage control (Fig. 4). The use of whole blood in this figure is slightly skewed because very little whole blood was used until the second half of the year.

The use of fresh whole blood is not a new concept. It has been used in almost every military conflict since World War I. The modern practice of blood transfusions was started in the 1930s when a Canadian surgeon, Norman Bethune, transported blood from donors to recipients on the front lines

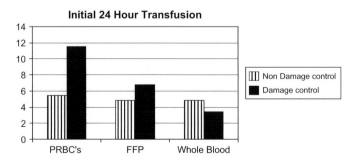

Fig. 4. Initial 24-hour transfusion (in units). FFP, fresh-frozen plasma; PRBCs, packed red blood cells.

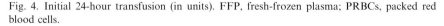

of the Spanish Civil War [16]. Component therapy is the standard for transfusion of blood products, but the process of separating these products results in the loss of half the platelets, and erythrocytes and clotting factors are diluted by 36%. The mixing of the components in a one-to-one ratio creates a unit of whole blood with a hematocrit of 29%, a platelet count of 88k, and 62% of the clotting activity [17]. The use of fresh whole blood has been described multiple times in situations where blood product components are limited or not available. During the battle of Mogadishu, 120 units of fresh whole blood were drawn, and 80 units were administered. These units were not tested and were transfused based on dog-tag information. The surgeons commented on the ability of the fresh whole blood to stop diffuse coagulopathy [16]. There were no known transfusion reactions or viral transmissions.

During the yearlong deployment, difficulty in obtaining adequate blood products in the correct distribution led to the development of a massive transfusion protocol. Massive transfusion commonly is defined as transfusions of 10 or more units of blood or the replacement of one blood volume in a patient. The massive transfusion protocol standardized the release of blood products including packed red blood cells, FFP, cryoprecipitate, and factor VIIa when initiated. At the same time, a call was made to the pre-screened walking donor pool within the hospital, the United States embassy, and the surrounding units for whole-blood donations. As the whole-blood donation was started, continued preparation of these standardized amounts of blood products was performed in an attempt to avoid delays in blood-product administration and to prevent the onset of coagulopathy. Identified donors were screened before donation for anemia with a copper sulfate test, and posttransfusion hematocrits were checked. One unit of whole blood was collected in a citrate phosphate dextrose adenine bag, and the sample was tested for HIV and hepatitis B and C, using ELISA if available. The entire process produced a steady supply of whole blood in 1 to 2 hours.

Although some believe that the extinction of whole blood use is imminent [18], the 31st CSH found it to be a vital part of its massive transfusion protocol. Although the retrospective evaluation of the use of whole blood is still ongoing, the surgical staff of the 31st CSH believed that fresh whole blood was the "magic bullet" that could help prevent physiologic exhaustion and also reverse it. Whole blood provided hemoglobin, clotting factors, and platelets in a prewarmed resuscitative fluid. The 31st CSH transfused 545 units of fresh whole blood to 86 severely injured trauma patients. There was one febrile nonhemolytic transfusion reaction; three were positive for hepatitis C virus, and one was indeterminate for HIV and human T-cell leukemia virus by Western blot [19]. The use of fresh whole blood was a vital part of the prevention or treatment of physiologic burnout in the severely injured trauma patient. The military is well suited for whole blood transfusions because of the presence of a large, prescreened walking donor pool that is at low risk for infectious transmission.

Factor VIIa

The use of activated blood coagulation factor VII in the treatment of OIF and OEF injured has increased steadily. Since its introduction for the treatment of hemorrhage in hemophilia patients who have antibodies to factor VIII, the use of activated factor VII has been described for prostatectomy, cardiac surgery, aortic aneurysm repair, polypectomy, postpartum bleeding, and bleeding complications in cirrhotic patients [20–23]. The first report of use for trauma injuries was from an Israeli group, and this report has been followed by several reports of success using activated factor VII for hemorrhage. In a retrospective review, Harrison and colleagues [24] compared the use of activated factor VII in 29 trauma patients with well-matched controls. He showed that there was no difference in mortality, but there were fewer packed red blood cell transfusions in the factor VIIA group (2.4 ± 6.2 versus 8.5 ± 9.6 units). This difference in transfusion requirements also held true with platelets and cryoprecipitate. There was no difference in FFP use. Patients who were given factor VIIa and survived had lower pHs than controls. Boffard and colleagues [25] reported similar results with a reduction in packed red blood cell transfusions after administration of factor VIIa. He also showed a 63% reduction in the need for massive transfusion. Thus, factor VIIa may play a role in the avoidance in the complications, including multiple organ failure, acute respiratory distress syndrome, and infectious complications, that are associated with massive transfusions [26–28].

The use of factor VIIa by the 31st CSH still is being reviewed. Approximately 600 doses of factor VIIa have been administered to 300 patients in Iraq. The protocol used calls for 90 μg/kg given immediately in the emergency room followed by an additional dose when the patient becomes normothermic. The use of factor VIIa in the acidotic patient is still a matter of controversy. Several studies have shown a decrease in the effectiveness of factor VIIA in the acidotic patient. The staff of the CSH found that in combination with massive resuscitation including crystalloid, bicarbonate, and other blood products, factor VIIa played a role in decreasing ongoing losses and reducing transfusion requirements. Additional research is required in this area to define further the effectiveness and possible strategies to reverse this effect, if present, and to allow the use of this product in the patients who may gain the most from it.

Future directions

The future may hold exciting changes in the use and position of blood products. Soldiers soon may carry units of their own freeze-dried blood or FFP on the same chain as the dog tags. If the soldier is injured, the blood and FFP may be reconstituted and given back to him. This technique would eliminate the need for blood typing, reduce preparation time, and prevent viral transmissions. FFP could be used as an initial resuscitative fluid administered by medics in the field. This technique would provide the casualty with volume and coagulation factors that mingt help to decrease additional bleeding. Blood stores may have the surface antigens removed by surface decoration to create a unit of universal blood that could be given to any patient without the delay of blood typing and prevent some transfusion reactions.

References

[1] Lewis. Tactical care combat casualty manual. First edition. Washington; 2005.
[2] Coupland RM, Molde A, Navein J. Care in the field for victims of weapons of war: a report from the workshop organized by the ICRC on pre-hospital care for war and mine-injured. Geneva (Switzerland): International Committee of the Red Cross; 2001.
[3] Husum HMD, Gilbert M, Wisborg T, et al. Letter to the editor. Journal of Trauma Injury Infection and Critical Care 2004;56(1):214–5.
[4] Dorlac WC, DeBakey ME, Holcomb JB, et al. Mortality from isolated civilian penetrating extremity injury. Journal of Trauma Injury Infection and Critical Care 2005;59(1):217–22.
[5] Lakstein D, Blumenfeld A, Sokolov T, et al. Tourniquets for hemorrhage control on the battlefield: a 4-year accumulated experience. J Trauma 2003;54(5 Suppl):S221–5.
[6] Beekley A. Outcomes after prehospital extremity tourniquet placement in Operation Iraqi Freedom. Presented at the meeting of the American Association for the Surgery of Trauma. Atlanta, Georgia, September 22, 2005.
[7] Sebesta D. Experience as the Chief of Surgery at the 67th Evacuation Hospital, Republic of Vietnam 1968 to 1969. Mil Med 1990;155(5):227–9.
[8] McManus J, Yershov AL, Ludwig D, et al. Radial pulse character relationships to systolic blood pressure and trauma outcomes. Prehosp Emerg Care 2005;9(4):423–8.
[9] Holcomb JB, Salinas J, McManus JM, et al. Manual vital signs reliably predict need for life-saving interventions in trauma patients. J Trauma 2005;59(4):821–8 [discussion: 828–9].
[10] Pringle JH. Notes on the arrest of hepatic hemorrhage due to trauma. Ann Surg 1908;48: 541–9.
[11] Feliciano DV, Mattox KL, Jordan GL Jr. Intra-abdominal packing for control of hepatic hemorrhage: a reappraisal. J Trauma 1981;21:285–90.
[12] Stone HH, Strom PR, Mullins RJ. Management of the major coagulopathy with onset during laparotomy. Ann Surg 1983;197:532–5.
[13] Eiseman B, Moore EE, Meldrum DR, et al. Feasibility of damage control surgery in the management of military combat casualties. Arch Surg 2000;135:1323–7.
[14] Jurkovich GJ, Greiser WB, Luterman A, et al. Hypothermia in trauma victims: an ominous predictor of survival. J Trauma 1987;27:1019–24.
[15] Sebesta J. Damage control surgery in Iraq: the experience of the 31st Combat Support Hospital. Presented at the meeting of the American Association for the Surgery of Trauma. Atlanta, Georgia, September 22, 2005.
[16] Mabry RL, Holcomb JB, Baker AM, et al. United States Army Rangers in Somalia: an analysis of combat casualties on an urban battlefield. Journal of Trauma Injury Infection and Critical Care 2000;49(3):515–29.
[17] Hess JR, Zimrin AB. Massive blood transfusion for trauma. Curr Opin Hematol 2005;12(6): 488–92.
[18] Hiippala S. Replacement of massive blood loss. Vox Sang 1998;74(Suppl 2):399–407.
[19] Spinella PC, Grathwohl K, Holcomb J, et al. Risks associated with fresh warm whole blood compared to PRBC transfusions during combat. 165-S. Crit Care Med 2005;33(12 Suppl): A44.
[20] Anantharaju A, Mehta K, Mindikogle AL, et al. Use of Activated recombinant human factor VII (rhFVIIa) for colonic polypectomies in patients with cirrhosis and coagulopathy. Dig Dis Sci 2003;48(7):1414–24.

[21] Friederich PW, Henny CP, Messelink EJ, et al. Effect of recombinant activated factor VII on perioperative blood loss in patients undergoing retropubic prostatectomy: a double-blind placebo controlled randomized trial. Lancet 2003;361:201–5.

[22] Tanaka KA, Waly AA, Cooper WA, et al. Treatment of excessive bleeding in Jehovah's Witness patients after cardiac surgery with recombinant factor VIIa. Anesthesiology 2003;98:1513–5.

[23] Wahlgren CM, Swedenborg J. The use of recombinant activated factor VII to control bleeding during repair of a suprarenal abdominal aortic aneurysm. Eur J Vasc Endovasc Surg 2003;26(2):221–2.

[24] Harrison T, Daniel DO, Laskosky J, et al. "Low dose" recombinant activated factor VII (rFVIIA) results in less packed red blood cell (PRBC) use in traumatic hemorrhage. Journal of Trauma Injury Infection and Critical Care 2004;57(6):1383.

[25] Boffard KD, Riou B, Warren B, et al, for the NovoSeven Trauma Study Group. Recombinant factor VIIa as adjunctive therapy for bleeding control in severely injured trauma patients: two parallel randomized, placebo-controlled, double-blind clinical trials. Journal of Trauma Injury Infection and Critical Care 2005;59(1):8–18.

[26] Young JS, Claridge JA, Crabtree TD, et al. Persistent occult hypoperfusion is associated with a significant increase in infection rate and mortality in major trauma patients. Journal of Trauma Injury Infection and Critical Care 1999;47(1):214.

[27] Sauaia A, Moore FA, Moore EE, et al. Early predictors of postinjury multiple organ failure. Arch Surg 1994;129(1):39–45.

[28] Moore FA, Moore EE, Sauaia A. Blood transfusion. An independent risk factor for postinjury multiple organ failure. Arch Surg 1997;132(6):620–4 [discussion: 624–5].

ELSEVIER
SAUNDERS

SURGICAL
CLINICS OF
NORTH AMERICA

Surg Clin N Am 86 (2006) 727–752

Surgical Support for Low-Intensity Conflict, Limited Warfare, and Special Operations

LTC Robert M. Rush Jr, MD[a,b,c,d],*

[a]Uniformed Services University of the Health Sciences, 4301 Jones Bridge Road,
Bethesda, MD 20814-4799, USA
[b]Department of Surgery, Madigan Army Medical Center, Building 9040
Fitzsimmons Drive, Tacoma, WA 98431-1100, USA
[c]Department of Surgery, University of Washington, 1959 NE Pacific Street, Box 356410,
Seattle, WA 98195-6410, USA
[d]Mayo Medical School, Mayo Clinic, 13400 East Shea Boulevard,
Scottsdale, AZ 85259, USA

The spectrum of warfare to which US forces must respond is wide, from large-scale invasions such as those in Vietnam and more recently in Iraq to small insertions of personnel for short, specific missions, as in Grenada, to peacekeeping operations in the former Yugoslavia and Haiti. In each case, special operations forces (SOF) were major participants, and directed, low-intensity battles played a part. This article describes how surgical support of special operations and low-intensity conflict differs from the support required by conventional brigade combat teams, such as those in action in Iraq at present and described elsewhere in this issue.

Defining special operations and low-intensity conflicts

To plan medical support for a training mission, combat operation, public sporting event, or other situation, one must know the specified and implied tasks of the event to be supported. For example, the specified task, "Seek

The views expressed in this article are those of the author and do not reflect the official policy of the United States Army, the Department of Defense, or the United States Government.

* Correspondence. Department of Surgery, Madigan Army Medical Center, Tacoma, WA 98431.

E-mail addresses: robert.rush@amedd.army.mil; robert.rush1@us.army.mil

0039-6109/06/$ - see front matter. Published by Elsevier Inc.
doi:10.1016/j.suc.2006.03.004

surgical.theclinics.com

out and incapacitate the al Qaeda terrorist organization in Afghanistan," carries with it an almost inconceivable number and breadth of implied tasks, only one of which is medical support. Fortunately for the US armed forces, a massive and intricate framework already is in place to assist with the planning and support that are described in detail in this issue. This organizational structure makes the US military especially responsive in defending the nation, assisting with peacekeeping, responding to natural disasters and delivering humanitarian aid, and protecting national borders, among other tasks. SOF missions generally require an even higher level of responsiveness, a wider range of possible scenarios, and sometimes a greater degree of sophistication, especially at the level of the individual soldier. Table 1 lists the requirements, missions, and capabilities of SOF personnel and units [1].

Table 1
Special Forces tasks for Operation Enduring Freedom as defined by the Congressional Record

Type of action/mission	Description
Direct action	Short-duration, small-scale offensive actions such as raids, ambushes, hostage rescues, and surgical strikes (eg, Operation Just Cause in Panama 1989)
Strategic (special) reconnaissance	Clandestine operations in hostile territory to gain significant information
Unconventional warfare	Advising and supporting indigenous insurgent and resistance groups operating in the territory of a common enemy (eg, Northern Alliance in Afghanistan)
Foreign internal defense	Assisting host nation military capabilities to forestall defeat by insurgent activities
Civil affairs	Promoting civil–military cooperation between US military forces and the foreign governments and populations within their area of operations (ie, "winning the hearts and the minds" of the people)
Psychological operations	Influencing the attitudes and behavior of the relevant populations to assist in accomplishing security missions
Counterterrorism	Operations conducted by special mission units to resolve or preempt terrorist incidents abroad and activities to assist or work with other counterterrorism-designated agencies within the United States
Humanitarian assistance	Providing rudimentary services to foreign populations in adverse circumstances (eg, de-mining, securing food delivery)
Theater search and rescue	Finding and recovering pilots and air crews downed on land or sea outside the United States, sometimes in combat or clandestine situations
Other	Other activities, at any time, with little or no notice, in any environment, as specified by the President or Secretary of Defense

Data from Bruner EF, Bolkom C, O'rourke R. Special operations forces in Operation Enduring Freedom: background and issues for Congress. CRS Report for Congress, CRS 1-CRS 6. Washington (DC): Library of Congress; 2001.

In addition to knowing what capabilities these units possess, it is essential to know the type and number of personnel to be supported. There are several tiers within the US special operations framework, with the more elite tiers involving service members from all four services (Army, Navy, Air Force, Marines) integrated in joint commands (Box 1) [2]. Tier one units are very specialized in counterterrorism, hostage seizure and release, and VIP security. Other levels involve service-specific units such as airborne/air assault units in the Army, force recon teams in the Marines, and special operations squadrons in the Air Force. Special forces, or the Green Berets, are tier one– or tier two–level assets that have wide-open missions. This article focuses, in the most part, on these units and their actions and on their Ranger and airborne/air

---

Box 1. Examples of special operations units and level of elite capability

For specific missions, units from varying services combine under temporary joint commands. Conventional forces also may be assigned temporarily to joint special operations task forces.

Joint Assets (tier one)
1st Special Forces Operational Detachment/D
Naval Special Warfare Development Group
160th Special Operations Aviation Regiment (Airborne)
16th Special Operations Wing

Army (tier two–three)
Special Forces Groups (Green Berets)
75th Ranger Regiment (Airborne)
160th Special Operations Aviation Regiment (Airborne)
18th Airborne Corps

Navy (tier two–three)
Special Boat Units
Sea Air and Land Teams (SEALS)
Mobile Communications Team

Air Force (tier two–three)
720th Special Tactics Group
23rd Special Tactics Squadron

Marine (tier two–three)
Force Reconnaissance
Marine Expeditionary Teams–Special Operations Capable

From Joint Special Operations Command (JSOC) Units. Available at: SpecialOperations.com. 2006. Accessed February 1, 2006.

assault brethren. Currently, it is estimated that there are 50,000 SOF person-nel, representing about 2% of the US armed forces. (This estimate does not include the 18th Airborne Corps assets.)

Elsewhere in this issue, Dr. Beekley describes large-scale conflict. Limited warfare involves fewer troops, sometimes for shorter periods of time, and generally does not interrupt a country's socioeconomic system. As defined by the US Joint Chiefs of Staff, "low intensity conflict is a political-military confrontation between contending states or groups below conventional war and above the routine, peaceful competition between states ... frequently in-volving protracted struggles of competing principles and ideologies ... rang-ing from subversion to the use of armed forces ... often localized, but contain regional and global security implications" [3]. For the purposes of this article, examples of low-intensity conflict are the invasion of Grenada in 1983, Panama in 1989, Somalia in 1993, and Operation Enduring Free-dom (OEF) in Afghanistan in 2001 to present. Initial actions in Northern Iraq at the outset of Operation Iraqi Freedom (OIF) also can be considered limited or low intensity because of the lack of conventional forces in that area of operations until well into May 2003. Another characteristic of spe-cial operations in Afghanistan and Northern Iraq were the relative isolation of these units, with no initial seaport or ground supply lines and the highly effective coordination of efforts with local militia so that militia forces did most of the fighting with SOF guidance and US Air Force, Navy, and Marine air support.

Medical/surgical support in special operations

The 18D "Eighteen Delta" Special Forces medic is the crux of medical support for Army Special Forces units. Navy independent duty corpsman, SEAL medics, and Air Force para-rescue jumpers are other service-specific equivalents, but the focus here is primarily on the 18D. Traditional Army Special Forces units are organized into Special Forces Groups that consist of three battalions, each battalion having 300 to 400 personnel [4]. Battal-ions are further subdivided into three companies of six "A" teams per com-pany. The "A" team, or "operational detachment alpha" (ODA), is the primary unit of action within Army Special Forces and is comprised of 12 members. In most cases the team commander is a captain who is assisted by an executive officer, usually a chief warrant officer; both of whom possess considerable experience in the army and usually are of infantry background. There are 10 other members of the team, all senior enlisted personnel. The primary specialties and number of these enlisted soldiers are one operations sergeant, one assistant operations and intelligence sergeant, two weapons sergeants, two engineer sergeants, two medical sergeants (18D), and two communications sergeants.

In addition to military training and experience received before entering Special Forces (all members usually have at least 3–6 years of experience with conventional or airborne/Ranger units), all personnel must go through an extensive selection process (a 3-week Special Forces Assessment and Selection course and 3 weeks of airborne/parachute school) and then attend a qualification course lasting approximately 1 year [5]. In this 1-year course, approximately 46 weeks are dedicated to medical training for the 18D. The 18D must master 381 major medical tasks from 30 different subject areas that encompass what medical students are taught in 4 years of medical school, albeit less in depth (Table 2) [6]. After this qualification, 18Ds are assigned to a Special Forces ODA team and go through further unit and individual training (SCUBA, free-fall and high-altitude parachute school, pathfinder school) lasting up to another year. All enlisted personnel are required to have a primary skill, as mentioned previously, a secondary skill, and also to be proficient in at least one foreign language in their battalion's area of responsibility on the world map.

This training completed, the 18D is prepared to provide complete medical services to the detachment and indigenous forces, in austere environments, without ancillary, physician, logistic, or medical evacuation support [5]. SOF units participate in large conventional wars, limited conflicts, peacekeeping operations, and disaster response. SOF units are particularly capable of rapid response to a wide variety of medical and tactical scenarios worldwide. In response to Hurricane Andrew in 1992, the 3rd Battalion, 11th Special Forces Group was activated with personnel in place within 24 hours, even though their headquarters was destroyed [7]. This unit proved to be ideal to augment existing medical care providers on short notice, bringing equipment, power generation, and supplies as well as

Table 2
18D Special Forces medic medical proficiency training main subject areas

Laboratory	Endocrinology
Administrative	Neurology
Basic medical skills	Psychiatry
Nursing	Communicable diseases
Preventive medicine	Parasitology
Dental	Vector-borne diseases
Veterinary medicine	Pediatrics
Dermatology	Trauma
Otolaryngology (HEENT)	Anesthesia
Cardiovascular conditions	Surgical procedures
Pulmonology	CMS (Central Material Supply)
Genitourinary conditions	NBC (Nuclear, Biological, Chemical)
Gastroenterology	Environmental medicine
Obstetrics and gynecology	Special Forces medic skills
Orthopedics	Senior Special Forces medic skills

Data from Soldiers manual/trainer's guide. MOS 18D Special Forces medical sergeant skill levels 3 and 4. STP 31–18D34-SM-TG. Washington (DC): Headquarters, Department of the Army; 2003.

providing command and control, security, needs assessments, and reconnaissance for locating victims in remote areas.

Part of the SOF mission entails performing military operations behind enemy lines for extended periods, where United States surgical/medical assets cannot be located easily or safely [8]. In this scenario, SOF personnel make special provisions to care for wounded and support guerilla force medical assets by forming clandestine hospitals [9]. These hospitals are very resource constrained, austere, and isolated and depend on camouflage, foraging, secrecy, and the ability to recruit local physicians and medical personnel (including available missionary and nongovernmental organization medical assets) for ongoing operations.

Despite extensive training, preparation for specific missions and refresher training are necessary and encouraged. In response to the analysis of casualties incurred in urban and modern conflict, such as seen in Somalia in the early 1990s, Butler and Hagmann [10] proposed that SOF change their treatment emphasis and algorithm. They found that combat prehospital protocols based on the traditional advanced trauma life support (ATLS) framework were not adequate for dealing with the casualties in the harsh reality of austere conditions that are often seen in the heat of battle. Their proposal that SOF medics be trained in the phases of (1) care under fire, (2) tactical field care, and (3) casualty evacuation care using short didactic sessions and case-based scenarios that required both medical and tactical decision making revolutionized training in and delivery of prehospital combat medical care [10]. A hybrid form of this training now is provided in both initial and refresher conventional US Army line medic training as the Tactical Combat Casualty Care course [11]. Under fire, only simple things can be done to save a life. Most often, the medic and others who are able return suppressive fire to the enemy to protect themselves and the injured. Obvious, exsanguinating external bleeding sometimes can be controlled in this environment. Once out of immediate danger, other interventions, such as airway management or the relief of a tension pneumothorax, can be performed, and the casualty is evacuated. Experienced 18D Special Forces medics provide most of the teaching cadre for this course with surgeon oversight. Other tactical and field medicine courses provide instruction on subjects ranging from disaster response to refresher war surgery courses, all emphasizing austere and unpredictable environmental and social conditions [10–14].

Additional, mission-specific training can be provided immediately before combat and other types of operations. Peoples and colleagues [15] describe the refresher training, in addition to far-forward surgical support, provided by surgeons and nurses of the 274th FST to 18D and SOF medical personnel in Uzbekistan before ODA teams entered Afghanistan in 2001 at the outset of OEF. OEF involved large numbers of SOF that entered Afghanistan, at first with no forward surgical or traditional medical evacuation assets provided in country (Fig. 1). Evacuation times ranged from 24 hours to 5 days at the outset of OEF [16,17], and the usefulness of a short didactic

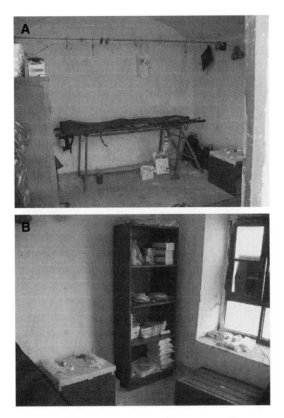

Fig. 1. (*A,B*) Special Forces austere but functional aid station in Afghanistan at the beginning of the war. These aid stations can be set up at any level. This one is aligned with the battalion headquarters (Operational Detachment Charlie [ODC]).

review covering field anesthesia, blood transfusions, and fracture management proved its worth in treating Northern Alliance soldiers, civilians, and enemy combatants as well as their own personnel.

Other medical assets within special operations groups consist of command surgeons (ie, medical officers, who usually are not surgeons, per se), who provide oversight and higher-level medical care and consultation for the 18D. There is one group surgeon, and there is a battalion surgeon for each of three operational battalions in the group. Each of the battalions also has a physician's assistant who provides most of the routine medical care for soldiers of the battalion. These physicians cannot be present in the far-forward area with each ODA team; battalion headquarters usually are hundreds of miles from some ODA teams and support a number of ODA teams in a widespread area, amplifying the need for advanced medical training for the 18D. Each group also has a support battalion containing a preventive medicine officer, several preventive medicine noncommissioned officers, a veterinarian (with dual responsibility as preventive medicine officer), a medical operations noncommissioned officer, and a medical logistician. These essential personnel mostly provide predeployment planning, ongoing assessments, and operational support but rarely are at the point of care on the battlefield where most ODA teams function.

Actual surgical support is provided to forward-deployed SOF by any of a number of surgical assets. Army forward surgical teams (FSTs) (units of approximately 20 persons with four surgeons), Air Force mobile forward surgical teams (six-person units with two surgeons), and Marine/Navy forward resuscitative surgical systems (eight personnel with two surgeons) can be assigned to Joint Special Operations Task Forces (JSOTF) for far-forward combat surgical support [17–21]. These assets most commonly are assigned to brigade/group base camps but can be prepositioned closer to combat action for short periods during battles and offensive campaigns. These small units depend to a varying degree on the unit to which they provide surgical support for supplies such as food, water, fuel beyond their basic combat load (the initial sustainment supplies with which a unit "goes to war"). While assigned to these missions, surgical teams may be the only unit with any type of hospital capability and sometimes are tasked with nondoctrinal missions such as limited sick call, treatment of infectious diseases, detainee care, and civil affairs and even can act as medical evacuation hubs.

Army forward surgical teams are especially robust, 20-person teams that often are placed in isolated areas to support combat casualty care of SOF soldiers and to provide synergistic care of civilian trauma and disease and so assist, along with 18D medics, in the SOF mission of "winning the hearts and the minds of the indigenous population." In 2002 and 2003, the 102nd FST served as the only trauma center in southern Afghanistan, taking on civilian and military casualties alike, regardless of mechanism [22]. In the opening rounds of OEF in Kandahar, the 250th FST treated as many patients for disease as for combat trauma and acted as the southern evacuation hub in sending more than 50% of trauma patients directly to Landstuhl Regional Medical Center in Germany (Fig. 2) [17]. Most FSTs can assemble and deploy anywhere in the world within 24 to 48 hours and in combination with a JSOTF can provide a robust military or disaster-response package capable of providing initial security, scene management, trauma/medical treatment, and civil affairs coordination. In addition to medical specialties, all members of the FST, including surgeons, are required to have at least two other duties. In many instances surgeons assisted the enlisted personnel in the unit with filling sand bags to improve force protection, standing guard, performing generator maintenance, and gathering supplies. It is absolutely necessary for the surgeons to be active in helping with these sometimes mundane tasks.

Ranger battalions, airborne brigades, air assault units, and mountain infantry brigades contain medical support that is similar to that of other, conventional forces, as pointed out in other articles in this issue. Combat medics

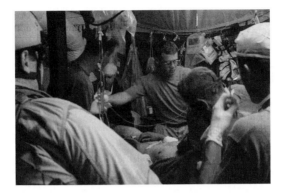

Fig. 2. The interface. Special operations force medics delivering injured to a Forward Surgical Team for far-forward surgical resuscitation in support of a joint special operations task force in Kandahar, Afghanistan in December 2001.

in elite units must have the additional skills of being airborne, air-assault or Ranger qualified. Ranger medics now obtain paramedic status before deploying on combat missions [23]. These units generally are busier than conventional units, especially in peacetime. Many of them are part of rapid deployment forces because they have lighter combat loads than mechanized infantry and armor heavy units. Each battalion has an aid station and can function as front-line ATLS providers, but there is no patient-holding capability. Forward support medical companies provide broader services, usually are at the brigade level, and are doctrinally where FSTs meld into the brigade medical support system as level two+ care. The FST and brigade aid station emergency sections provide parallel support with life-threatening hemorrhagic/central nervous system/airway injuries being triaged to the FST, usually from a common triage area. The Marines have a similar system in that one or more forward resuscitative surgical systems can integrate with the organic shock/trauma platoon of a brigade-sized marine expeditionary unit for far-forward battlefield trauma support.

Environmental factors, situational awareness, and injury/disease prevention

Environmental conditions such as terrain, weather, and location can have a significant effect on the success of a mission as well as on the medical support provided. Often, SOF missions occur in isolated areas, sometimes behind enemy lines, in austere conditions with unpredictable weather and lines of communication. The supporting medical/surgical assets do not always have the luxury of training with the units with whom they go to war, nor are they always located with the units to be supported before deploying [15,17]. These factors require maximum communication between all aspects of support for SOF missions, and particularly for reserve medical units. In these circumstances, the supporting medical unit commander/ group/individual augmentee must communicate with the unit to be supported ensure that the medical/surgical support is appropriate for the combat unit's mission and that the personnel of the medical unit are prepared adequately on a personal readiness level (ie, with appropriate immunizations for the area of operations, weather-appropriate clothing, conditioning, medical and food supplies, and hygiene material).

Before parachuting into northern Iraq at the beginning of OIF, the 250th FST had 48 hours to link with leaders and medical support personnel of the 173rd Airborne Brigade and Joint Special Operations Task Force–North (JSOTF-N) at Aviano Airbase, Italy [20]. Planning continued after the jump and through air-land operations. Educating brigade medical planners about FST capabilities and employment was extremely challenging, because no modern-era FST had supported a combat jump. The FST was broken into echelons for 24 hours, per protocol. Because of soft conditions on the drop zone (the jump was preceded by approximately 24 hours of rain), the unit sustained only 10 injuries, the most serious being one soldier who had a tibia–fibula fracture and another who had bilateral shoulder dislocations. ATLS procedures were performed on the drop zone by first-echelon elements, as had been done in Operation Just Cause in Panama. On the second night the FST second echelon landed as planned, and the unit reformed for full operational capability. In all operations, conditions on the battlefield can change on a daily basis, and evacuation and injury patterns, casualty flow, and a unit's own capabilities can change in an instant; thus, constant reassessment is required.

Embarking from stateside bases to areas of operation for immediate combat action in markedly different climatic conditions must be planned for. Most Rangers and paratroopers participating in Operation Just Cause in Panama (December 1989), including support and medical personnel, went from bases in North Carolina, Georgia, and Washington, where at that time of the year the temperature was cold and wet (30°–40°F), to a hot and humid jungle environment (>90°F) and were thrust immediately into combat [24]. Many of the paratroopers consumed their recommended two canteens (1 quart each) of water during the flight, leaving none available for strenuous combat operations on the ground. Eleven soldiers (4% of those injured) were evacuated from the theater emergently because of heat injuries [25]. Probably, more were treated and kept in country, for whom data were not published. Prevention of heat injuries involves the addition of CamelBak® (CamelBak Products, LLC, Petaluma, California) personal water blivets, frequent and available resupply points, larger canteens (the newer, 2-quart canteen), and a command emphasis on continued hydration.

Altitude plays a major role in mountainous military operations. The recent campaign to crush al Qaeda and Taliban forces on the frontier ranges of the Hindu Kush Mountains of Afghanistan during OEF have shown that altitude is particularly relevant to current military missions where SOF assets are exposed to the possible effects of the hypoxia, low barometric pressure, and freezing temperatures of high altitude. High altitude is defined as 1500 to 3500 m (4921–11,483 feet), very high altitude as 3500 to 5500 m (11,483–18,045 feet), and extreme altitude as over 5500 m (18,045 feet) [26]. Most US military special operations that occur at altitude take place at heights defined as high altitude. The most frequent occurring syndrome of high altitude in US troops is acute mountain sickness (AMS). Presenting symptoms of AMS include headache, dyspnea, nausea, insomnia, anorexia, cough, emesis, and dizziness. Symptoms usually occur between 6 and 96 hours after arrival at high altitude [27]. Almost all symptoms and syndromes of AMS resolve upon returning to lower elevations. In military special operations, however, this return is not always possible because of mission constraints. To define better the incidence of AMS among regular troops, Pigman and Karakla [27] reported that in a 638-man Marine battalion landing team performing a routine training mission at 8200 feet, 9 (1.4%) presented with incapacitating symptoms of AMS, 7 of whom required treatment. These men were taken directly to altitude without acclimation. For subsequent missions at high altitude, the authors recommend prophylaxis only for those who have a history of AMS.

Operation Anaconda at the beginning of OEF (March 2–14, 2002) occurred in the Shah-i-Kot Mountains in Afghanistan at an average altitude of 10,000 feet. There are several reports of soldiers developing mild and incapacitating AMS during this battle [16]. In the only published study reporting numbers, Midla [28] reports on prophylaxis given to 120 soldiers using acetazolamide, 250 mg by mouth twice daily for 24 hours before going to altitude, and then changing to 125 mg by mouth twice daily for 4 days while remaining at altitude. None in this group experienced AMS, and all were exposed to the rigors and stress of combat conditions. If AMS develops, a descent of 500 to 1000 feet may be all that is necessary for treatment. In lieu of descent, the treatment for AMS consists of giving supplemental oxygen. Administration of acetazolamide may slow the process but is not definitive. High-altitude pulmonary edema is the most commonly lethal of the altitude syndromes. When it is recognized early, a descent of 500 to 1000 feet can correct the condition. When descent is not possible because of mission constraints, supplementary oxygen or a hyperbaric bag are adequate treatments. The alternative medical treatments were based on the treatment of common overload pulmonary edema using a diuretic and morphine. Calcium-channel blockers such as nifedipine (10 mg sublingually at once, followed by 30 mg sustained release by mouth every 12–24 hours) reduce pulmonary hypertension and thus pulmonary edema without the untoward effects of dehydration and decreased sensorium [29]. High-altitude cerebral edema is the severe form of AMS and, like high-altitude pulmonary edema, is fatal if not quickly recognized and treated. Symptoms start with a more severe headache than AMS and progress to confusion, ataxia, and irrational behavior. Rapid descent and oxygen administration are the treatments of choice, and dexamethasone is started (8 mg at once by mouth or intramuscularly, then 4 mg every 6 hours) to temporize and treat the condition [29]. Letting the patient "sleep off" these symptoms may result in coma or death by the next day.

Injuries caused by cold have plagued armies since the beginning of recorded history. SOF are especially vulnerable because of their wide range of missions in variable and frequently harsh climates and environments, sometimes on extended patrol from base camps and with limited supplies. These injuries fall into three main categories: nonfreezing and freezing tissue injuries and systemic accidental hypothermia (as opposed to secondary hypothermia after severe injury, which Dr. Beekley has addressed in another article). Although hypothermia occurs more often at high altitudes and cold temperatures, it can occur at any altitude and temperature and can be magnified by emersion into cold or cool water (defined as $< 77°$ F) [30]. In 1995, four US Army Ranger candidates died from hypothermia because of immersion while traversing a Florida swamp on a training mission in February. Factors contributing to this event were unplanned and abnormally high water levels, lack of knowledge of how to perform jungle/swamp extraction by medics on the ground, adverse weather conditions inhibiting rotary wing extraction, and lack of adequate fuel supply for medical evacuation helicopters [31]. Classic accidental hypothermic symptoms begin at core temperatures below 89.6°F (32°C) that manifest as vague fatigue, hunger, nausea, and dizziness. Cold temperatures and exhaustion precipitate hypothermia. Early physical findings include tachycardia and signs of dehydration that lead to bradycardia and hypotension if the process is not reversed. Treatment involves passive and active rewarming. Prehospital rewarming consists of mostly passive external methods: ensuring the patient is dry to prevent evaporative heat loss and placing warm chemical bags, sleeping bags, and hot water bottles next to the casualty [32]. Active external rewarming consists of forced heated air and either total (difficult in most settings) or partial immersion in warm water (placing extremities in warm water baths of 104°F). Active internal rewarming in the field setting usually consists of warmed intravenous fluids. In the first hospital setting, whether the FST or combat support hospital, active internal rewarming consists of ventilation with warmed humidified oxygen, body cavity lavage with warmed isotonic saline, and femoral–femoral bypass with a fluid warmer in circuit (such as a level-one intravenous fluid warmer).

Nonfreezing injuries such as trench and immersion foot are characterized by long-term exposure to cold water (0–10°C). Prolonged wearing of wet boots and socks and exposure to water in life rafts are the usual mechanisms. The extremity looks white, is cold to the touch, and is numb. Afterwards an initial period of hyperemia and urticaria is followed by tissue sloughing and pain. Treatment consists of careful drying, elevation, and passive rewarming through increasing core body temperature [33]. Non–weight bearing and avoidance of repeated cold exposures are essential for weeks to months afterward. Frostbite currently is the most common injury sustained from cold exposure, especially among SOF personnel operating in austere conditions [34]. Freezing injuries result from the crystallization of water molecules in cells and the interstitial spaces leading to decreased blood flow and ischemia. Frostbite occurs in degrees from erythema and numbness to full-thickness tissue loss and gangrene. Treatment consists of removing the victim from the cold. If there is any chance of further cold exposure (as in prolonged transport or walking through snow), no rewarming efforts should occur, because it worsen the extent of injury [35]. Victims should be transported with injured areas padded and dry and blisters left intact. No massaging should be performed. At a treatment facility rapid rewarming is initiated by treating systemic hypothermia and associated trauma. Then extremities are warmed rapidly by immersion in strictly regulated 104° to 108°F baths with gentle circulation. To prevent the progression of cell death, ibuprofen is administered to inhibit arachidonic acid–stimulated fibrinolysis, thus opening capillaries at the tissue injury interface [36]. Débridement should not be performed unless tissue cellulitis exists, the patient becomes septic, or there is lack of progression of healing at the skin–gangrene interface. Tetanus prophylaxis is mandatory for both types of tissue injury patterns. This treatment usually is not necessary in US forces because of the mandatory immunization protocol but must be administered to all others unless accurate history dictates otherwise. Frostbite, trench foot, hypothermia, and heat injuries are all command-reportable incidents; that is, physicians diagnosing and treating these conditions must report the incident to their higher military chain of command, because all commanders in the US Army can be held accountable for these injuries occurring in troops in their unit. Education of combat leaders and soldiers in preventing these injuries is the key to treatment [34].

Indigenous diseases and hazards in areas of operation are too numerous to address fully in this article. A few deserve comment here, because these diseases affect many current missions worldwide. Insect-borne diseases have the potential to incapacitate an entire unit. Malaria is endemic to most current SOF areas of operation. Wallace and colleagues [37] reported the following risk factors associated with malaria transmission in operation Restore Hope in Somalia (1992–1993): noncompliance with recommended chemoprophylaxis, failure to use bed nets, and failure to keep sleeves rolled down. Minimizing risks and effects of any insect-borne disease requires pre-deployment education, immunization where necessary and available, bite avoidance, chemoprophylaxis, rapid diagnosis, and command emphasis that ensures soldier mass participation [38]. Insect netting and insect repellants are maximally important to deter vectors from transmitting parasites. Permethrin is an insect repellant impregnated on all clothing and netting to deter mosquitoes and sand flies, the vector for Leishmnaiasis. Diethyltoluamide (DEET) can by applied to exposed areas of skin but not to mucous membranes [39]. Prophylaxis is mandatory and depends on the endemic malarial species. Chloroquine-based regimens (500 mg by mouth weekly) are adequate for regions with *Plasmodium vivax*. Mefloquine (250 g by mouth weekly) usually covers the more virulent *P falciparum* species. Daily doxycycline (100 mg by mouth) is an alternative, especially for pilots, because the other regimens can have side effects related to sleep deprivation. Doxycycline also increases skin sensitivity to UV radiation, however. Once the soldier is out of the endemic area, the previous medications are continued for 3 weeks, and primaquine is given for the second and third weeks after returning. Many recommend that people who have glucose-6-phosphate dehydrogenase deficiency should not take primaquin because of the increased risk of hemolysis. Symptoms of malaria include fatigue, daily temperature spikes, and detection of organisms on peripheral blood smears. Treatment of malaria once symptoms become clinically relevant involves daily does of chloroquine, mefloquin or higher daily doses of doxycycline than used for prophylaxis, and primaquine. Personal protection, chemoprophylaxis, and vector control at base camps, when possible, act synergistically to combat vector-borne diseases.

Diarrheal illnesses and gastroenteritis are common in a deployed environment especially when food is obtained by foraging. Symptoms include vomiting, cramping abdominal pain, fever, and diarrhea. In deployed US military troops, viruses cause most diarrheal diseases, most notably the Norwalk-like virus and rotavirus [40–44]. Bacterial diarrhea usually is watery and bloody and is associated with a higher white blood cell count and fever. Generous administration of intravenous fluids is sometimes required. Pharmacologic treatment of bacterial diarrhea consists of ciprofloxacin, 500 mg by mouth two times per day, in most cases. Loperamide HCl can reduce symptoms and allow soldiers to continue working with almost full combat effectiveness in some cases but must be used with caution, especially in bacterial diarrhea. There are no known regimens for the prevention of diarrheal illnesses, but correspondence with members of 250th FST supports the author's experience that effects can be minimized by taking 500 mg of ciprofloxacin before and again on the day after consuming a meal from local food sources [40,45,46]. The Department of Defense has long implemented an aggressive immunization program that is tracked on the local unit and national levels. Compliance is mandatory. All service members are immunized against typhoid, typhus, yellow fever, tetanus, pertussis, diphtheria, polio, influenza, and hepatitis to minimize combat ineffectiveness resulting from disease. Other immunizations are used for region-specific missions. Although they are not specifically included in the field manual for forward surgical teams, the 250th FST included an entire chest of sick-call type medicines for treatment of assigned members. This precaution was especially helpful in augmenting SOF unit command elements who became ill at base camps and required both inpatient and outpatient care.

Psychologic stress of special operations and low-intensity conflicts occurs, although the incidence is lower in SOF than in conventional forces

[47]. Dissociation is the most likely mechanism in individuals exposed to acute, uncontrollable stress. SOF personnel do not dissociate as much as conventional troops, indicating that previous exposure to and successful negotiation of previous stressful events, both in training and combat, inoculate these soldiers against detrimental stress responses. Combat stress injury is more prevalent in those who have poor relationships at home before deploying, who are wounded more than once, who have friends wounded in action, or who feel guilty about the death of a friend or patient [48]. This observation suggests that predeployment screening for those at risk may help identify potential combat stress casualties so that preventative interventions can be instituted. In addition, it is recommended that critical-event debriefings be held for situations involving mass casualties, both for the unit sustaining the casualties and for the medical personnel treating them [49]. During OEF these debriefings were held routinely as part of the 250th FST's internal after-action reviews of all mass casualty incidents.

In addition to the information provided here, several publications concisely and systematically outline preventive and environmental medicine topics for physicians and small-unit leaders in rapid deployable small-unit surgical teams of any sort [39,50,51].

Combat injury patterns, mechanisms, and far-forward surgical support in special operations and low-intensity conflict

Since Vietnam the United States has been involved in many low-intensity conflicts throughout the world. Areas of special interest are those with more significant troop involvement: Grenada (1983), Central America (1984–1990), Panama (1989), Somalia (1993), Afghanistan (2001–present), Philippines (2002–present), Colombia (2003–present), and northern Iraq (2003). Exact injuries and mechanisms are not well documented in the literature for all missions. Table 3 depicts casualty rates for the major SOF operations for which data have been recorded and made available.

Operation Urgent Fury in Grenada involved large numbers of SOF, Army Rangers, airborne units, and Marine amphibious landing teams. In

Table 3
Casualty rates from recent US special operations missions*

Operation	Total troops	Killed in action	Died of wounds	Wounded in action	Total casualties	Casualty rate (%)
Grenada	5000	18	1	116	135	3.3
Panama	26,000	23	0	323	346	1.3
Somalia (Mogadishu)	1640	14	4	58	76	4.6
Afghanistan (2001–May 2002)	20,000	17	0	86	103	0.5

* This table does not include casualties who were treated and returned to duty on the same day.

addition to battalion aid stations, the assault involving approximately 5000 troops was supported by an airborne clearing company's alpha echelon consisting of 27 personnel including one general surgeon, one orthopedic surgeon, one nurse anesthetist, and one general medical officer [52]. These surgeons, having been taken from a local military hospital on the base from which a majority of the troops deployed, were not regularly assigned to the unit supported and had not trained with the unit. After most hostilities ceased, the unit was augmented with additional surgical support. Data from the first echelon revealed an 88% extremity injury rate with a 19% amputation rate [53]. Islinger and colleagues [53] report that all injuries resulted from gunshot wounds, clearly a different type of battle than seen at present in OIF and OEF. The use of fragmentary devices may have been limited for fear of collateral damage, because the mission involved rescuing US civilians as well as overthrowing communist rule on Grenada. Also noted was the absence of radiology capability for the entire mission that may have hampered treatment of some orthopedic injuries. There were only 28 disease/nonbattle injuries listed, 4 of which were accidental deaths by drowning suffered by one SEAL team because of heavy combat loads and high seas during their attempted insertion [54]. Most of the severely injured were transferred offshore by rotary-winged aircraft to a Naval amphibious warship with operating capability, were stabilized, and then were brought back to the island for fixed-winged transport to a naval hospital in Puerto Rico or to the continental United States.

Operation Just Cause in Panama in 1989 involved 26,000 troops. At about 0100 on December 20, a jump force of 3900 Rangers, airborne, and SOF soldiers performed a surprise nighttime drop on Panamanian Defense Forces led by General Manual Noriega. Surgical support was more detailed than in the invasion of Grenada, with several surgical elements (two surgeons and one certified registered nurse anesthetist) actually jumping with the initial Ranger and SOF assault waves to provide drop-zone resuscitation in the event of impossible evacuation, which did not occur (COL Stephen Hetz, personal communication, 2006). Resuscitations were performed on the drop zone but consisted mainly of ATLS procedures as recommended in the FST field manual for trauma care during "hot" combat jumps and experienced in other campaigns [20,23,55]. Casualties were taken quickly from the point of injury to a level two surgical complex by helicopter. There were two forward surgical slices (precursors of the forward surgical teams developed in the 1990s) positioned at the United States–occupied Howard Air Force Base, along with a medical clearing company and an Air Force evacuation team [24]. During the first few waves of casualties, surgical teams in direct support of the jumps accompanied casualties being evacuated from the front lines; they augmented the forward surgical slice at Howard Air Force Base for the remainder of the conflict. At Howard Air Force Base rotary-wing and ground ambulance could drop incoming wounded 20 feet from the entrance to the facility. C130 fixed-wing evacuation aircraft could come within 30 feet to transport casualties to Wilford Hall Air Force Medical Center and Brooke Army Medical Center, both in San Antonio, Texas. Some casualties arrived in San Antonio within 12 hours form the time of injury.

Of the 253 casualties evacuated from Panama to San Antonio for whom records were available, McBride and colleagues [25] report the primary cause of injury was fragmentary munitions (29%), followed closely by jump-related injuries (28%), gunshot wounds (23%), accidents (11%), heat exhaustion (4%), and other (6%). Of 378 total injuries in the 253 evacuated casualties, 70% were extremity wounds, 11% head and neck, 10% thorax, 4% abdomen, 4% pelvis, and 1% spinal injuries. Most of those injured (80%) required some type of orthopedic treatment or operation. Data on specific injuries and procedures performed are not reported. Injury severity scores (ISSs) were calculated for the 253 casualties evacuated. Seventy-two percent of the casualties had an ISS between 1 and 5, 13% had an ISS between 6 and 10, and 13% had an ISS higher than 10, indicating that most injuries were of low severity. Jacob and colleagues [56] performed an analysis of 37 open fractures sustained during Just Cause, 35 of which were available for this study. The most significant finding was the reduced infection rate reported on severe open fractures that were washed out and débrided immediately in Panama (22%) as opposed to those washed out after transfer to tertiary-care facilities in the United States (66%). These data support the role of débriding moderate and severe soft tissue injuries and fractures at the FST or level two + arena.

Comprehensive casualty data for the battle of the Black Sea occurring in Mogadishu, Somalia, (July 1993) is well documented by Mabry and colleagues [57]. This mission used SOF personnel from multiple tiers to perform a combined air-assault and ground-assault mission to attempt the capture of the Somali warlord, Aidid. Within 48 hours, two general surgeons and one orthopedic surgeon performed 56 surgical procedures on 34 patients/operative cases (three patients required two operations) at the 46th Combat Support Hospital. As pointed out by Hetz elsewhere in this issue, the patient-care capability of combat support hospitals is 3 to 10 times greater than that at an FST. This extra capability, however, may not be in the form of surgeons but in the increased holding capability, radiology, and laboratory services, and largely in nursing and ICU care. Injury rates by location of wounds were similar to those seen in Panama: 75% extremity, 14% head and neck; 7% thorax; and 3% abdomen. In this study, injuries from gunshot wounds (42%) and fragment wounds (43%) were almost equal, followed by blunt injury (13%) and burns (2%). Mabry and colleagues [57], however, point out that, when also accounting for the mechanisms of those killed in action in this urban battlefield, the wounding rate was higher from bullets (at 55%) than from fragmentary munitions (at 31%). Thirty-six percent of deaths in Somalia were the result of penetrating head injuries, which is close to historical data, despite the use of the Kevlar

(DuPont, Wilmington, Delaware) helmets. One of the most important observations in dealing with intense urban warfare is that, despite the close proximity of medical facilities, casualty evacuation times from the battlefield can be delayed. For combat medics, 18Ds, Air Force para-rescuemen (or parajumpers), and navy independent-duty corpsmen, these situations are as austere as those in the jungles of Panama or the mountains of Afghanistan. Delays in evacuation equate to longer periods of care under fire and tactical field care of seriously wounded casualties, for which they must be prepared.

The opening phases of OEF in Afghanistan involved unprecedented numbers of SOF that aligned with and assisted Northern Alliance fighters to oust the ruling Taliban and the al Qaeda terrorists they harbored. Because of operational and tactical considerations, surgical support at the beginning of this mission involved the initial stabilization of casualties by Special Forces medics and transportation of most casualties out of country to surgical assets outside Afghanistan in Oman, Uzbekistan, and Germany [19]. Evacuation times from point of injury to operation averaged more than 12 hours. Both the 274th and 250th FSTs then were sent into Afghanistan for far-forward surgical support of all missions in the country. After the FSTs were moved to Bagram (274th) and Kandahar (250th), the time to operation decreased significantly to less than 3 hours, slightly better than the Soviet experience in Afghanistan [17,58]. Combined data from the 274th and 250th FSTs show that the mechanisms for wounds that required major surgical interventions (not including detainee cases) during the initial special operations assault in OEF (October 2001–May 2002) were fragments (57, 57%), gunshot wounds (21, 21%), disease, non-battle injury (14, 14%), and aircraft crash 7 (7, 7%) [17,19]. This injury distribution is markedly similar to experience in other wars. Here also, extremity wounds (58%) greatly outnumbered wounding to other body locations. Body armor used by US forces was found to change the injury distribution in favor of less lethal extremity wounds [20].

Forward surgical units deployed in support of the initial assaults in OEF and OIF encountered many issues. An important lesson learned is that Army FSTs can be deployed in echelon fashion for short periods of time but ideally not longer than 24 to 48 hours. Both the 274th and 250th FSTs performed longer periods of split operations during the initial phases OEF because of operational constraints in the support of SOF. The 250th entered Iraq in echelons, with the nine-man alpha echelon participating in the 173rd Airborne Brigade's combat jump at Bashur in March 2003. FST members were prepared to perform lifesaving operations on the drop zone, but forward care in this arena consists mainly of ATLS and MARCH (*M*assive hemorrhage, *A*irway, *R*espiration, *C*irculation, *H*ead injury/hypothermia) procedures because of severe operational constraints. Damage-control techniques performed included temporary intraluminal shunting of vascular injuries, pelvic sheeting, pelvic and long bone external fixator placement, abbreviated laparotomy, and many prophylactic fasciotomies. Although they are not doctrinally mandated, FSTs performed reoperations on many casualties because of the lack of available higher-echelon medical care in country. In nondoctrinal missions, especially in support of special operations, evacuation of casualties can be erratic because of weather, terrain, and mission constraints. Scenarios may develop in which patients routinely are held in the recovery room/ICU at an FST for prolonged periods, and mass civilian casualties that include children and babies occur. These situations will stress existing logistic and personnel limitations, and these shortages must be planned for. When evacuating critically injured patients from an FST in a remote area, the use of critical care air transport (CCAT) teams is mandatory. FST personnel cannot be afforded to accompany patients to the next higher echelon because of the possible degradation of capabilities that could occur in their absence. Augmenting forward surgical elements with blood technicians, radiographic equipment, and portable ultrasound also was found to extend the capabilities of these units in a special operations environment when medical companies cannot colocate with them at the far-forward area [19,59].

Airborne operations and insertions

An important aspect of special operations involves airborne assaults into hostile enemy areas, often behind enemy front lines. Although other types of insertions are used (ie, air assault or fast-roping, helicopter or air-landing, ground and waterborne insertions) airborne (parachute) operations are considered the most exciting, thrill provoking, and potentially dangerous. Historically, modern combat parachute operations carry a 2% injury rate [23]. Many factors, among them wind speed, combat load, height of jump, conditions and terrain on the drop zone, and experience of the jumper, influence this injury rate. Wind speeds greater than 13 knots are found to increase jump-related injuries significantly. To avoid and minimize inherent risks, commanders perform a detailed cost–benefit analysis and risk assessment of the combat situation before embarking on an airborne assault as a course of combat action.

The invasion of Panama was the largest modern combat parachute assault, and although the paratroopers encountered resistance in the form of firefights almost immediately upon landing, the jump-related injury rate remained low at 2% [25]. Table 4 displays the largest of the most recent combat parachute operations. An acceptable attritional injury rate for combat parachute missions is 2% to 3%. Kotwal and colleagues [23] provide an excellent analysis of jump injuries incurred on four Army Ranger combat parachute missions in OEF and OIF. Although they do not report the numbers of paratroopers participating in individual missions, they do report that there was a slightly higher rate of attritional injuries in parachute assaults into Iraq. This increased rate was thought to result from a higher combat

Table 4
Known jump-related injury data from three recent parachute missions or groups of missions[*]

Operation	Total jumpers	Total injured	Number of injured evacuated	Injury rate[a] (%)	Condition of drop zone	Most frequent injury	Height of jump (feet)
Panama 1989	3900	-	71	2	Hard/even (landing strip)	Ankle	500
Rangers in Afghanistan and Iraq[b]	634	76	27	4	Hard/even (landing strip)	Foot	800
173rd ABN Brigade in northern Iraq	954	18	4	0.4	Soft/uneven (fields after rain)	Hypothermia	800

Abbreviation: ABN, Airborne.

[*] Injuries sustained by hostile enemy activity are not included. All jumps were at night and were conducted into enemy territory.

[a] Based on the number of jumpers evacuated.

[b] Data combine four similar missions (exact numbers of paratroopers participating in each jump were not given). *Data from* Kotwal RS, Meyer DE, O'Connor KC, et al. Army Ranger casualty, attrition, and surgery rates for airborne operations in Afghanistan and Iraq. Aviat Space Environ Med 2004;75:833–40.

load secondary to the need for MOPP (chemical-protective gear) and obstacles on the drop zone. In contrast, the 173rd Airborne Brigade working with JSOTA-N in Iraq, performed a combat jump with an extraordinarily low injury rate (0.4%). Excluding injuries from hypothermia, there were only 10 injuries: three bicep static-line injuries, four ankle sprains (one thought to be a tibia–fibula fracture on the drop zone), one herniated disc, one soldier who had bilateral shoulder dislocations, and one knee (anterior cruciate ligament) injury (MAJ John DeVine, personal communication, 2005) [20]. Three of the injured were evacuated using back-haul technique on the night following the injury when the rest of the brigade began air landing at the secured airfield. Back-hauling of casualties from an airhead occurs when a plane lands, drops off its load of troops, supplies, and equipment, and the casualties are loaded back on the plane for evacuation. For efficient and safe back-hauling, CCAT teams must be present on the aircraft identified for back-hauling. The paratrooper with the anterior cruciate ligament injury was evacuated several days later.

Other insertion methods carry dangers as well. Several Rangers in the battle of Mogadishu sustained fast-roping injuries while performing an air assault (repelling from helicopters) onto the objective. Having aircraft in close proximity of the ground during daylight operations in a combat setting can be inherently dangerous. Four of those killed in action in that same battle sustained fatal blunt trauma from two of the helicopters being shot down, and several others were injured [57].

Special operations and civil affairs

The credos, "Wining the hearts and the minds" and "Free the oppressed," are phrases that Special Forces live by. These words express a dedication to helping those who are left as bystanders and accidental victims of combat actions, tyrannical rule, and natural disasters. There are succinct guidelines in the Special Forces medical handbook and field manuals for civil actions before, during, and after bullets fly [6,8].

Humanitarian demining operations are a significant part of SOF civil and military actions [60]. Injuries from landmines (LM) and unexploded ordinance (UXO) are a major public health risk worldwide. LMs are placed in strategic positions for defensive purposes to prevent the enemy from attacking an objective or base camp easily or to channel an enemy force that is on the offensive into a location that supports an easy counterattack or ambush. A significant threat exists from LMs and UXO to both combatants and noncombatants alike. The International Committee of the Red Cross reported that over 70 million LMs are placed in more 70 countries and that during a 1-year period in Afghanistan 1636 people were treated for LM/UXO injuries (a number that does not include immediate deaths or insignificant injuries) [61]. Data from the 250th FST in the opening phases of OEF in Kandahar show that 20% of those injuries and deaths

were caused by LMs or UXO [17]. Characteristics of anti-personnel LMs include severe mangling of the impact limb, usually the foot, with associated
injuries of the opposite great toe and one or both hands (Fig. 3). Care under
fire and tactical field care consists of removing the casualty and uninjured
from the danger area. Removal is very difficult in some cases because of
the detailed measures needed to minimize risk to rescuers negotiating the
suspected LM field, especially if still under enemy fire. External hemorrhage
is stopped using any means necessary and available (direct pressure, tourniquet, hemostatic dressing). Casualties are resuscitated and evacuated. Antibiotics can be given in the field or at the aid station or surgical asset level.
Débridement is performed to minimize infection and may include amputation. Amputations in the far-forward area should be done only to the level
where all necrotic tissue is removed, and the skin should be loosely approx-
imated over gauze to prevent retraction. No formal amputation should be
attempted at this level or as a first procedure. All Special Forces ODA teams
are trained and equipped for demining operations, mostly in support of SOF
combat operations and humanitarian missions [62].

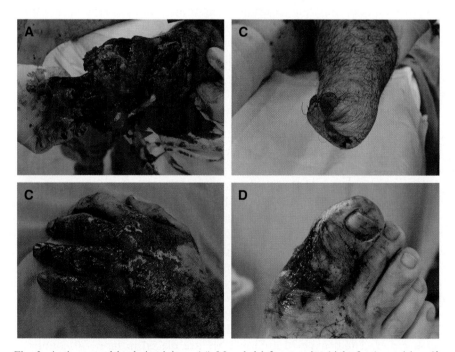

Fig. 3. Antipersonnel landmine injury. (*A*) Mangled left extremity (right foot) requiring débridement and below-knee amputation. (*B*) Débrided injury with skin placed on tension to
avoid retraction so that formal revision can take place at higher echelon of care. (*C*) Left
hand injury (soldier was carrying weapon out in from of him when impact occurred). (*D*) Concomitant left toe injury (peritoneal injuries can coexist).

Other civil affairs actions include rebuilding schools, assessing the host nation medical infrastructure, resuppling and rebuilding as well as establishing clinics to care for refugees, and providing expedient natural disaster response. SOF provide third-world nations with military advisors for training and civil protection. In support of the credos given previously, forward surgical elements assist Special Forces A teams in caring for local militia fighters and noncombatants. The 102nd, 250th, and 274th FSTs cared for numerous Northern Alliance fighters in the opening and subsequent phases of OEF [16,17,22]. Approximately half of the 250th's workload consisted of caring for local militia, civilians, and enemy combatants. In support of JSOTF-N and Task Force Bayonet in the early phase of OIF, medical assets from the 173rd Airborne Brigade and the 250th FST assisted local Iraqi efforts in rebuilding the medical infrastructure in Kirkuk [20]. One hundred five joint cases were performed at local Iraqi hospitals, surgical grand rounds and education were re-established, and the Kirkuk emergency medical system was retrained. More than 200 emergency medical technicians, nurses, and paramedics underwent this training and have been seen to use this knowledge in actual mass-casualty scenarios (LTC Benjamin Starnes, personal communication, 2004). Additional assets to rebuild disaster-stricken or war-torn nations are available through nongovernmental organizations. These entities are diverse. Some are willing to work side-by-side with the US military, and some are not, depending on organizational structure, goals, and visions. Regardless of the reason for deployment, all US military actions involve some sort of civil affairs opportunities, and these opportunities should be planned for ahead of time.

Summary

This summary is intended to provide a snapshot framework for some of the issues faced by surgeons supporting special operations and missions in austere environments in support of low-intensity conflicts. Many significant changes in prehospital, surgical, and evacuation support of special operations missions have occurred in a short period of time. One of them is the creation of dedicated and cohesive forward surgical teams that are able to perform lifesaving surgery at or near the front lines of battle in the austere conditions and with the underdeveloped logistic support chains that often are found in special operations and low-intensity conflicts. Another innovation is the development of Air Force CCAT teams. Because of the CCAT teams, casualties were transported from Kandahar directly to Germany and other medical facilities outside Afghanistan without sacrificing inherent patient-care ability at the FST. Without the expanded capability of the 18D Special Forces medics and their dedication to and expertise in the care of the combat soldier, civilian, and enemy combatants at the point of injury, there would be no need for higher echelons of care.

References

[1] Bruner EF, Bolkom C, O'rourke R. Special operations forces in Operation Enduring Freedom: background and issues for Congress. CRS Report for Congress, CRS 1-CRS 6. Washington (DC): Library of Congress; 2001.

[2] Joint Special Operations Command (JSOC) units. Available at: SpecialOperations.com. Accessed February 1, 2006.

[3] Field manual 100–20. Military operations in low intensity conflict. Washington (DC): Headquarters, Department of the Army; 1990.

[4] Army Special Forces Command US. (Airborne). Available at: SpecialOperations.com. Accessed December 16, 2005.

[5] Moloff AL, Bettencourt B. The Special Forces medic: unique training for a unique mission. Mil Med 1992;157:74–6.

[6] Soldiers manual/trainer's guide. MOS 18D Special Forces medical sergeant skill levels 3 and 4. STP 31–18D34-SM-TG. Washington (DC): Headquarters, Department of the Army; 2003.

[7] Godbee DC, Odom JW. Utilization of Special Forces medical assets during disaster relief: the Hurricane Andrew experience. Mil Med 1997;162:92–5.

[8] Medical aspects. In: Field manual 3–05.201, Special Forces unconventional warfare operations. Washington (DC): Headquarters, Department of the Army; 2003. p. C-1-C-10.

[9] Cloutier MG. Medical care behind enemy lines: a historical examination of clandestine hospitals. Mil Med 1993;158:816–20.

[10] Butler FK Jr, Hagmann J, Butler EG. Tactical combat casualty care in special operations. Mil Med 1996;161(Suppl):3–16.

[11] Sohn VY, Rush RM Jr, Miller JP, et al. From the combat medic to the forward surgical team (FST): the Madigan model for improving combat trauma readiness of brigade combat teams fighting the global war on terror [abstract]. J Surg Res 2006;130:249.

[12] Ciccone TJ, Anderson PD, Gann CA, et al. Successful development and implementation of a tactical emergency medical technician training program for United States federal agents. Prehospital Disaster Med 2005;20:36–9.

[13] Navein JF, Dunn RL. The Combat Trauma Life Support course: resource-constrained first responder trauma care for Special Forces medics. Mil Med 2002;167:566–72.

[14] Butler FK Jr, Hagmann JH, Richards DT. Tactical management of urban warfare casualties in special operations. Mil Med 2000;165:1–48.

[15] Peoples GE, Gerlinger T, Budinich C, et al. The most frequently requested precombat refresher training by the Special Forces medics during Operation Enduring Freedom. Mil Med 2005;170:31–7.

[16] Peoples GE, Gerlinger T, Craig R, et al. Combat casualties in Afghanistan cared for by a single Forward Surgical Team during the initial phases of Operation Enduring Freedom. Mil Med 2005;170:462–8.

[17] Place RJ, Rush RM Jr, Arrington ED. Forward surgical team (FST) workload in a special operations environment: the 250th FST in Operation Enduring Freedom. Curr Surg 2003;60: 418–22.

[18] Chambers LW, Rhee P, Baker BC, et al. Initial experience of US Marine Corps forward resuscitative surgical system during Operation Iraqi Freedom. Arch Surg 2005;140: 26–32.

[19] Peoples GE, Gerlinger T, Craig R, et al. The 274th Forward Surgical Team experience during Operation Enduring Freedom. Mil Med 2005;170:451–9.

[20] Rush RM Jr, Stockmaster NR, Stinger HK, et al. Supporting the global war on terror: a tale of two campaigns featuring the 250th Forward Surgical Team (Airborne). Am J Surg 2005; 189:564–70.

[21] Pratt JW, Rush RM Jr. The military surgeon and the war on terrorism: a Zollinger legacy. Am J Surg 2003;186:292–5.

[22] Beekley AC, Watts DM. Combat trauma experience with the United States Army 102nd Forward Surgical Team in Afghanistan. Am J Surg 2004;187:652–4.

[23] Kotwal RS, Meyer DE, O'Connor KC, et al. Army Ranger casualty, attrition, and surgery rates for airborne operations in Afghanistan and Iraq. Aviat Space Environ Med 2004;75: 833–40.

[24] Vermillion CL. Operation just cause. Aviat Space Environ Med 1996;67:87–8.

[25] McBride JT Jr, Hunt MH, Hannon JP, et al. Report and medical analysis of personnel injury from Operation Just Cause. Institute Report # 468. Presidio of San Francisco (CA): Letterman Army Institute of Research, Division of Military Trauma Research; 1991. p. 1–90. Ref Type: Report.

[26] Hackett PH, Roach RC. High-altitude medicine. In: Auerbach PS, editor. Wilderness medicine. 4th edition. St. Louis (MO): Mosby; 2001. p. 2–43.

[27] Pigman EC, Karakla DW. Acute mountain sickness at intermediate altitude: military mountainous training. Am J Emerg Med 1990;8:7–10.

[28] Midla GS. Lessons learned. Operation Anaconda. Mil Med 2004;169:810–3.

[29] Tan SS, Chee VWT. Common high altitude medical problems. Available at: http://www.priory.com/anaes/altitude.htm. Accessed February 2, 2006.

[30] Steinman AM, Giesbrecht GG. Immersion into cold water. In: Auerbach PS, editor. Wilderness medicine. 4th edition. St. Louis (MO): Mosby; 2001. p. 197–225.

[31] Kempthorne D, Byrd RC, Dornan RK, et al. Army Ranger training—safety improvements need to be institutionalized. GAO/NSIAD-97–29. Washington (DC): United States General Accounting Office; 1997.

[32] Danzl DF. Accidental hypothermia. In: Auerbach PS, editor. Wilderness medicine. 4th edition. St. Louis (MO): Mosby; 2001. p. 135–77.

[33] Hamlet MP. Non-freezing cold injuries. In: Auerbach PS, editor. Wilderness medicine. 4th edition. St. Louis (MO): Mosby; 2001. p. 129–34.

[34] Schissel DJ, Barney DL, Keller R. Cold weather injuries in an arctic environment. Mil Med 1998;163:568–71.

[35] McCauley RL, Smith DJ, Robson MC, et al. Frostbite. In: Auerbach PS, editor. Wilderness medicine. 4th edition. St. Louis (MO): Mosby; 2001. p. 178–96.

[36] Vaughn PB. Local cold injury—menace to military operations: a review. Mil Med 1980;145: 305–11.

[37] Wallace MR, Sharp TW, Smoak B, et al. Malaria among United States troops in Somalia. Am J Med 1996;100:49–55.

[38] Houston DJ, Tuck JJ. Malaria on a military peacekeeping operation: a case study with no cases. Mil Med 2005;170:193–5.

[39] A guide for staying healthy in Central Asia. USACHPPM. Deployment information. Available at: http://chppm-www.apgea.army.mil/deployment/stayinghealthy.asp. Accessed February 22, 2006.

[40] Matson DO. Norovirus gastroenteritis in US Marines in Iraq. Clin Infect Dis 2005;40:526–7.

[41] Thornton SA, Sherman SS, Farkas T, et al. Gastroenteritis in US Marines during Operation Iraqi Freedom. Clin Infect Dis 2005;40:519–25.

[42] Farkas T, Thornton SA, Wilton N, et al. Homologous versus heterologous immune responses to Norwalk-like viruses among crew members after acute gastroenteritis outbreaks on 2 US Navy vessels. J Infect Dis 2003;187:187–93.

[43] Sharp TW, Thornton SA, Wallace MR, et al. Diarrheal disease among military personnel during Operation Restore Hope, Somalia, 1992–1993. Am J Trop Med Hyg 1995;52:188–93.

[44] Bourgeois AL, Gardiner CH, Thornton SA, et al. Etiology of acute diarrhea among United States military personnel deployed to South America and West Africa. Am J Trop Med Hyg 1993;48:243–8.

[45] Thornton SA, Wignall SF, Kilpatrick ME, et al. Norfloxacin compared to trimethoprim/sulfamethoxazole for the treatment of travelers' diarrhea among US military personnel deployed to South America and West Africa. Mil Med 1992;157:55–8.

[46] Scott DA, Haberberger RL, Thornton SA, et al. Norfloxacin for the prophylaxis of travelers' diarrhea in US military personnel. Am J Trop Med Hyg 1990;42:160–4.

[47] Morgan CA III, Hazlett G, Wang S, et al. Symptoms of dissociation in humans experiencing acute, uncontrollable stress: a prospective investigation. Am J Psychiatry 2001;158:1239–47.

[48] Chemtob CM, Bauer GB, Neller G, et al. Post-traumatic stress disorder among Special Forces Vietnam veterans. Mil Med 1990;155:16–20.

[49] Pearn J. Traumatic stress disorders: a classification with implications for prevention and management. Mil Med 2000;165:434–40.

[50] Auerbach PS, editor. Wilderness medicine. 4th edition. St. Louis (MO): Mosby; 2001.

[51] Sustaining soldier health and performance in operation Support Hope: guidance for small unit leaders. US Army Research Institute of Environmental Medicine. USARIEM Technical Note 94–3. 1994. Fort Detrick (MD): US Army Medical Research, Development, Acquisition and Logistics Command; 1994.

[52] Nolan DL. Airborne tactical medical support in Grenada. Mil Med 1990;155:104–11.

[53] Islinger RB, Kuklo TR, McHale KA. A review of orthopedic injuries in three recent US military conflicts. Mil Med 2000;165:463–5.

[54] Bolger DP. Special operations and the Grenada campaign. Parameters 1998;18:49–61.

[55] Field manual 4–02.25. Employment of Forward Surgical Teams; tactics, techniques, and procedures. Washington (DC): Headquarters, Department of the Army; 2003.

[56] Jacob E, Erpelding JM, Murphy KP. A retrospective analysis of open fractures sustained by US military personnel during Operation Just Cause. Mil Med 1992;157:552–6.

[57] Mabry RL, Holcomb JB, Baker AM, et al. United States Army Rangers in Somalia: an analysis of combat casualties on an urban battlefield. J Trauma 2000;49:515–28.

[58] Grau LW, Jorgensen WA. Handling the wounded in a counter-guerilla war: the Soviet/Russian experience in Afghanistan and Chechnya. Army Medical Department Journal 1998;8–16.

[59] West BC, Bentley R, Place RJ. In-flight transfusion of packed red blood cells on a combat search and rescue mission: a case report from operation enduring freedom. Mil Med 2004;169:181–3.

[60] New United States policy on landmines: reducing humanitarian risk and saving of United States soldiers. Available at: http://www.state.gov/t/pm/rls/fs/30044.htm. Accessed December 16, 2005.

[61] Bilukha OO, Brennan M, Woodruff BA. Death and injury from landmines and unexploded ordnance in Afghanistan. JAMA 2003;290:650–3.

[62] US Army Special Forces. Humanitarian demining fact sheet. Available at: http://www.specialoperations.com/Army/Specialforces/HumanitarianDemining/Factsheet.htm. Accessed December 16, 2005.

SURGICAL
CLINICS OF
NORTH AMERICA

ELSEVIER
SAUNDERS

Surg Clin N Am 86 (2006) 753–763

Peacekeeping and Stability Operations: A Military Surgeon's Perspective

LTC Benjamin W. Starnes, MD

Vascular and Endovascular Surgery Service, Department of Surgery, Madigan Army Medical Center, 7521 53rd St Ct W, University Place, Tacoma, WA 98467, USA

The imperfect instruction to students with no experience to guide them, leads to a perpetuation of error, and when such men enter the Medical Corps they are tinctured with the fundamental error that what they have seen, and been taught concerning (surgery) in civil life, is a reliable and safe guide for military practice.

C.B.G. De Nancrede [1]

This quotation by the late Major and Chief Surgeon C.B.G. De Nancrede was written nearly 100 years ago and still holds true today. Standard surgical curriculum and training in the civilian western world bears little resemblance to that which is encountered by military surgeons during deployments to resource-constrained and often hostile environments. Recent events have focused a considerable amount of attention on the role of the military medical system in response to actions other than war or terrorism. The role of the military medical system in response to humanitarian crises, peacekeeping and stability operations, and natural disasters has become increasingly complex. Military surgeons are often tasked to perform leadership and administrative functions and clinical practices outside the scope of their training to support such missions. The purpose of this article is to explore the unique features of a surgeon's role in the support of these missions.

Background

United Nations peacekeeping forces are employed by the World Health Organization to maintain or re-establish peace in an area of armed conflict.

Dr. Starnes has had three combat deployments in support of medical teams providing lifesaving and resuscitative surgery during peacekeeping operations in Kosovo and combat operations in Iraq.

E-mail address: bwstarnes@comcast.net

The United Nations initially took on the task of sending observers to monitor the armistice between Israel and the Arab states in 1948. Since then, 109 peacekeeping missions have been performed [2]. The fall of communism and the end of the Cold War brought about an increased requirement for peacekeeping missions throughout the world, and the United States has contributed heavily to the military medical support of many of these events. The United States military and specifically, military surgeons have been actively engaged in an organized response to crises since the Civil War [3].

The modern paradigm of military intervention involves a relatively brief period of active fighting followed by a long commitment of peacekeeping and nation building. Surgical support during active fighting is relatively simple: casualties are characteristically few, and the support of an expeditionary force is well known to our military medical units [4]. When "peacemaking" ends and peacekeeping begins, the provision of comprehensive care becomes problematic. Military medical units are not equipped to provide prolonged humanitarian aid or civilian health support [4,5].

Military surgeons are a diverse group of practitioners from a variety of backgrounds. Recruitment of surgeons into the United States military occurs through several different mechanisms and includes Reserve Officer Training Corps and Health Profession Scholarship Program scholarships. The Uniformed Services University of the Health Sciences in Bethesda, Maryland, is also a robust source of well-trained military surgeons. A term of obligation is incurred by these trainees for education funded by the federal government. A large population of surgeons serving during the active phases of conflict may be called from reserve duty to active duty. As such, these surgeons have standard surgical and trauma education most often obtained from civilian institutions. Although exposed to some military training during their careers that emphasized the treatment of the acutely injured soldier on the battlefield, most surgeons are not prepared to care for patients outside the realm of standard surgical practice (Fig. 1). Tremendous experience is obtained during the active phases of war, but in the period between wars, the average active-duty military surgeon practicing in a community-based hospital-type environment has a limited opportunity to maintain trauma expertise [5]. The military surgeons at military trauma centers, however, are able to maintain skills commensurate with that of a major urban trauma center [6].

The initial burden of casualty care for any conflict lies on the military and the existing host nation medical infrastructure. This infrastructure is often severely disrupted, so the military bears the burden of caring for large numbers of the sick and wounded [6]. Others trained to provide long-term humanitarian care include physicians from regional countries, supranational agencies such as the United Nations, and nongovernmental organizations including the International Committee of the Red Cross/Red Crescent. The United States military and its existing infrastructure are the best poised to rapidly respond to such crises. Strengths of this response include air

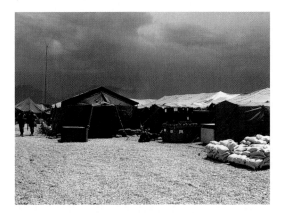

Fig. 1. 212th Mobile Army Surgical Hospital in Tirana, Albania, in April 1999 in support of peacekeeping missions during the war in Kosovo. (Photo courtesy of LTC Benjamin W. Starnes, MD.)

evacuation and cargo transport capability, communications, engineering, logistics, and most important, security [7]. Nongovernmental organizations and humanitarian aid agencies often have strong reservations about any involvement with the military because they seek to maintain neutrality. Current postconflict scenarios may present an unacceptable level of threat to these agencies in the form of terrorist threats, kidnap, or murder. The military has been suggested to be the best fit for coordinating these humanitarian efforts until a satisfactory level of security is obtained [8].

The surgeon's response to natural disasters has become a topic of renewed interest since the devastation and evacuee crisis recorded with Hurricane Katrina and the October 8, 2005 earthquake in Pakistan measuring 7.6 on the Richter scale.

Planning for the mission

The United Nations has maintained records of the fatalities incurred during peacekeeping deployments over the past 57 years. Through October 31, 2005, 2058 fatalities have been recorded during the course of 109 different peacekeeping missions [9]. Forty-one percent were accidental deaths, 30% were due to hostile acts, and 29% were due to "illness/other" [2]. Projections of casualties from military planners is a part of any preparation for modern armed conflict. Casualty projections during peacekeeping and stability operations allow medical planners to assess in advance the medical resources needed to support such operations [9]. These forecasts can be fraught with uncertainty. The types of casualties for which medical resource planning is needed include nonbattle injuries, disease occurrences endemic to the region of interest, psychiatric illness, and wounds sustained as a result of hostilities. In a review of 188 peacekeeping incidents, Blood and colleagues [9] determined an estimated mean wounded-in-action rate for these operations of 3.16 per 1000-strength per year and a mean killed-in-action rate of just 0.709 per 1000-strength per year.

The mission: treating the peacekeepers

The primary mission for any military medical unit deployed in support of peacekeeping and stability operations is to care for the deployed force, whether it be active military units, United Nations personnel, or contract civilian workers supporting the mission. Military medical units must deploy with a thorough knowledge of the host country, including endemic infectious diseases encompassing HIV/AIDS, tuberculosis, malaria, typhoid fever, cholera, and certain endemic parasitic infections (ie, ecchinococcal infection) [10]. Protective measures must be employed by military medical personnel for care providers and peacekeepers. Some investigators have advocated a policy of mandatory malaria protection, with an impressive rate of zero malarial cases during deployment [11].

Many casualties often present to the treatment area with full body armor and armed with weapons or other ordnance. Knowledge in the safe removal of this body armor and safe disarmament and storage of weapons and ordnance remains of paramount importance in protecting the casualty and the health care provider from grave injury.

Unlike combat operations in which injury patterns are heavily concentrated with penetrating and blast type injuries, wounding mechanisms during peacekeeping and stability operations can be diverse. In a review of injury patterns sustained during the war in Kosovo, MAJ George Appenzeller [3] described a 63% incidence of blunt trauma versus a 37% incidence of penetrating trauma. Motor vehicle accidents made up 72% of the blunt trauma encountered and 45.5% of trauma overall. Of 404 trauma patients treated during an 18-month period, 277 (nearly 70%) were civilian casualties (Fig. 2). In a review of surgical experience during the same peacekeeping mission over a longer period of time, MAJ Steven Grosso [12] found that over a 46-month period, 676 major operations were performed while supporting nearly 30,000 troops in the Balkans (Fig. 3), corresponding to a mean of 2.13 operations performed per surgeon per month.

Unlike conventional warfare, which features a daily or near-daily casualty stream, peacekeeping missions and peace-enforcement operations not only have lower casualty rates but also have a much lower percentage of days in which casualties are sustained. In peacekeeping operations, sometimes weeks or even months can pass without the occurrence of a single casualty [9]. Such a low casualty rate calls into question the volume of surgical procedures required to maintain a surgical skill set for any well-trained surgeon [6]. For example, the operative experience of the 10th Combat Support Hospital over a 7-month period while deployed to Bosnia in 1999 consisted

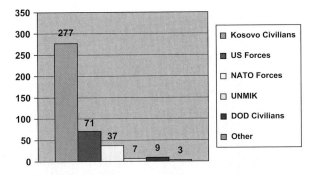

Fig. 2. Patient demographics. DOD, Department of Defense; UNMIK, United Nations mission in Kosovo. (*From* Appenzeller GN. Injury patterns in peacekeeping missions: the Kosovo experience. Mil Med 2004;169(3):187–91; reprinted with permission of *Military Medicine: International Journal of AMSUS.*)

of five operative trauma cases and seven emergency operations (five appendectomies, one extremity abscess, and one ectopic pregnancy) between two general surgeons, two orthopedic surgeons, and a gynecologist.

The overwhelming percentage of injuries cared for on the battlefield are extremity in nature, whereas the injury pattern encountered during peacekeeping and stability operations is somewhat different. During the war in Kosovo, extremity injuries predominated (54%) (Fig. 4); however, when evaluating isolated extremity injuries, the rate was approximately one-half that of previous conflicts (33%) [3].

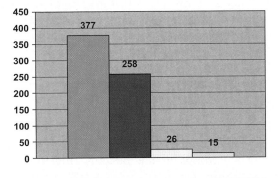

	Number of Operative Cases
General Surgery	377
Orthopedic Surgery	258
Plastic/ENT/Oral Surgery	26
Obstetrics/Gynecology	15

Fig. 3. Distribution of cases. ENT, ear, nose, and throat (Otorhinolaryngology). (*From* Grosso SM. US Army surgical experiences during the NATO peacekeeping mission in Bosnia-Herzegovina, 1995 to 1999: lessons learned. Mil Med 2001;166(7):587–92; reprinted with permission of *Military Medicine: International Journal of AMSUS.*)

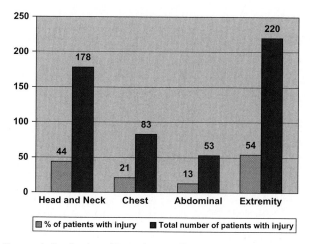

Fig. 4. Overall wound distribution. (*From* Appenzeller GN. Injury patterns in peacekeeping missions: the Kosovo experience. Mil Med 2004;169(3):187–91; reprinted with permission of *Military Medicine: International Journal of AMSUS*.)

Combat stress is another important aspect in the care of any deployed force. Extreme and sometimes mentally disturbing circumstances are often encountered during armed conflict. It is estimated that between 2% and 8% of service members, including surgeons deployed on combat operations, United Nations peacekeeping tasks, and humanitarian and disaster relief operations, present with one or more stress disorders within 3 years of deployment [13]. Military surgeons are sometimes exposed to cases involving dismemberment, torture, severe starvation, extensive burns, and beheading. Surgeons are by no means immune to combat-related stress.

The reality: treating the victims

The true impact of conflict on noncombatant civilians and local nationals is difficult to surmise. Estimates state that between 35% and 80% of the casualties of war are civilians including women, young children, the infirm, and the elderly [14]. In a recent review of injury patterns during peacekeeping missions in Kosovo, 69% of those cared for by a military medical unit were civilian [3]. Adding to the complexities of managing these patients are language barriers and diverse cultural mores. Casualties often have a delayed presentation, with severe underlying comorbidities that have gone untreated or are advanced at the time of presentation.

Landmines and unexploded ordnance are found in several parts of the world, with heavy concentrations in Southeast Asia, the Balkan region, and Afghanistan. These weapons are usually left over from conventional warfare, but the resultant casualties of these devices are usually civilians and returning refugees. In an analysis of 390 health facilities over a 14-month period in Afghanistan, 81% of mine-related injuries were sustained by civilians [15]. Antipersonnel mines are exceedingly uncommon in the United States and Europe, and as such, many surgeons trained in these countries are unfamiliar with the proper management of the resulting war wounds.

Military surgeons deployed in support of peacekeeping operations are sometimes required to operate outside their scope of standard practice. The author has personal experience involving the surgical correction of a tracheoesophageal fistula on a 2-hour old infant girl born during the early phases of nation building in Iraq in late 2003 (Fig. 5). Local surgeons were not prepared to remedy this life-threatening condition and the only solution was to proceed with repair within a local Iraqi hospital. The surgery was ultimately acknowledged by local physicians as the first successful tracheoesophageal fistula repair in the history of Kirkuk, Iraq, which has a population of 1 million persons. This experience is illustrative of the fact that conventional surgical training only serves to bolster the capabilities of deployed military surgeons in support of these peacekeeping and stability operations.

Additional unique circumstances for military surgeons include the opportunity to practice with surgeons from other supporting nations or the host nation itself. These liaison relationships foster a sense of collegiality that is difficult to reproduce in civilian life (Fig. 6). Not all standards of practice among those involved are equivalent, which must be recognized by the visiting military surgeon. Understanding that there are always differing perspectives with regard to patient care renders the visiting surgeon more capable of providing good counsel and good care with available limited resources. The author was fortunate to round with the Chief of Surgery of Skopje Military Hospital in 1999 during the peacekeeping phase of the war in Kosovo. At 9:00 AM on a rainy Monday morning in July, after rounding on 35 patients, the Chief and author retired to the Chief's office. The Chief offered the author a drink. "What would you like?" "I'll have whatever you are having" was the response. The Chief pulled out a bottle of

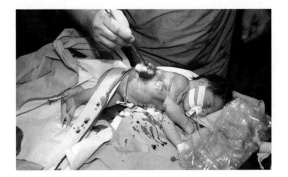

Fig. 5. Two-hour-old "Baby Ayat," an infant girl born with a congenital tracheoesophageal fistula that was successfully repaired in an Iraqi hospital in Kirkuk, Iraq, in December 2003. (Courtesy of LTC Benjamin W. Starnes, MD.)

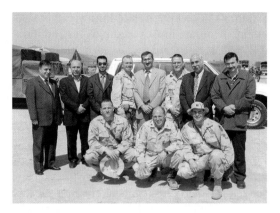

Fig. 6. American and Iraqi surgeons posing for a picture in Bashur, Iraq, in April 2003. (Courtesy of LTC Robert M. Rush, MD.)

Macedonian whiskey, poured a full glass, and offered it to the visiting surgeon. Glasses were raised and a strong friendship was fostered. Flexibility in the consideration of cultural traditions is a unique and often underappreciated requisite in the practice of military medicine.

Response to natural disasters

Private sector physicians who have a military background have long been regarded as having a great depth of experience and understanding in atypical threats involving large numbers of people. In a survey assessment of the Eastern Association for the Surgery of Trauma on the level of preparedness for mass casualty incidents in May, 2004, Ciraulo and colleagues [16] concluded that "across all variables, physicians with military training were significantly better prepared for response to catastrophic events." In response to natural disasters such as hurricanes, tsunamis, and earthquakes, military surgeons must possess the capability to handle a wide variety of patient presentations. The training and skill of surgeons makes them especially suited for the rapid decision making required by large casualty burdens following natural disasters [17]. The response to such disasters requires a paradigm change—from the civilian application of unlimited resources for the greatest good of each patient to the military allocation of limited resources for the greatest good of the greatest number of casualties [17].

Surgeons responding to natural disasters must have expert knowledge in the management of crush injuries and crush syndrome, hypothermia and exposure, concomitant burns, and massive soft tissue injury. In a review of an Israeli military medical response to an earthquake in Turkey in 1999, Wolf and colleagues [18] noted that over 50% of operations were for debridement and often amputation or closure of soft tissue injuries.

Hurricanes Katrina and Wilma have brought to center stage the role of the federal government in response to natural disasters. In a thorough review of the use of military hospitals after hurricanes, Weddle and Prado-Monje [19] described the history of the military medical response; specifically, problems encountered while attempting to dovetail the military into standard local and state government disaster relief plans. To significantly affect mortality from any natural disaster, trauma surgery must be available within minutes or hours because overall surgical needs fall off after the initial 72 hours [19]. In 1980, a review of the military response to a cyclone in Sri Lanka in 1978 concluded "there is a strong tendency for medical personnel to rush into disaster areas and generate more difficulties in terms of support than they actually contribute" [20]. This report was referenced in a 1994 review that concluded "simply sending military clinics and hospitals will rarely provide the appropriate medical support" [21].

Landfall for Hurricane Katrina was on August 29, 2005. LTG Russel Honoré, Commander of Joint Task Force Katrina, stated in an interview that a request for additional military assistance went out on the same day that the hurricane hit New Orleans [22]. The USS Bataan, an 844-foot ship with hospital facilities including six operating rooms and beds for 360 patients happened to be in the area 5 days after weathering out the storm in the Gulf of Mexico [23]. Much criticism was directed at the federal response in not effectively using this military medical facility in New Orleans. The reality was that there was only one nonsurgeon physician on board this vessel and most of its resources were being used for search and rescue missions. LTG Honoré later dispatched this naval craft to Biloxi, Mississippi, where it could be better used [22].

In the early days after Katrina, the Louis Armstrong New Orleans International Airport became a makeshift field hospital and served as a triage facility before evacuation of patients to other health care facilities around the country [24]. The USS Comfort, a floating naval hospital with 250 beds was due to arrive in New Orleans on September 9, 2005, 11 days after the Katrina landfall. At the time of this writing, it is too early to determine the impact of this deployment of medical resources to a disaster zone.

It is the author's belief that surgeons can be used effectively in response to natural disasters. Military surgeons, however, are often too late to arrive to affect a significant impact in the acute phase. The power of the military in response to these disasters is in providing shelter, command and control, security, and search and rescue and in restoration of infrastructure including electricity and communications. The most useful impact of a surgeon in the early phases after a natural disaster is wound debridement, amputation, and control of infection. Each disaster is a learning event for preparation for future disasters.

Summary

Military surgeons serve a unique role in peacekeeping and stability operations and in response to natural disasters. Military medical units are the best medical resource to respond early in times of crisis but are often less equipped for prolonged missions and the subsequent requirements for managing the chronic health care needs of the masses. Most traumatic injuries during peacekeeping and stability operations are a result of blunt mechanism and accidental deaths in a largely civilian population. Because endemic and host nation diseases often add complexity and variety to the management of many of these cases, military surgeons are often tasked with performing operations outside the scope of their usual civilian practice. The primary medical mission of any peacekeeping and stability operation is to treat the peacekeeping force, but the reality lies in eventually treating the refugees and victims of hostile conflict including women, small children, and the elderly. The role of the military surgeon in response to natural disasters is often delayed beyond the true effectiveness of the deployment. The military is probably best used to establish order out of chaos—for security, transportation, command and control, logistics, and restoration of urban infrastructure—and ultimately leaving urban medical facilities to bear the burden of the ongoing medical mission.

References

[1] De Nancrede CBG. Experience versus theory in the explanation of the nature and treatment of gunshot wounds, especially those inflicted by modern military small-calibre projectiles. Military Surgeon 1910;26–27:14–41.

[2] Department of Peacekeeping Operations (United Nations). Available at: http://www.un.org/Depts/dpko/fatalities/totals.htm. Accessed October 31, 2005.

[3] Appenzeller GN. Injury patterns in peacekeeping missions: the Kosovo experience. Mil Med 2004;169(3):187–91.

[4] Eiseman B, Chandler JG. Sheriff's surgeon's alert: a trauma surgeon's responsibility. J Trauma 2003;54(1):156–60.

[5] Rumbaugh JR. Operation Pacific Haven: humanitarian medical support for Kurdish evacuees. Mil Med 1998;163(5):269–71.

[6] Place RJ, Porter CA, Azarow K, et al. Trauma experience comparison of army forward surgical team surgeons at Ben Taub Hospital and Madigan Army Medical Center. Curr Surg 2001;58(1):90–3.

[7] Baker MS, Ryals PA. The medical department in military operations other than war. Part I. Planning for deployment. Mil Med 1999;164(8):572–9.

[8] Court BV. The role of the military in post-conflict situations. J R Soc Health 2004;124(6): 259–61.

[9] Blood CG, Zhang J, Walker GJ. Implications for modeling casualty sustainment during peacekeeping operations. Mil Med 2002;167(10):868–72.

[10] Dubois BJ, Anderson IB, Brown RJ. Echinococcal disease and the provision of humanitarian surgical aid in Bosnia. Mil Med 1998;163(9):656–60.

[11] Houston DJ, Tuck JJ. Malaria on a military peacekeeping operation: a case study with no cases. Mil Med 2005;170(3):193–5.

[12] Grosso SM. US Army surgical experiences during the NATO peacekeeping mission in Bosnia-Herzegovina, 1995 to 1999: lessons learned. Mil Med 2001;166(7):587–92.

[13] Pearn J. Traumatic stress disorders: a classification with implications for prevention and management. Mil Med 2000;165(6):434–40.

[14] Meddings DR. Civilians and war: a review and historical overview of the involvement of non-combatant populations in conflict situations. Med Confl Surviv 2001;17(1):6–16.

[15] Bilukha OO, Brennan M, Woodruff BA. Death and injury from landmines and unexploded ordnance in Afghanistan. JAMA 2003;290(5):650–3.

[16] Ciraulo DL, Frykberg ER, Feliciano DV, et al. A survey assessment of the level of preparedness for domestic terrorism and mass casualty incidents among Eastern Association for the Surgery of Trauma members. J Trauma 2004;56(5):1033–9.

[17] Frykberg ER. Disaster and mass casualty management: a commentary on the American College of Surgeons position statement. J Am Coll Surg 2003;197(5):857–9.

[18] Wolf Y, Bar-Dayan Y, Mankuta D, et al. An earthquake disaster in Turkey: assessment of the need for plastic surgery services in a crisis intervention field hospital. Plast Reconstr Surg 2001;107(1):163–8.

[19] Weddle M, Prado-Monje H. The use of deployable military hospitals after hurricanes: lessons from the Hurricane Marilyn response. Mil Med 2000;165(5):411–7.

[20] Byrd TR. Disaster medicine: toward a more rational approach. Mil Med 1980;145(4):270–3.

[21] Sharp TW, Yip R, Malone JD. US military forces and emergency international humanitarian assistance. Observations and recommendations from three recent missions. JAMA 1994; 272(5):386–90.

[22] United States Department of Defense Official Website. Available at: http://www.defense link.mil/transcripts/2005/tr20050901-3843.html. Accessed November 13, 2005.

[23] Hedges SJ. Chicago Tribune. Available at: http://www.chicagotribune.com/news/nationworld/ chi-0509040369sep04,1,4144825.story?coll=chi-news-hed&ctrack=1&cset=true.

[24] Miles D. United States Department of Defense Official Website. Available at: http:// www.defenselink.mil/news/Sep2005/20050907_2633.html. Accessed November 13, 2005.

ELSEVIER
SAUNDERS

SURGICAL
CLINICS OF
NORTH AMERICA

Surg Clin N Am 86 (2006) 765–777

Caring for Non-Combatants, Refugees, and Detainees

COL Ronald J. Place, MD

Landstuhl Regional Medical Center, CMR 402, Box 1756, APO, AE 09180, USA

Rules of warfare are almost as old as recorded civilization. The ancient Chinese forbade their troops to injure already wounded combatants or to otherwise mistreat prisoners [1]. In 1625, Hugo Grotius, considered by many to be the father of international law, devoted an entire chapter in his book on the law of war to "Moderation in Regard to Prisoners of War" [2]. The first record of arrangements being made between opposing commanders for reciprocal care of wounded and protection of hospitals and medical staff was in 1759. At L'Ecluse, the French and British commanders signed an agreement forbidding the taking of physicians or apothecaries as prisoners of war (POWs) and mandating the care of wounded enemy soldiers [3]. Four years later, the Red Cross movement began in Geneva, where the parties resolved to establish national committees to aid military medical services during war and that belligerents should consider hospital, ambulance, and medical personnel, and the wounded completely neutral [4].

Medical care for displaced persons (DPs), including POWs, detained personnel, refugees, or other noncombatants is remarkably similar. Except for the amount of personal freedom the patient is allowed, medical care is essentially no different. One principal difference is the attitude of military commanders toward medical care. Combatant commanders generally view medical assets as existing for coalition use. The medical assets can be "loaned out" for humanitarian missions but can be redirected by the military commander at any time. Although that may be the case for some refugee situations, the detaining power has the obligation to care for captured soldiers as if they were their own. In addition, an occupying power has a duty to ensure that the medical needs of the local civilian population are met [5].

The views expressed in this article are those of the author and do not reflect the official policy or position of the Department of the Army, Department of Defense, or the United States Government.

E-mail address: Ronald.Place@US.Army.Mil

doi:10.1016/j.suc.2006.02.004   *surgical.theclinics.com*

Care for DPs can be an emotionally difficult task. Medical caregivers are asked to disregard any feelings of animosity toward members of enemy forces in providing appropriate medical care. Whether the goal of neutrality is attainable is a difficult question. A survey of 600 United States military physicians deployed to the Persian Gulf during Operation Desert Storm (ODS) examined combat medical ethics [6]. Of the respondents, 84% indicated that they were familiar with the 1949 Geneva Conventions guidelines and 60% stated that they had read the actual documents. One third disagreed with the statement, "the only criteria used for triage should be medical status (need)," and 22% agreed that "POWs, no matter how severe their injuries, should only be treated after all allied forces are treated." While there is no direct evidence, it is possible that there have been rare instances where medical care givers did not act immediately to protect DPs or report injuries [7].

The Geneva Conventions

1864 Geneva Conventions

The 1864 Geneva Conventions primarily dealt with the Amelioration of the Condition of the Wounded in Armies in the Field. This document was the first to specifically address the protection of medical services during war. The first two Articles stated that hospitals, ambulance, and persons employed in them were neutral and exempt from attack [8]. When a hospital is overrun by an enemy force, Article 3 states that the medical personnel should be given the option of withdrawing immediately to their own units or continuing their patient care efforts and then returning when their medical work is completed. This convention also imposed on belligerents the obligation to care for the sick and wounded. Commanders were given the authority to deliver wounded and sick soldiers to the outposts of their enemy if both belligerents agree (Article 6). Finally, the distinctive emblem of medical service was declared to be the red cross, the reverse of Switzerland's national flag, to honor the Convention's country of origin of (Article 7) [8].

1906/1929 Conventions

One shortcoming of the 1864 convention was that it applied only to land warfare. A second convention convened in 1906 to adapt maritime warfare to the principles of the 1864 Geneva Conventions [9]. In a departure from the practice of the eighteenth and nineteenth centuries, captured wounded and sick (but not medical workers) became POWs. Finally, medical staff personnel were given the right to carry weapons of self-defense or for defense of the sick and wounded.

The lessons of World War I induced further changes in the Geneva Conventions. The 1929 convention recognized medical aircraft for the first time (Article 18). Additionally, the convention gave legal recognition to Iran's use of the red lion and sun and other Arabian countries' use of the red crescent in lieu of the red cross as the emblem of medical service (Article 19).

1949 Conventions

During World War II, euthanasia, experimentation, and exterminations were performed on German nationals, civilian populations of occupied countries, and DPs. This treatment made it clear that existing protections, although significant, were inadequate. In the 1949 Geneva Conventions, therefore, changes were made and discussed in four separate conventions, each addressing a separate issue: (1) the sick and wounded (Geneva I), (2) the shipwrecked wounded and sick (Geneva II), (3) POWs (Geneva III), and (4) the protection of civilian populations (Geneva IV) [10].

The 1949 conventions are what most people refer to when they quote the Geneva Conventions. Geneva I specifically defined medical personnel as those individuals "exclusively engaged in the search for, or the collection, transport, or treatment of the wounded or sick, or in the prevention of disease, (and) staff exclusively engaged in the administration of medical units and establishments" (Geneva I, Article 24) [3]. These personnel could not be made POWs but could be retained only if the health status and numbers of existing POWs made it necessary. In contrast to rules set in prior conventions, medical personnel were not to be returned as soon as militarily possible, but retained if they were needed to care for the belligerents. Israel attempted to add a reservation to article 38 of Geneva I to use the red Star of David as its distinctive emblem. Although this failed by one vote, it has since been accepted by customary law and has thereby gained equal status [3]. The four Geneva Conventions of 1949 have been signed by essentially every nation (with a few minor exceptions); in fact, these conventions have more partisans than the United Nations has members [11].

The policies of the US Government echo those of the Geneva Conventions, stating that care for the sick and wounded shall be based on need and not gender, race, religion, politics, nationality, or any other similar criteria. Additionally, the policy of the US Department of Defense is that health care personnel of the armed forces and Department of Defense should make every effort to comply with "Principles of Medical Ethics Relevant to the Rule of Health Personnel, Particularly Physicians, in the Protection of Prisoners and Detainees Against Torture and Other Cruel, Inhuman or Degrading Treatment or Punishment" adopted by the United Nations General Assembly Resolution 37/194 of December 18, 1982 [12].

Medical care

Standard of care

One of the most difficult adjustments for any physician to make is to the appropriate standard of care in a combat environment with limited resources.

Many countries involved in combat operations have limited medical care-givers and supplies even before overt hostilities erupt. That standard at which western physicians are accustomed to practicing, especially in the United States, is extremely difficult to approximate in a wartime scenario. The overall devastation of war on civilian and military populations can contribute to a provider's frustration and their perception that they are unable to make a noticeable difference, especially among their own soldiers, sailors, airmen, or marines. The minimum standard of practice to achieve is that of the sur-rounding medical community, were it not involved in conflict. A higher stan-dard is desirable if it can be achieved. Physicians should render the highest quality of care available, regardless of the status of the patient [13].

A physician's first duty is to do no harm. In that vein, those responsible for the health of DPs must be separate from the interrogation process. If patients are receiving medications that significantly alter their level of con-sciousness, intelligence-gathering questions should be avoided. Interroga-tors do not have the right to examine the patient's medical record. The reasons for these recommendations are twofold. Primarily, the attending physician is the advocate for the patient. Also, physicians should not do anything that may put them, the hospital staff, or the physical structure in danger of losing the Geneva Convention's guarantee of protection. How medical personnel should act during war so they do not lose their protec-tions is important. When health care workers are complicit in the interroga-tion process, the hospital is no longer a protected facility. Hiding intelligence-gathering military actions behind medical insignia and a hospital can be viewed as a war crime [14].

Medical in-processing

Every prisoner who comes into the DP camp is medically screened. Those who require urgent care are quickly searched by their captors and then taken directly to the same resuscitation department as are friendly forces (or one for prisoners that is of equal capability). Routine in-processing can be very time consuming because DPs are closely searched by nonmedical workers for hidden weapons or other potentially dangerous materials before seeing a health care worker. They are separated into officer and enlisted com-pounds and should be separated according to different armies if that is an issue. During medical ingress at United States facilities, every DP undergoes a complete medical history, physical examination, dental examination, and chest radiograph, and children up to age 14 receive a tuberculin skin test. Demographic information should also be obtained. Less obvious injuries, such as tympanic membrane rupture and postconcussive head injuries, should receive particular attention [14].

The resources required for medical in-processing of DPs can be signifi-cant, and may become staggering when care for the sick and wounded is in-cluded. The United States captured approximately 425,000 prisoners during

World War II, and 105,000 during the Korean Conflict. More than 62,000 DPs were captured by Allied Forces during ODS [15]. During the 1-week ground war, 308 DPs underwent treatment in US Military medical facilities. Within 1 month after the ground war ended, nearly 9000 DPs were treated. In those areas where civilian facilities were damaged, the volume may have been even higher. During the United States–backed coalition advance on Baghdad during Operation Iraqi Freedom (OIF), most of the injured Iraqi combatants were treated at local hospitals. On April 6, 2003, Yarmouk Hospital in Baghdad received 100 new casualties per hour [16]. Because enemy militaries may perform little or no medical screening before conscription [14], chronic medical problems such as hypertension, diabetes mellitus, and chronic gastrointestinal disorders and surgical problems such as inguinal hernias, anorectal disease, and chronic wounds occur frequently.

Physician and other health care workers who believe they must perform unnecessary examinations or unethical duties should ask to be recused. If necessary, an independent arbitrator such as an inspector general can be used to resolve differences of opinion. Similar to the advice given to service members, DP duty limitations should be communicated to the guards or chain of command, and the report should include a notation as to when the DP is "cleared for all interrogation." This medical recommendation only concerns the health of the DP; the detention facility commander performs the interrogation.

Daily sick call

During internment, daily sick call must be staffed. This task includes medication dispensing, wound care, and indicated operative procedures. Although many casualty reports focus on surgical care, one study showed dental disease to be the most common condition, reported by 24% of patients with a health-related complaint [15]. Dental issues included extensive caries, fractures, and periodontal infections. In the same study, commonly treated medical conditions included upper respiratory infections (12.4%), headache (11.7%), urinary tract infections (9.6%), and dermatologic conditions (8.2%).

The daily prisoner census in ODS camps varied from 115 to more than 19,000, whereas the daily sick call ranged from 11 to 692 [16]. When the detainee population was low, nearly 20% of the DPs went on sick call. The percentage dropped to around 2% when the population was higher. Although the cause of this discrepancy has not been determined, several theories are possible: (1) the DPs may have been less willing to wait for care of minor problems when a larger number of patients needed to be seen; (2) the guards may have performed a sort of triage, determining who was sick enough to go on sick call, and (3) those who were captured early, before the ground war was completed, may have had significant medical problems or injuries and could not escape, or surrendered to get care from United States health care workers. Those captured after the war were less likely to be sick or injured. Both heat and cold casualties were seen. Other international groups found that malnutrition and chronic diarrhea were epidemic among children; infectious diseases such as typhoid, cholera, polio, hepatitis, tetanus, and meningitis worsened; and medicines to treat these diseases and infant formula were in short supply [17].

During Operation Enduring Freedom (OEF), multiple units from the US Army, Navy, and Air Force participated in the care of POWs at Kandahar Airfield, Afghanistan. From December 2001 through April 2002, 646 personnel were held in a detention facility at this site (Ronald J. Place, MD, unpublished data, 2002). Of those detained, 109 (17%) experienced dental problems (large caries, abscesses, or fractures) and 135 (21%) had combat-related injuries requiring continuing surgical care. The prisoners often requested treatment for wounds experienced long before any hostility with the coalition forces. Because of the age of the wounds, combined with differences in clothing and protective gear, wounds seen in DPs can be much different from those seen in friendly forces. All OEF DPs had their hair clipped and were deloused by health care personnel before they were transferred to a definitive confinement facility in Cuba. The DPs received little medical or dental care from their own forces before capture. In addition, troops did not seem to undergo any medical screening before entering the military of the Taliban government. Finally, malingering was believed to be a significant problem among those requesting medical care.

For those who stay in the detention facility longer than 1 month, repeat examinations, including monthly patient weigh-in, must be performed. During egress (whether for transfer or repatriation), another medical examination should be performed and any ongoing medical, surgical, or wound care problems should be documented. If ongoing simple medical issues exist, such as duty limitations or medications, clearly written instructions should be given to the guards and a copy kept in the patient's medical records.

Inpatient care

Surgical issues are often the leading cause of admission in DP facilities. Fragment wounds accounted for 42% of the patients admitted, whereas 21% required treatment for fractures at one of the two United States hospitals caring for DPs in ODS [18]. The most common admission diagnoses included gunshot wounds, soft tissue injuries, and burns. More than 90% of the admissions were to the surgical service. Almost 30% of admissions required surgical procedures. The most common operations were wound debridement, open reduction and internal fixation of fractures, exploratory laparotomy, and incision and drainage of abscesses.

Wound care is a significant portion of the workload for DPs. Standard procedures should be written to ensure consistent wound care. This practice will help improve efficiency when prisoners are incoming. Although practice variations will always exist, a standardized wound-care protocol makes the job of the nursing staff easier and helps minimize patient neglect. All patients who have incisions or wounds encased in plaster must have the date of the casting or procedure clearly marked on the dressing with an indelible pen. Additionally, wounds may be caused by devices rarely seen in civilian practice, such as nuclear, biologic, and chemical wounds. In these cases, having the causal factor identified on the dressing may also be helpful. DPs who have contagious diseases, severe mental diseases, or other illnesses determined by the physician staff should be isolated from other patients.

Medical supplies

Depending on the size of the medical unit, the medical supply section may range from a medic who has other duties to a full fledged logistical staff. In addition to determining what is needed in an initial or "push" pack, the length of time required to receive medical re-supply must be ascertained so that adequate supplies are maintained. In addition, basic laboratory and radiograph equipment is needed. Regulated shipping to a reference laboratory may be necessary for testing other than basic analysis. An appropriate blood bank section should be part of any surgical care unit.

Of all ODS medical providers, 47% felt that maintaining adequate supplies for the treatment of DPs was a problem [18]. Another study of Bosnian health care workers found that medical supplies were the most effective form of refugee assistance, followed by nonmedical material assistance (eg, fuel, food, blankets) [19]. In the same study, most providers (82%) also believed that the largest obstacle to providing care to the refugees was a lack of infrastructure, such as heating, potable water, and edible food. Large volumes of analgesics, antibiotics, dermatologic preparations, and gastrointestinal medications should be anticipated. Special equipment is often needed for clipping hair, delousing, and treating parasites. Field hygiene supplies and environmental protection measures, such as insect netting and sunscreen, can be essential. Common vaccines should be available for preventing communicable disease. Although United States and coalition casualties are generally evacuated for definitive fracture management, DPs are not. Plans must include local facilities or the personnel and supplies to perform this function in theater.

Medical staffing

The medical staffing should be similar to what would be required to definitively treat a similar number of friendly casualties. Personnel required to serve in DP facilities should be carefully selected. Tensions can develop between the prisoners and members of the medical unit, and therefore plans to deal with these tensions, including the use of psychologists and psychiatrists, should be considered. Physicians should have the time to evaluate all patients at the same frequency whether they are friendly or DP. Captured physicians and nurses can perform sick call for their compatriots in conformity with the Geneva Conventions. Their familiarity and experience with local diseases, such as cutaneous leishmaniasis in Iraq, can be extremely useful [8]. Gifts may not be accepted from DPs, even from their professional staff.

Although deployed medical facilities will usually not perform rehabilitation services, DPs often require physical therapy, occupational therapy, physiatry, and prosthetic services. More than 50% of landmine victims die from the initial blast, but those who survive have acute disabling injuries that require significant ongoing medical treatment [20]. Because chronic pain has been reported in up to 73% of former DPs, staff to evaluate and treat this condition should be considered [21]. Many DP populations, especially refugees, have a high incidence of burned children. Plastic/reconstructive surgeons and pediatricians should be strongly considered in this situation. As shown in Afghanistan, where dental disease is a common problem in detention facilities, the need for robust dental capabilities should be anticipated.

Staff education

Health care workers should be instructed in the tenets of the Geneva Conventions and all other related documents pertaining to DP care before deployment. A text favored by deploying United States medical caregivers, *Emergency War Surgery Handbook,* has a new chapter on the care of DPs and other internees [22]. For example, current United States military health care staff deployed to OEF and OIF receive predeployment instruction on the Geneva Conventions and Medical Rules of Engagement. This practice is further codified in the 44th Medical Command (Airborne) Rule of Conduct for Medical Personnel Providing Detainee Medical Care (COL J. Giddens, personal communication, 2005). Additional measures should be considered for staff protection, such as instruction in self-defense and hostage avoidance.

Medical administration

Facilities

Medical leaders involved with mission planning should be aware of the cost of damage to the medical infrastructure for enemy forces, and therefore should make contingency plans for each mission. The war in the former Yugoslavia underscores the trend in 21st-century warfare of targeting civilians and exploiting them for military gain. One study found that hospitals were among the first targets to be destroyed and the last to be rehabilitated [23]. For example, the number of hospital beds in the former Yugoslavia decreased by 35%, whereas infant mortality doubled.

Hospital planners should also consider the care of patients who have disabilities before constructing any medical facilities. Preventive medicine should support the facility by performing pest management, field sanitation, waste disposal, and potable water management, among other requirements. Veterinary services or an equivalent should provide food inspection services. The hospital command team should develop a close working relationship with the civil affairs team if one is present. This partnership would focus on the development of a local or government-sponsored medical infrastructure, including sanitation, hospitals, and medical education.

Patient administration

The patient administration system needs some changes. Special DP medical records are often required because the standard medical forms may not cover all necessary issues. The medical records in United States DP facilities belong to the US Government. DPs are entitled to copies of their records on request. DPs are given an identification number using the Prisoner of War Information System (PWIS). In addition to the standard history and physical examination, DP records should annotate wounding mechanisms, initial treatments and treatment location, time to initial treatment, time to treatment at the DP facility, operative procedures, and postoperative care. All DPs who require amputation or have already undergone an amputation or major wound debridement at another facility should be clearly photographed for legal purposes. All radiographs or digital images obtained for these patients should be kept in a separate area and remain available for medicolegal purposes.

Clear standard operating procedures (SOPs) should be made. For example, security measures of guard placement, weaponry, and restraining methods, including isolation, should be standardized. Before any interrogation occurs, the DP must be medically cleared by the attending physician. Guidelines for SOPs can be found in Army Regulation 190-8, the set of Army regulations governing Enemy Prisoners of War, Retained Personnel, Civilian Internees, and other Detainees [24].

Interpreters

Interpreters always seem to be scarce. In most cases, the DPs do not know any language but their own. Medical planners should include basic foreign language training as an essential part of predeployment training. Additionally, medical phrase books in most languages are available through the Department of Defense, such as DA PAM 40-3 [22]. Language barriers in communicating with the DPs at their initial medical ingress and treatments may be overcome using the translational skills of captured health care workers. However, simulation of mental illness by captured DPs is a potential technique for evading interrogation, especially when they are paired with a captured interpreter [25].

Because local nationals must often be contracted to serve as interpreters, their safety must be assured through methods such as using aliases and blindfolding patients during communication. Health care workers should be careful when using blindfolds on DPs to ensure that the sensory (ie, sight) deprivation is performed only to protect staff identity and cannot be misinterpreted as torture.

Medical maintenance

The battlefield or natural disaster environment, and therefore DP locations, are often extreme and can be hard on sensitive medical equipment. In addition to methods to protect the equipment from the heat, cold, sand, and dust, qualified medical maintenance technicians should be available. Additionally, life-cycle management should be part of a long-term planning and budget analysis program.

Security

One of the first responsibilities of POW medical care is the safeguarding of the facility site. The military authority should situate medical facilities "in a manner that attacks against military objectives cannot imperil their safety" (Geneva I, Article 19) [10]. Facility preparations should include basic heating and cooling, bathing, and nutritional elements that are consistent with the likely religious tenets of the DPs. Copies of the Geneva Conventions written in local languages should be posted in all treatment areas.

Infantry or military police units often provide physical security. Medical staff are exposed to an element of danger in treating DPs. The entire medical staff should insist that the security routine always be maintained. Security personnel should accompany medical providers in treatment areas of a detention facility. If the hospital building is separate from the detention facility, armed guards should accompany the patient at all times. Medical equipment should rarely enter the detention facility for security reasons. Security personnel should investigate all medical interpreters before they are hired.

Communications

The medical and main DP facility must have good communication. Effective communication lines at every level are essential between the medical providers and security members. Physicians who suspect any abuse or maltreatment of a DP should report it to the appropriate chain of command. Additionally, physicians should report any communicable diseases, such as tuberculosis and cholera, to lessen the risk for other DPs and staff.

In many cases, a shortage of bandwidth for communications systems will occur. Internet and worldwide telephone access are extremely helpful because they allow providers to contact subspecialty experts for consultation. For smaller facilities, digital images of radiographs can be sent to radiologists at central sites.

Legal

Signed permission should be obtained for all surgical or invasive procedures, when possible. DPs have the right to refuse any surgical procedure, even if the refusal is deemed detrimental to their health. The refusal should be documented as completely as possible [5]. DPs often have high rates of illiteracy, and therefore arrangements should be made for those who cannot read or write. For medicolegal purposes, a high-quality camera is important for photodocumentation. In contrast to civilian medical photography, the patient's identity should be absolutely clear in each photograph [26]. This disclosure is invaluable if a claim of unnecessary surgery or amputation is made; clearly identifiable photographs can show the state of a patient's wound. However, photography is prohibited within the medical facility for anything other than medical or legal purposes. Only information necessary to supervise the general health, nutrition, and cleanliness of DP facilities is releasable.

Deaths besides those from natural causes are investigated in military facilities by the US Army Criminal Investigative Command for the DP facility commander. If the cause of death is unknown, this should be noted by the attending physician. When the cause of death is determined, a supplemental report may be filed.

The sick and wounded may not be repatriated against their will during hostilities. For military patients, AR 190-8 specifically delineates how sick or wounded DPs may be repatriated or sent to a neutral country during hostilities [24].

Plans should be made for made for those prisoners who go on hunger strikes and those who refuse treatment. Providers should be prepared for the possibility that the only life-saving therapy is contrary to a patient's religious or cultural norms, especially for a patient who is incapacitated. Physicians should consider what would happen if another DP or the DP's government learned about the treatment, or lack thereof. In some cases, either choice could result in media problems or even a charge of war crimes. These scenarios require the involvement of the Judge Advocate General or other legal officer and the detention facility commander.

Article limitations

Research on the care of enemy DPs is scarce, for several possible reasons. The stain of DP abuse at the Nazi concentration camps, especially in camps that purportedly performed the "medical research" that led to the 1949 Geneva Conventions, may make the study of DP care politically difficult to support. Another potential reason is that medical research would show that the care of DPs does not meet the standard of care for the detaining power. At least part of the reason is undoubtedly the strict international laws governing this research. Medical research on DPs can have only minimal risk and be only an inconvenience to the DP. Research involving prisoners is carefully scrutinized for a potentially retributive or extrapunitive purpose or nature [27]. Therefore, essentially all published research on DP care consists of observational cohort studies.

Summary

An episode of extreme violence often leads to POWs or refugees. Developing a sense of order, providing comfort, and caring for the sick and wounded in DP camps is the job of the health care system, whether at home or deployed, military or civilian. An optimal outcome requires tremendous amounts of planning, staff selection and education, and resource allocation.

References

[1] Sun Tzu. The art of war. Oxford: Oxford University Press; 1963. [Griffith SB, Trans.]
[2] Grotius H. De Jure Belli Ac Pacis. Libri Tres. In: Scott JB, editor. The classics of international law. Oxford: Clarendon Press; 1925.
[3] Vollmar LC. Development of the laws of war as they pertain to medical units and their personnel. Mil Med 1992;157:231–6.
[4] Schindler D, Toman J, editors. The Laws of Armed Conflict. 1863 Resolutions of the Geneva International Conference. Dordrecht (The Netherlands): Martinus Nijhoff Publishers; 1988.
[5] Baer HU, Kaar JF. Teaching the International Law of Armed Conflict to a wide military community. Mil Med 2002;167(8 Suppl):20–5.
[6] Carter BS. Ethical concerns for physicians deployed to Operation DESERT STORM. Mil Med 1994;159:55–9.
[7] Available at: http://www.armymedicine.army.mil/news/detmedopsrprt/detmedopsrpt.pdf. Accessed May 3, 2006.
[8] Friedman L, editor. 1864 Red Cross convention for the amelioration of the condition of the wounded in armies in the field. The Law of War. New York: Random House; 1972.
[9] Convention (II) with respect to the laws and customs of war on land and its annex: regulation concerning the laws and customs of war on land, 26 Martens Nouveau Recueil (ser.2) 949, 187 Consol. T.S. 429, entered into force Sept. 4, 1906.
[10] Robers A, Guelff R, editors. 1949 Geneva Convention IV relative to the protection of civilian persons in time of war. Documents on the Laws of War. Oxford: Clarendon Press; 1989.
[11] Meron T. The Geneva Convention as customary law. Am J Int Law 1982;81:348–70.
[12] Convention against Torture and Other Cruel, Inhuman or Degrading Treatment or Punishment (1984). Available at: http://www.ch/html/menu3/b/h_cat39.htm. Accessed May 28, 2005.
[13] Keung YK, Lau S. Medical care of prisoners: controversial or not? South Med J 1998;91: 991–2.
[14] Keenan WF. Non-surgical medical care of enemy prisoners of war during Operation Desert Storm. Mil Med 1991;156:648–51.
[15] Longmire AW, Deshmukh N. The medical care of Iraqi enemy prisoners of war. Mil Med 1991;156:645–8.
[16] Dyer O. Baghdad hospitals struggle to cope with war wounded. BMJ 2003;326:799.
[17] Gunby P. Another war…and more lessons for medicine to ponder in aftermath. JAMA 1991; 266:619–21.
[18] Wintermeyer SF, Pina JS, Cremins JE, et al. Medical care of Iraqis at a forwardly deployed US Army hospital during Operation DESERT STORM. Mil Med 1996;161:294–7.

[19] Van Rooyen MJ, Eliades MJ, Grabowski JG, et al. Medical relief personnel in complex emergencies: perceptions of effectiveness in the former Yugoslavia. Prehosp Disast Med 2001;16:145–9.

[20] Meier RH, Smith WK. Landmine injuries and rehabilitation for landmine survivors. Phys Med Rehabil Clin N Am 2002;13:175–87.

[21] Hermansson AC, Thyberg M, Timpka T, et al. Survival with pain: an eight-year follow-up of war wounded refugees. Med Confl Surviv 2001;17:102–11.

[22] Emergency War Surgery Handbook—Third United States Revision. Washington (DC): Borden Institute; 2004.

[23] World Bank Document. Bosnia-Herzegovina country overview. Washington, DC: World Bank Group; 1997.

[24] Army Regulations. Enemy prisoners of war, retained personnel, civilian internees and other detainees. Available at: http://www.au.af.mil/au/awc/awcgate/.law/ar190-8.pdf. Accessed May 28, 2005.

[25] Cappucci DT. Medical observations of malingering in Iraqi enemy prisoners of war during Operation DESERT STORM. Mil Med 1994;159:462–4.

[26] Westreich M, Waron M. Guidelines for a prisoner of war medical treatment center in a civilian hospital. Mil Med 1988;153:549–54.

[27] Stone TH. Discussing minimal risk in research involving prisoners as human subjects. J Law Med Ethics 2004;32:535–7.

ELSEVIER
SAUNDERS

SURGICAL
CLINICS OF
NORTH AMERICA

Surg Clin N Am 86 (2006) 779–785

Index

Note: Page numbers of article titles are in **boldface** type.

0039-6109/06/$ - see front matter © 2006 Elsevier Inc. All rights reserved.
doi:10.1016/S0039-6109(06)00063-6
surgical.theclinics.com

Moving?

Make sure your subscription moves with you!

To notify us of your new address, find your **Clinics Account Number** (located on your mailing label above your name), and contact customer service at:

E-mail: elspcs@elsevier.com

800-654-2452 (subscribers in the U.S. & Canada)
407-345-4000 (subscribers outside of the U.S. & Canada)

Fax number: 407-363-9661

Elsevier Periodicals Customer Service
6277 Sea Harbor Drive
Orlando, FL 32887-4800

*To ensure uninterrupted delivery of your subscription, please notify us at least 4 weeks in advance of move.

ELSEVIER